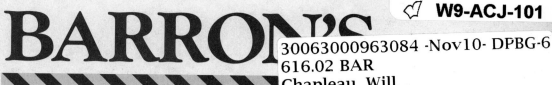

BARRON'S

EMT
EMERGENCY MEDICAL
TECHNICIAN EXAM

EDITION

...u, EMT-P, RN, TNS
...port Program, American College of Surgeons

..r, Ed.D. (abd), NREMT-P
...ny, University of New Mexico

BARRON'S

DEDICATION

First, I'd like to dedicate this book to all of the students and EMS professionals that have trusted me enough to use my books over the years and given me the opportunity to continue in the work I love in constantly evolving ways. I must also thank my wife, Kathy, my sons, Paul and Alex (now a paramedic firefighter in Chicago Heights), and my daughter, Abby, her husband, Alfie (also a paramedic firefighter in the Heights), and my grandsons, Rocco and Santino. They have all shared time that should have been theirs in service to my chosen profession. **WC**

   To my EMT and paramedic students over the past 18 years who have constantly kept the student's perspective fresh in my mind; and to the new generation of EMS providers. **MA**

© Copyright 2008, 2003 by Barron's Educational Series, Inc.

All inquiries should be addressed to:
Barron's Educational Series, Inc.
250 Wireless Boulevard
Hauppauge, NY 11788
www.barronseduc.com

ISBN-13: 978-0-7641-3937-6
ISBN-10: 0-7641-3937-1

Library of Congress Catalog Card No. 2007031516

Library of Congress Cataloging-in-Publication Data
Chapleau, Will.
   EMT basic exam / Will Chapleau, Melissa Alexander. -- 2nd ed.
      p. ; cm.
   Includes index.
   Rev. ed. of: Barron's how to prepare for the EMT exam / Will Chapleau. c2003.
   ISBN-13: 978-0-7641-3937-6 (alk. paper)
   ISBN-10: 0-7641-3937-1 (alk. paper)
 1. Emergency medicine—Examinations, questions, etc. 2. Emergency medical technicians—
Licenses—United States—Study guides. I. Alexander, Melissa. II. Chapleau, Will. Barron's how
to prepare for the EMT basic exam. III. Title.
   [DNLM: 1. Emergency Medical Services—methods—Examination Questions. 2. Emergencies—
Examination Questions. 3. Emergency Medical Technicians—Examination Questions.
WX 18.2 C464e 2008]

   RC86.9.C426 2008
   616.02'5076—dc22   2007031516

PRINTED IN THE UNITED STATES OF AMERICA
9 8 7 6 5 4

Contents

Preface   vii

About the Authors   ix

1 Introduction to the EMT Exam   1

Purpose of Testing   1
Preparing for Written Examinations   2
Test Formats and Strategies   6
Test Anxiety   7
Preparing for Practical Examinations   8
What You Can Find on the National
  Registry Web Site   9
Summary   9
Key Terms   10
How to Interpret and Use Learning
  Objectives   11

2 Introduction to Emergency Care   13

Objectives   13
Emergency Medical Services Systems   14
Health Care System   14
Public Safety Personnel   14
Roles and Responsibilities of the EMT   15
Personal Attributes   16
Medical Direction   17
State and Local Legal Issues   17
Scenario   17
Review Questions   18
Answers to Review Questions   24

3 Well-Being of the EMT   29

Objectives   29
Emotional Aspects of Emergency Care   30
Stressful Situations   31
Stress Management   31

Friends and Family   31
Critical Incident Stress Debriefing (CISD)   32
Scene Safety   32
Scenarios   34
Review Questions   35
Answers to Review Questions   41

4 Medical, Legal, and Ethical Issues   45

Objectives   45
Scope of Practice   46
Do Not Resuscitate Orders and
  Advance Directives   46
Consent   47
Assault and/or Battery   47
Refusals   47
Abandonment   47
Negligence   48
Duty to Act   48
Confidentiality   48
Special Situations   48
Scenarios   49
Review Questions   50
Answers to Review Questions   56

5 The Human Body   59

Objectives   59
Anatomical Terms   60
The Skeletal System   60
The Respiratory System   63
The Circulatory System   64
The Nervous System   65
The Endocrine System   65
The Muscular System   66
The Skin   66
Scenarios   66
Review Questions   67
Answers to Review Questions   72

6 Baseline Vital Signs and SAMPLE History   75

Objectives   75
General Information   76
Vital Signs   76
SAMPLE   78
Medical Identification   78
Scenarios   79
Review Questions   80
Answers to Review Questions   85

7 Lifting and Moving Patients   89

Objectives   89
Body Mechanics   90
Types of Moves   91
Patient Positioning   93
Scenarios   93
Review Questions   94
Answers to Review Questions   98

8 Airway   101

Objectives   101
Anatomy Review   102
Opening the Airway   103
Suctioning   103
Artificial Ventilation   104
Airway Adjuncts   104
Oxygen   105
Scenarios   106
Review Questions   107
Answers to Review Questions   113

9 Patient Assessment   117

Section 1—Scene Size-Up   117
Objectives   117
Section 2—Initial Assessment   118
Objectives   118
Section 3—The Focused History and
    Physical Exam: Trauma Patients   120
Objectives   120
Section 4—The Focused History and
    Physical Exam: Medical Patients   121

Objectives   121
Section 5—Detailed Physical Exam   122
Objectives   122
Section 6—Ongoing Assessment   123
Objectives   123
Scenarios   123
Review Questions   125
Answers to Review Questions   130

10 Communications   133

Objectives   133
Scenarios   135
Review Questions   136
Answers to Review Questions   139

11 Documentation   141

Objectives   141
Scenarios   142
Review Questions   143
Answers to Review Questions   146

12 General Pharmacology   149

Objectives   149
Scenarios   150
Review Questions   151
Answers to Review Questions   154

13 Respiratory Emergencies   157

Objectives   157
Inadequate Breathing   158
Artificial Ventilation   159
Scenarios   160
Review Questions   161
Answers to Review Questions   164

14 Cardiac Emergencies   167

Objectives   167
Anatomy and Physiology Review   169
Emergency Care for Cardiac Patients   170
Scenarios   171
Review Questions   172
Answers to Review Questions   176

15 Diabetes/Altered Mental Status 179

Objectives	179
Diabetes	180
Seizures	180
Scenarios	181
Review Questions	182
Answers to Review Questions	184

16 Allergies and Poisoning/Overdose 187

Section 1—Allergies	187
Objectives	187
Section 2—Poisoning/Overdose	188
Objectives	188
Scenarios	189
Review Questions	190
Answers to Review Questions	193

17 Environmental Emergencies 195

Objectives	195
Types of Environmental Emergencies	196
Scenarios	198
Review Questions	199
Answers to Review Questions	202

18 Behavioral Emergencies 205

Objectives	205
Behavior	206
Scenarios	207
Review Questions	208
Answers to Review Questions	211

19 Obstetrics/Gynecology 215

Objectives	215
Anatomy	216
Delivery	216
Scenarios	218
Review Questions	219
Answers to Review Questions	224

20 Bleeding and Shock 229

Objectives	229
The Circulatory System	230
Bleeding	230
Scenarios	231
Review Questions	232
Answers to Review Questions	235

21 Dealing with Injuries 239

Section 1—Soft Tissue Injuries	239
Objectives	239
The Skin	241
Section 2—Musculoskeletal Injuries	241
Objectives	241
Scenarios	242
Review Questions	244
Answers to Review Questions	248

22 Injuries to the Head and Spine 251

Objectives	251
Injuries to the Spine	252
Injuries to the Head	253
Scenarios	253
Review Questions	254
Answers to Review Questions	258

23 Infants and Children 261

Objectives	261
Developmental Phases	262
Problems in Infants and Children	263
Scenarios	264
Review Questions	265
Answers to Review Questions	269

24 Ambulance Operations   273

Section 1—Always Ready   273
Objectives   273
Section 2—Gaining Access   275
Objectives   275
Section 3—Hazards, Casualties,
  and Disasters   276
Objectives   276
Scenarios   276
Review Questions   277
Answers to Review Questions   281

25 Final Exams   283

Exam 1   287
Answers to Exam 1   308
Exam 2   319
Answers to Exam 2   338

Glossary   347

Appendix   359

Index   391

Preface

Prehospital care is a relatively young profession. Over the last 30 years, the profession has evolved from what was a transportation service provided by responders with limited training or none at all, to specially trained professionals ranging from First Responders to Advanced Life Support.

Emergency Medical Technicians, or EMTs, form the backbone of the U.S. Emergency Medical System (EMS) and comprise the largest number (over 500,000) of EMS Responders.

EMT is a pre-requisite for employment with ambulance services all over the United States and many police and fire departments. Most employment projections show EMTs and paramedics as a growing profession with shortages in many urban areas. Salaries are rising and many employers create benefit packages to attract and retain employees.

This book is intended to help the EMT candidate prepare for the licensure or certification examination. **The intent of this book is to provide a review and emphasis on key points. The book should be used in concert with the text and materials used in your EMT course.** Each chapter begins with a listing of the U.S. Department of Transportation (DOT) curriculum objectives and a review of the material they cover. While the latest guidance from the DOT moves away from detailed objectives, we feel they provide reference to the material in each chapter of the book.

To improve this book as we moved into this second edition, we listened to the users of the first edition and enhanced the review questions. We accomplished this through the efforts of Melissa Alexander, who joined me on this edition. The multiple-choice questions are drawn from the objectives and are intended to give you an opportunity to practice the type of questions you are likely to face in the licensure or certification exam. Melissa also designed fill-in-the-blank-type questions to encourage guided study in preparation for the exams. To enhance comprehension of the material we provide rationales or explanations for the correct answers to all questions. Melissa provides guidance in the new Chapter 1, which gives advice on preparing for the examination.

Throughout the book there are also scenario questions to give you a chance to apply what you have learned to lifelike situations. It is our hope that this book will assist you in your preparation to become an EMT.

About the Authors

Will Chapleau is the manager of the Advanced Trauma Life Support Program for the American College of Surgeons. He has been a paramedic for over 30 years and a trauma nurse specialist for 19 years. He has worked on ambulances, in fire departments, and in hospitals over the length of his career, served as fire chief for 6 years, and has worked as an educator in prehospital, nursing, and physician programs. Will has been the chair of the Prehospital Trauma Life Support for NAEMT since 1996, and serves on the board of directors of the National Association of EMTs, the National Association of EMS Educators, and the Society of Trauma Nurses. He has authored numerous texts and articles on EMS and emergency services and has lectured on these topics all over the world.

Melissa Alexander is the director of the EMS Academy in the Department of Emergency Medicine at the University of New Mexico. She has been in EMS since 1982, spending most of her clinical career in Indianapolis, Indiana. Her undergraduate degree in Community Health Education is from Purdue University, with a master's degree in Health Sciences Education from Indiana University. She is completing a doctorate in Human and Organizational Learning at The George Washington University. Melissa has worked as a consultant in EMS education both domestically and abroad. She has published a number of articles in trade journals, and has published a text on EMS education. She is a contributor to numerous EMS textbooks and frequently develops instructor resource materials and test banks for EMS texts. Melissa's research interests are in the areas of adult learning in EMS and in EMS workforce issues.

Introduction to the EMT Exam

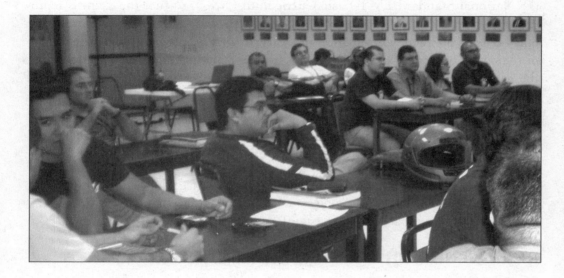

This chapter is designed to guide your preparation for both the written and practical Emergency Medical Technician (EMT) examinations. Whether you are preparing for a class final, a state-level examination, or the **National Registry of EMTs** exam, you will find this chapter useful. This chapter gives insight into the purpose of testing, how exams are constructed, and how to use learning objectives to guide your study, study habits, and learning styles. By learning more about testing and test taking, you will feel more confident and be better prepared for the **high-stakes testing** ahead of you.

PURPOSE OF TESTING

No doubt by now you are aware of the tremendous trust placed on the shoulders of EMTs by the public, and the tremendous ethical obligation EMTs have to provide the best patient care possible. The general purpose common to all testing in Emergency Medical Services (EMS) is to assess the degree to which you have achieved the **competencies** that are essential to safe practice as an EMS provider. During an EMT class, the instructor can also use the results of exams to provide feedback to you and your classmates so that you can learn from your mistakes. Course final exams are used to determine whether students have met the **objectives** of the EMT course. Students who meet or exceed the minimum standards have met one of the conditions for eligibility to test at the state or National Registry level.

State-level testing is used to determine your eligibility for **licensure** or **certification** by the state. Some states use the National Registry exam as evidence of having met the minimum competencies required for licensure. Other states have their own examination process to establish a minimum level of competence for licensure.

The purpose of the National Registry examination is to assess whether you meet the minimum competencies for EMS practice, as established by a **practice analysis** based on the input of a national sample of EMTs. The practice analysis is a comprehensive document that establishes the important aspects of the job of an EMT. It includes items that EMTs perform frequently, as well as items that are performed infrequently, but are critical in nature. The practice analysis is cross-referenced with the **National Standard EMT-Basic Curriculum** (NSC), so that the exam is representative of the skills and knowledge taught at the national level. Therefore, there may be items on a state examination that exceed what is taught at the national level; or there may be items that are not taught in your state that you may be tested on at the national level. The National Registry Practice Analysis for EMTs can be found in the Appendix.

Passing the National Registry exam does not, in and of itself, give you permission to practice as an EMT. Only the state in which you work can grant you permission to practice. However, the exam does assess whether you meet the minimum competencies established by the national practice analysis. The more states that recognize National Registry testing as evidence of competence, the easier it will be for EMTs to take their careers from one state to another. States that currently recognize National Registration are listed on page 10.

PREPARING FOR WRITTEN EXAMINATIONS

Preparing for a high-stakes written examination produces some level of anxiety in most students for at least two reasons. The first is obvious: it is a high-stakes exam, meaning that there is a lot riding on the outcome. You have made an investment of time, and probably money, in your efforts to become an EMT. Your career, or at least the ability to move up in your career, may depend on the outcome of the exam. The second reason for anxiety is that the purposes and processes related to the exam are often unknown, and the unknown always provokes some anxiety, especially when the consequences are important to you. We cannot change the high-stakes nature of the exam, but in this section we will provide you with information that takes away some of the unknown.

Content of the Exam

High-stakes examinations are often different from the instructor-created exams you are used to. For one, they are obviously more comprehensive in nature. But second, high-stakes examinations are created using sophisticated principles of test construction and input from EMS community **stakeholders** and are subject to statistical analysis to improve their **validity** and **reliability**.

Often, students become used to test items that come directly from their instructors' lectures or from the specific content of the textbook required for their EMT class. They want to know, "Should I study from my notes or from the text?" Students may pressure the instructor to state specifically what will and will not be on class exams. These practices may result in a good grade in the class, but may not prepare you well for high-stakes testing. High-stakes testing does not rely on a specific textbook or the particular things that your instructor, program, or geographical region emphasizes. Instead, high-stakes exams are developed and reviewed with input from a variety of people and sources.

The review material and practice tests in this book are designed according to the same principles, sources of information, and guidelines used for high-stakes examinations. The review material and content of the practice tests are based on the National Registry Practice Analysis for EMTs and the EMT NSC.

Difficulty of the Exam

A frequently heard complaint about high-stakes exams is that they seem to be much more difficult than the exams students are used to. High-stakes exams are designed to have a mix of items that are easy, moderately difficult, and difficult. Many instructor-made exams have more items that test lower-level knowledge, and fewer items that test critical thinking and problem solving. Students may get good grades on their in-class exams and feel very confident about their knowledge, only to be disappointed by their performance on a state or National Registry exam. The good news is that the best way to learn problem-solving and critical thinking is to create opportunities to practice both. This book allows you the opportunity to solve difficult problems and provides feedback for improvement by explaining the reasoning behind the correct answers. Another way to prepare for more difficult items is to understand the learning objectives behind the items.

Learning objectives are statements of the intended outcomes of the learning process. They are found at the beginning of most textbook chapters, and may be discussed or distributed by your instructor. Unfortunately, students are generally given little guidance about how to use the objectives and instead tend to use them as a content outline of the chapter or lecture.

The key to every learning objective is the verb that describes the expected behavior of the learner. The verb must be interpreted properly, not just used as a guide to content. We provide examples on page 11 to help you learn to analyze the objective and determine what it is really asking you to do.

Studying for the Exam

GENERAL APPROACH

The key to studying for the exam is to not study for the exam. What we mean by this is, do not try to figure out what specific questions may be on the exam and focus your studying on only those questions. You are sure to be disappointed in the outcome. Even if you are successful in figuring out what questions are likely to be on the exam, you will have learned only the limited amount of information that can be placed on the exam. The patient whom you fail to treat properly will not be satisfied with the answer, "I was never tested on that."

A good examination samples your learning, but cannot possibly test everything that is important for you to know to be a good EMT, unless it contains hundreds, or even thousands, of items. Think of it this way: When your physician wants to know what your cholesterol level is, he or she relies on a small but representative sample of your blood to provide information about the entire volume of blood in your body. It is the same with testing your knowledge. We rely on a relatively small number of questions that are representative of the kinds of things you need to know to tell us the state of your overall competence in EMT practice.

SOURCES OF INFORMATION FOR STUDYING

It is a good practice to have more than one source of information from which to study. But avoid having so many sources that it becomes impractical to spend enough time studying each concept. You already (wisely!) chose this study guide to help focus on critical information. A second source of information is the EMT text-book used for your course. All of the EMT texts by the major publishers very closely follow the EMT NSC. If you are preparing for a class final or a state exam, you should be aware of any areas in which your scope of practice (SOP) exceeds the national standards. For example, in some areas, EMTs are allowed to administer the drug naloxone (Narcan®) for narcotic overdoses. In this case, you may want to study from protocols or SOP documents.

LEARNING STYLES

Learning style refers to the way an individual prefers to receive and process infor-mation. Usually, the preferred style is the most useful style for an individual, but not always. Regardless of our preferences, we all can, and do, learn in a variety of ways. There are multiple categories of learning styles and several instruments for testing learning styles. You may have already done such an assessment of your learn-ing style. If not, there are a variety of sources online that can be found through an Internet search for "learning style assessment." Your college or employer may also offer learning style assessments. But remember: Your learning style is only one aspect of what is required to successfully prepare for an exam, and learning style assessments are most useful when the results are accompanied by suggestions for how to maximize the use of your preferred style.

STUDY HABITS

There truly are different strokes for different folks when it comes to study habits. There is no single prescription for what will work. If you are satisfied with the results you have gotten with your current study habits, stick with your plan. If you are less than satisfied with previous results, we offer some suggestions. Begin by asking yourself some questions about your practices. You may not have thought about whether what you do really works best for you.

If you study in a group, is the group productive? Or does each meeting tend to become a social gathering rather than a study group? Group study is not for every-one. Students who are not outgoing may not like studying with others. Students who are outgoing may have difficulty refraining from social conversation. Also, the group's learning needs may not be the same as yours.

Think about what time of day allows you the most productivity. Some people are morning people, and others are night owls. What time of day do you feel most energized and motivated? Are there times when you are easily distracted or find it difficult to maintain interest in your studies? Try to arrange study time when you are at your peak ability to concentrate.

What kind of setting do you find most conducive to productive study? Do you need absolute quiet for concentration? Or do you prefer some kind of background noise, such as music or television? It is common to see students of all types studying in coffeehouses and cafes that offer Internet access, but the atmosphere may be too busy for some people. Have you chosen a place to study that is relatively free of interruptions? If you can, turn off pagers and cell phones. What kind of lighting do you prefer? Does lamplight, rather than overhead lighting, make you comfortable so you can focus on your studies? Or does it relax you too much and decrease your motivation to study? Are you more productive in a comfortable easy chair, or at a desk? Finally, do you find it helpful to have food or drink available?

There are some general suggestions that tend to be helpful for most people. First, take regular breaks from studying to give your brain time to process what you are concentrating on and store it in your long-term memory. Studying for 20 to 50 minutes, then taking a 5-to-10-minute break allows you to take in "chewable chunks" of information. Cramming is not effective. Hopefully, you purchased this text in plenty of time to allow you to pace your learning effectively.

Our brains are programmed to want to find the answers to questions we have. Try converting the section headings and key terms in your reading into questions, and then answer them in your own words. This will let you know what your progress is in learning the material. You may also want to write down the answers to these questions, because writing forces us to clarify information that we may gloss over if we simply think to ourselves. If you study with a partner, you can take turns explaining concepts, in detail, aloud.

Repetition is a key strategy in learning. After a break, ask yourself the same questions again. The more times we access the information, the better established the mental path to that information becomes. Also, asking for the same material in different ways establishes more pathways to the information so that we can recall it in a variety of circumstances.

Summarizing the information in your own words and creating tables and diagrams to explain concepts to yourself can help you be an active, and more effective, learner. And do not forget: A picture is worth a thousand words. Pay attention to the diagrams and tables provided in texts. Often, studying these first, before undertaking a full reading of a chapter or section, provides a mental framework for organizing the more detailed content of the chapter.

Finally, assess the strengths and weaknesses in your knowledge using the review questions in this text. Prioritize areas in which you need the most study—but do not forget to review information you are comfortable with from time to time.

TEST FORMATS AND STRATEGIES

Tests are available in different formats. Your written exam may be computer-based or printed on paper. If the exam is on paper, you may write your answers on the exam, or be required to use a separate answer sheet. We will provide a brief discussion of each format.

Computer-Based Testing

The National Registry of EMTs is transitioning to computer-based testing (CBT) in a particular format known as computer adaptive testing (CAT). This format offers several benefits. One benefit is that the turnaround time for test results is very short. No more waiting for the mail to arrive each day, week after week, while you hold your breath and keep your fingers crossed! Another benefit is that the results of CAT are very accurate. The test is individualized so that those who show competence with fewer questions will answer fewer questions. CBT also allows students to test individually, so that there is less likelihood of having a schedule conflict with the exam. However, with computerized tests, you cannot change your mind after you submit the question. There is no way of going back and changing your answer as some students do on paper-and-pencil tests. Make sure you double-check your answer before moving on! The CBT for the National Registry is offered through test centers. You can find out more about CBT, the locations of test centers, and how to register for the exam on the National Registry's Web site (*www.nremt.org*). Many of the suggestions in the next section also apply to CBT.

Paper-and-Pencil Testing

When taking a paper-and-pencil test, there are a few key strategies to keep in mind. Instructions may be delivered orally by an exam proctor, in writing on the exam, or both. Make sure that you completely understand the instructions and follow them during the exam. The entire test may be timed, and sections within the test may be timed. It is a good practice to glance over the exam, if allowed, or the section of the exam you are working on, so that you can budget your time. Also, know whether you are allowed to use scratch paper or calculators, write on the exam, or leave the room during the exam. It is a good practice to bring as little as possible with you into the exam room, and to place anything you do bring in a location where it could not be thought that you were making reference to notes. Particularly books, notebooks, cell phones, cameras, and electronic devices should not be brought to the exam. Think how disappointing it would be to pass the exam but be disqualified because instructions were not followed.

Very often, instructors hear students say, "I had the right answer the first time, but I changed it!" If you are unsure of the answer, stick with your first choice. However, you should change your original response if: 1) You clearly mismarked your answer, or 2) you misread the question and a second reading makes it clear that your first choice was wrong.

If possible, first answer easy questions, then come back to the hard ones. Be careful, though; skipping around on the exam may increase the likelihood that you overlook items, or place your answers in the wrong place on the answer sheet. Resist the temptation to leave as soon as you have finished the exam. Take a few minutes to review in order to establish that you have not inadvertently skipped over items and that the answer for each item is in the right place.

Other frequently heard statements from students who have taken a high-stakes examination are, "Most of the questions had two right answers," and "None of the answers were right." While it may seem this way, it is probably not the case. Most high-stakes exams are designed to have a certain proportion of very difficult questions, but they are also thoroughly reviewed. If two alternative answers seem correct, compare and contrast the alternatives to find the difference between them. It is the difference between the two answers that makes one correct, or "more" correct, than the other. In cases where there seems to be no right answer, or where all the answers seem to be right, choose the *best* answer.

Finally, there is no magic formula for how long you should spend trying to answer an item with which you are having difficulty. Keep the following in mind: 1) Consider the importance of that item in relation to items you have not yet answered. In other words, better to miss one question because you do not know the answer than to miss five questions because you ran out of time, and 2) sometimes moving on and answering other questions will trigger something that makes you think of the right response for the item you were struggling with. At the other end of the spectrum, make sure you spend enough time to actually understand what the question is asking. You may "sight recognize" an item that seems familiar when, in fact, it is written slightly differently. Even if the question seems familiar, take the time to read it carefully before answering; likewise with the possible responses. One response may seem to jump out at you, but be sure to try out the stem (main part) of the question with each possible response before making a final decision.

TEST ANXIETY

Everyone experiences a level of anxiety about a high-stakes examination. A normal level of anxiety actually increases our performance. But, when anxiety levels are too high, our performance can suffer. You may have test anxiety if you experience physical symptoms of stress, such as excessive perspiration, rapid heart rate, or muscle tension. People with test anxiety may have trouble reading and understanding the questions being asked, difficulty organizing their thoughts, or "draw a blank" on some questions, only to remember the answer after the exam is over. Some of the things that contribute to test anxiety can be controlled. These include your level of preparation, and worry about the consequences of failing an exam.

First, study so that you know the material well enough that you can remember it under stress. Build your confidence with practice tests, like the ones in this study guide. Do not allow yourself to become overwhelmed and succumb to negative thoughts about your performance. If needed, put your pencil down, take a deep breath, and relax before proceeding with the exam. Do not worry about how much or how little time it is taking others to finish the exam. As a final point, take the exam one item at a time, without worrying about how many questions you have answered or how many remain to be answered.

If you are in a college or university program, take advantage of the counseling services offered for test anxiety. If you are in a program without such resources, there are a variety of college and university academic support or student services centers that have great online help for dealing with test anxiety. These can be found using an Internet search for "test anxiety." When selecting a source of information on test anxiety, remember that college and university Web sites generally use ".edu," rather than ".com" or ".org."

The evening (or day, if the exam is offered later in the day) before your exam should not be spent trying to learn new material. While a review of main points is important, the time for learning new material has passed. Follow your normal routine as much as possible, eat well, and get a full night's (6 to 8 hours) sleep.

PREPARING FOR PRACTICAL EXAMINATIONS

Much of what you learned about the purposes of written examinations is true for practical examinations as well. The purpose of a practical examination is to establish whether or not you can perform critical skills at the level of accuracy and rate of speed required of entry-level EMTs. However, do not forget that it is not only the **psychomotor skills** that count in a practical examination. You need to know such things as what an appropriate flow rate of oxygen is for a given patient, and what the indications and contraindications are for the use of medications and devices. In many cases, you will also need to interact appropriately with your patients in scenarios.

Typically, the examiners for the practical skills examination are not the instructors or assistants who have evaluated your skills during class. Many students worry that the expectations for performance will be different than what they became used to in class. This is an understandable worry. Sometimes instructors put too much emphasis on their preferences for how a skill should be performed, and too little emphasis on the principles for performing the skill. For example, if an instructor teaches that the straps or fasteners for a particular piece of equipment must be connected in a certain order when, in fact, there may not be a principle behind the practice, students may become unnecessarily concerned with details that will not matter to the examiner. If the instructor followed a different set of criteria for teaching the skill than the criteria on which students will be tested, students may miss a critical step that the examiners are looking for. The solution to this is to ensure that you practice using the same criteria for performing the skill that will be used when you are tested.

The National Registry skill sheets are available on the National Registry's Web site at *www.nremt.org* and in many EMT textbooks. You can also find the National Registry basic-level skill sheets in the Appendix. If you will be tested according to other standards, those standards should be made available to you. If your practical examination is not based on the National Registry, be sure to ask your instructor where you can find the standards that will be used.

In addition to practicing the skills that will be on the exam, you may want to view "expert" performances of the skills. Many EMT textbooks now come with CDs, DVDs, or companion Web sites that have video clips of skills being performed. These videos have been carefully produced in order to show the skills being performed properly.

During practical testing, the use of personal protective equipment (PPE) or body substance isolation (BSI) equipment, and doing an actual scene size-up all count toward your score. We recommend, rather than trying to remember to say, "I am wearing BSI," when you enter the testing station, that you actually put on gloves and have a pair of goggles with you so that there is no question as to whether this step was taken. Not needing to remember to verbalize "BSI" will be one less thing to stress about during the exam. In some stations, the instructions given will inform you that the scene is safe. If not, avoid simply asking, "Is the scene safe?" You may be answered with, "I don't know. What are you looking for?" You must know what types of potential dangers are likely. For example, if the scene is a motor vehicle collision (MVC), ask specific questions such as, "Is the vehicle stable?" "Are there any indications of fire or spilled fluids?" "Is there a crowd?" "Are there power lines down?" and so forth.

Another area of concern for students who are being tested on practical skills is the interaction, or rather, lack of interaction, between them and the examiner. You may be used to the encouraging nods, subtle corrections, and other verbal and non-verbal feedback of your instructor. This interaction is an important part of teaching, but is not a part of testing. Nonetheless, it is somewhat disconcerting to students that the examiner has no reaction, either encouraging or discouraging, during their performance of the skill. You will not likely be told whether you passed or failed the skill station until you have completed the entire exam. Remember, it is nothing personal; the evaluator is just doing his or her job.

WHAT YOU CAN FIND ON THE NATIONAL REGISTRY WEB SITE

The National Registry testing process and requirements are well outlined on their Web site. The Web site contains a wealth of information and guidance to help you properly register for the exam, and help you gain more knowledge about their processes. If you are taking a state-level examination, check with your instructor or the state EMS office for guidance on registering for the exam.

SUMMARY

High-stakes testing is an important part of all health care professions. As formidable a hurdle as the testing may seem, we are sure that you understand its importance. Nonetheless, we also know that the anticipation of testing and of waiting for results can be agonizing. Our goal is to help reduce the anxiety and stress associated with this process by offering insights into the testing process, and providing helpful strategies, topic summaries, and practice tests for preparation that will help you feel confident on exam day.

KEY TERMS

Certification is a process by which a party attests that an individual has met certain standards. In some states, certification is used in place of licensure.

Competency is a statement of a proficiency required to perform a particular job or occupation.

High-stakes testing refers to any examination process in which the outcome is used as a criterion for licensure, registration, or certification of competence.

Learning style is the way in which an individual prefers to receive and process information. There are a variety of different schemes for classifying learning styles.

Licensure is the granting of permission by a governmental agency to engage in an occupation.

The National Standard EMT Curriculum is a document published by the National Highway Traffic Safety Administration that outlines the competencies and minimum required content of EMT-Basic courses.

The National Registry of EMTs is a national certification agency that establishes uniform standards for training and certification of emergency medical services personnel.

Practice analysis is a process that determines the critical components of a job and results in the documentation of those components, which may include knowledge, skills, and attitudes.

Psychomotor skill is a coordinated, goal-directed, physical activity.

Reliability refers to the consistency of performance of an examination or test.

Stakeholders are parties who have a vested interested in the activities of an organization or profession, and whose input is required to make sure their needs are met by the organization or profession.

Validity refers to whether an examination actually tests what it is supposed to test.

NATIONAL REGISTRY EMT STATES

Alabama	Illinois	Montana	Rhode Island
Arizona	Iowa	Nebraska	South Carolina
Arkansas	Kentucky	Nevada	South Dakota
Colorado	Louisiana	New Hampshire	Tennessee
Connecticut	Maine	New Jersey	Texas
Florida	Michigan	North Dakota	Vermont
Georgia	Minnesota	Ohio	West Virginia
Hawaii	Mississippi	Oklahoma	Wisconsin
Idaho	Missouri	Oregon	Wyoming

How to Interpret and Use Learning Objectives

Objective	Explanation	Possible Test Item
Identify the airway anatomy of infants, children, and adults.	This objective uses the verb "identify." This simply means being able to recognize something when you see it.	A typical test item for this objective is to have students list the names of the airway structures on a picture or model of the airway.
Differentiate between the airway anatomy of infants, children, and adults.	This objective uses the verb "differentiate." In this case, the desired behavior is to discern differences between things that also have similarities.	A typical test item might have students write several sentences to state in what ways the pediatric airway is different from the adult airway. The objective could also be tested with true/false or multiple choice items. For example: Which of the following is true of the pediatric airway, but not the adult airway? (A) The trachea is more flexible. (B) The left lung has three lobes. (C) The tongue is relatively small. (D) The epiglottis is firm.
List possible scene hazards.	This objective uses the verb "list." This simply means to provide an inventory of items.	A typical question would be: List four possible hazards that you might encounter on an EMS call.
Determine if a scene is safe to enter.	This objective uses the verb "determine." To determine something means to find out, establish, or verify.	This item is best tested in a lab scenario, but could also be tested using a written description of a scene. This is much different from, and requires a higher level of thinking, than the objective above. This illustrates why you must read the objective, rather than just seeing "scene safety" and assuming that you have to know something about scene safety. The two objectives, while both involving knowledge about scene safety, ask for two very different behaviors, and should be tested in different ways.

Introduction to Emergency Care

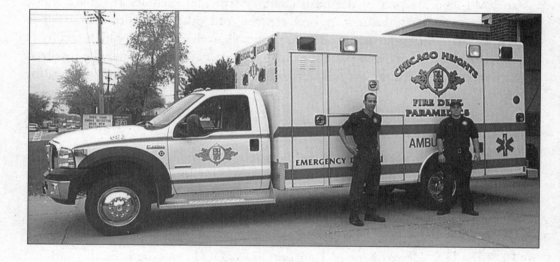

CHAPTER 2

OBJECTIVES

This chapter and the review questions will help readers determine if they are able to

1. define Emergency Medical Services (EMS);

2. differentiate the EMT's roles and responsibilities from other prehospital care providers;

3. describe the roles and responsibilities related to personal safety;

4. discuss the EMT's roles and responsibilities regarding the safety of patients, crew, and bystanders;

5. define quality improvement and the EMT's role in the process;

6. define medical direction and the EMT's role in the process;

7. state the specific statutes and regulations in your state regarding the EMS system.

EMERGENCY MEDICAL SERVICES SYSTEMS

Prehospital care providers work within EMS systems to provide emergency care to people all over the world that suddenly become sick or injured. This system is built on the training of the Emergency Medical Technician. EMTs are trained to assess, stabilize, and transport patients to appropriate medical facilities to receive definitive care. You will interact with other health care professionals that include advanced EMTs, paramedics, doctors, and nurses.

HEALTH CARE SYSTEM

As an EMT you are part of the health care system that includes trauma centers, burn centers, pediatric centers, poison centers, and other specialty centers. It is important that you understand the local protocols in determining which facility is appropriate to transport your patient to in an emergency. You also may be involved in nonemergency transport or transfers of patients between these facilities and/or patients' homes.

PUBLIC SAFETY PERSONNEL

EMTs also work closely with other public safety personnel, such as police and fire personnel. Close communication and cooperation with these agencies will be imperative to ensure the safety of EMTs, their teammates, and their patients.

Standards and Attributes

In 1973 the U.S. Department of Transportation (DOT) standardized the national curriculum all EMT courses follow. The National Highway Traffic Safety Administration (NHTSA) technical assistance standards are the components essential to any EMS System. These include regulation and policy, resource management, human resources and training, transportation, facilities, communications, public information and education, medical direction, trauma systems, and evaluation. These standards were revised into 14 attributes in the EMS Agenda for the future (also funded and published by NHTSA) in 1996. The 14 attributes are:

1. Integration of Health Services
2. EMS Research
3. Legislation and Regulations
4. System Finance
5. Human Resources
6. Medical Direction
7. Education Systems
8. Public Education
9. Prevention
10. Public Access
11. Communications Systems
12. Clinical Care
13. Information Systems
14. Evaluation

In order for EMS to function, the community served by EMS must understand what the system is designed to do, how it is used appropriately, and how to best facilitate its ability to serve them.

Access to EMS across much of the United States is through 911 systems. Callers into 911 systems have the potential for important information stored within the system to be available to the responders dispatched to care for them. There are areas of the country, however, that are not covered by 911 dispatch centers and may still use conventional phone numbers to access EMTs for response. An important part of your education will be orienting your community to the communication and dispatch system that covers them.

The care given by prehospital care providers has four levels of care. First Responders or Emergency Medical Responders (EMRs) give initial care which might include bleeding control or cardiopulmonary resuscitation (CPR); they typically do not transport patients. EMTs provide basic life support at the scene and during transport to the hospital. EMT-Intermediates (EMT-I) or Advanced EMTs provide some advanced life support care like intravenous (IV) fluid administration, limited medications, and in some cases, defibrillation. Paramedics provide advanced life support, which includes advanced airway control such as intubation, defibrillation, cardioversion and pacing capabilities, intravenous fluids, medications, and invasive techniques for airway support and control.

As you enter an EMT course, you must have a physical examination and review of your immunization records. This is to ensure that you are physically up to the job and that you are protected against exposure to diseases for which vaccines are available. Suggested immunizations are:

✔ tetanus
✔ hepatitis B
✔ verify immune status to common diseases such as measles, chicken pox, and mumps
✔ TB testing
✔ seasonal flu vaccines and others that may be available to you

ROLES AND RESPONSIBILITIES OF THE EMT

The roles and responsibilities of the EMT include

✔ personal safety;
✔ safety of your crew;
✔ patient assessment;
✔ patient care based on assessment findings;
✔ lifting and moving patients safely;
✔ transport/transfer of care;
✔ record keeping and data collection;
✔ patient advocacy (patient rights), patient as a whole.

The EMT's primary responsibility is personal safety. The EMT first determines the safety of a scene and takes proper precautions to protect against exposure to any patient body fluids. Training to lift and move patients safely enables you to move patients while minimizing the risk of injury to yourself. This is a very important part of your practice as back injuries are the most common career-ending injury. Determining whether the scene is safe includes making sure that other responders (like police or fire) have done their job to make the scene safe and secure before the EMT enters. This also includes protection from blood-born pathogens, by wearing HEPA or N95 masks, eye proteciton, and gloves. The EMT's safety is the priority. You can be of no help to the sick and injured if you become a patient yourself.

You will be called on to make assessments of the sick and injured and treatments will be based on the needs of your patient determined through this assessment. Special situations may call for special clothing such as hazmat suits or self-contained breathing apparatus (SCBA).

PERSONAL ATTRIBUTES

To ensure confidence and convey an image of well-trained professionals, EMTs should work to maintain a neat, clean, and positive image. It is also the responsibility of the EMT to attend continuing education and refresher courses as required to maintain licensure and to their keep skills and knowledge base up to the highest levels possible. It is also important to remember that in caring for patients, their needs must always be the priority. This priority is met only if it can be done without placing the EMT in jeopardy. The EMT also needs to keep up-to-date with local, state, and national issues that affect EMS. EMS is affected by the activities of a variety of legislative and commercial entities and it is important for EMTs to know what is going on that will affect their ability to care for patients.

Quality Improvement

The DOT curriculum defines quality improvement as "A system of internal/external reviews and audits of all aspects of an EMS system so as to identify those aspects needing improvement to assure that the public receives the highest quality of prehospital care."

The roles of the EMT in quality improvement include

- ✔ documentation;
- ✔ run reviews and audits;
- ✔ gathering feedback from patients and hospital staff;
- ✔ conducting preventative maintenance;
- ✔ continuing education;
- ✔ skill maintenance.

MEDICAL DIRECTION

A physician is responsible for the clinical and patient care aspects of an EMS system and every ambulance service must have physician medical direction. This medical direction is provided in two ways.

Online Medical Direction

This is direct medical direction over patient care during an EMS run via phone or radio communication.

Off-line Medical Direction

Medical direction is also provided through establishing protocols and standard operation guidelines/orders.

The medical director is also responsible for reviewing quality improvement. The EMT's relationship with his or her medical director is important, as the EMT is the agent of the medical director. As an extension of the medical director, the EMT carries out the medical director's orders by following protocols, standard guidelines, or direct orders.

STATE AND LOCAL LEGAL ISSUES

In each state, a law is in place that establishes the practice of prehospital care. Associated with that law are rules and regulations that dictate how EMTs are to be trained and licensed. The regulations also describe the authority of the medical director and what the minimum practice levels are for EMTs throughout the state.

Scenario

You are called to a scene of an industrial accident to treat a man who is bleeding profusely from his right forearm. As an EMT, what should you do as you approach this scene?

SOLUTION

Scene safety is first. The EMT should first make sure that the hazard that created the injury, or any other hazard, has been secured. The EMT should also be wearing any special equipment (helmet, goggles, etc.) that this industrial situation requires. Scene safety also includes BSI and at the very least, the EMT should be wearing gloves and protective eye covering. Masks or gowns may be necessary in particularly messy situations.

Review Questions

EXERCISES

The exercises in this review are designed to help reinforce your knowledge of the objectives for this chapter. If you find it difficult to meet any of the objectives stated, go back and review those materials again.

1. List and give an example of each of the 14 attributes that are essential to any EMS system. (Objective 1)

Attribute	Example

2. Describe the roles and responsibilities of EMTs and other prehospital care providers. (Objective 2)

Provider	Roles and Responsibilities
First Responder or Emergency Medical Responder (EMR)	
Emergency Medical Technician (EMT)	
EMT—Intermediate or Advanced EMT	
Paramedic	

3. You have been dispatched to a scene of a motor vehicle collision with injuries. Describe specific behaviors that will help you maintain personal safety. (Objective 3)

_____

_____

_____

_____

4. You have been dispatched to an office building where several people have become ill after an exterminator sprayed for insects. (Objective 4) Describe how you will maintain the safety of

Your crew:

_____

_____

Your patients:

_____

_____

Bystanders:

_____

_____

5. How is quality improvement defined by the DOT curriculum?

_____

_____

Give examples of how you can fulfill each of the following roles in quality improvement. (Objective 5)

Documentation:

_____

_____

Reviews and audits:

_____

_____

Gathering feedback from patients and hospital staff:

_____

_____

Conducting preventative maintenance:

_____

Continuing education:

_____

_____

Skill maintenance:

_____

_____

6. What is online medical direction?

_____

_____

What is off-line medical direction?

_____

_____

As an extension of the medical director, the EMT carries out the medical

director's orders by _____

_____.

(Objective 6)

7. Specific state laws establish the _____ of prehospital care. The

rules and regulations also dictate _____

_____.

(Objective 7)

MULTIPLE-CHOICE QUESTIONS

1. The purpose of a system of emergency medical services is to care for sick and injured patients by providing all of the following EXCEPT
   (A) assessment.
   (B) definitive care.
   (C) transportation.
   (D) stabilization.

2. EMTs may transport patients from _____ to _____ .
   (A) the hospital; the patient's home
   (B) the scene of an emergency; the hospital
   (C) one hospital; another hospital
   (D) all of the above

3. According to the NHTSA technical assistance standards, which of the following is an essential component of an EMS system?
   (A) ambulances
   (B) physicians
   (C) policies
   (D) all of the above

4. The level of EMS provider that gives initial emergency care but does not usually transport patients is
   (A) First Responder (Emergency Medical responder).
   (B) EMT.
   (C) EMT-Intermediate (Advanced EMT).
   (D) Paramedic.

5. The EMT's first responsibility is
   (A) complying with medical direction.
   (B) caring for the patient.
   (C) maintaining personal safety.
   (D) following the employer's policies.

6. Which of the following is NOT an example of medical direction?
   (A) standing orders
   (B) protocols
   (C) following paramedics' verbal orders
   (D) following physicians' radio orders

7. The primary reason the EMT must use body substance isolation (BSI) or universal precautions is to
    (A) protect the patient from infectious diseases carried by the EMT.
    (B) prevent contamination of equipment after contacting patients.
    (C) protect the EMT from contracting diseases from patients who have known infections.
    (D) prevent the EMT from exposure to blood and body fluids that may contain potentially infectious material.

8. The most important responsibility of the EMT in providing public information and education is to inform the public regarding
    (A) how to access the communication and dispatch system if EMS is needed.
    (B) which illnesses and injuries require an EMS response, and which do not.
    (C) the cost of being transported by ambulance.
    (D) comprehensive health and wellness programs.

9. Which of the following is an important personal attribute of EMTs?
    (A) being informed about local, state, and national issues in EMS
    (B) maintaining a neat, clean, positive image
    (C) placing the patient's needs above all else, except personal safety
    (D) all of the above

10. The laws that govern the practice of EMS are typically enacted at the _____ level of government.
    (A) federal
    (B) state
    (C) county
    (D) city

ANSWERS TO REVIEW QUESTIONS
Exercises

1.

Attribute	Example
Integration of Health Services	Use of evidence-based protocols that are consistent from the field through in-hospital care
EMS Research	Scientific review of prehospital treatment and patient outcomes
Legislation and Regulations	Federal and state laws, such as laws governing licensure and scope of practice; rules that apply the law to practice
System Finance	Budgeting and funding the provision of EMS in a variety of environments using diverse delivery models
Human Resources	Providers of prehospital care; paid or volunteer.
Medical Direction	Active involvement of physicians knowledgeable in EMS
Education Systems	Educational systems to provide training for prehospital care personnel
Public Education	Educating the public on how to access EMS and how EMS works
Prevention	Education to encourage prevention of illness and injury
Public Access	Universal access to EMS through 911 dispatch centers
Communication Systems	Radio and cellular systems linking EMS providers with dispatch centers, other response agencies, and hospitals
Clinical Care	Actual patient care guided by evidence-based protocols
Information Systems	Systems to provide information crucial to EMS personnel and to record EMS activity including paper, electronic, and wireless applications
Evaluation	Data collection and setting and assessing performance benchmarks

2.

Provider	Roles and Responsibilities
First Responder or Emergency Medical Responder	Gives initial care, such as bleeding control or CPR. Typically does not transport patients.
EMT	Provides basic life support at the scene and during transportation to the hospital.
EMT—Intermediate or Advanced EMT	Provides some advanced life support, such as defibrillation, IVs, and a limited number of medications.
Paramedic	Provides advanced life support, including intubation, defibrillation, cardiac pacing, and medications.

3. Important considerations include having the appropriate immunizations, driving safely, assessing the scene for hazards, such as downed power lines and unstable vehicles, parking in a safe location, using appropriate personal protective equipment, and using safe lifting techniques.

4. Your crew:
The crew should not enter the area if a chemical hazard exists, and should use protective gear to prevent contamination of the skin and clothing by the insecticide.
Your patients:
The patients should be removed to fresh air to prevent further exposure to the insecticide.
Bystanders:
Bystanders should not be allowed to gather in the area where there may be a chemical hazard.

5. "A system of internal/external reviews and audits of all aspects of an EMS system so as to identify those aspects needing improvement to assure that the public receives the highest quality of prehospital care."
Documentation:
It is critical to be accurate and complete in documentation.
Reviews and audits:
Attending reviews and audits of EMS calls allows your calls to be critiqued to identify areas of strength and weakness.
Gathering feedback from patients and hospital staff:
This practice allows continual improvement by learning the perspective of patients and hospital personnel.

Conducting preventative maintenance:
Making sure equipment and vehicles are in top working order prevents complications in patient treatment due to equipment failure, or delays in response or transportation.
Continuing education:
Attending regular continuing education offerings and reading journals allows you to be as up to date as possible on issues in prehospital care.
Skill maintenance:
Practicing skills, such as ventilation skills, ensures that the patient is cared for efficiently and skillfully when the time comes.

6. **On-line medical control** is the direct medical oversight of patient care by a physician via telephone or radio contact.
Off-line medical control is provided by the physician's written protocols or standing orders.
As an extension of the medical director, the EMT carries out the medical director's orders by **following protocols, guidelines, or direct orders.**

7. Specific state laws establish the **practice** of prehospital care. The rules and regulations also dictate **how EMTs are to be trained and licensed, and describe the authority of the medical director and what the minimum practice levels are for EMTs throughout the state.**

Multiple-Choice Answers

1. **(B)** Objective 2
Definitive care can only be provided in a hospital equipped to manage the patient's condition. EMS personnel are responsible for assessing the patient, providing initial stabilization, and transporting the patient to a facility that can provide definitive care.

2. **(D)** Objective 2
While the role of the EMT that receives the most attention in the media is that of transporting ill and injured patients from the scene of an emergency to a hospital, EMTs are also frequently responsible for transporting patients from a hospital to their homes and from one hospital to another.

3. **(D)** Objective 1
All of these elements are critical to the operation of an EMS system.

4. **(A)** Objective 2
First responders play a critical role in getting to the scene of an emergency quickly and providing initial life-saving care. However, the first level of EMS provider who may transport patients is the EMT.

5. **(C)** Objective 3
While providing patient care under medical direction and within the policies of the employer is critical, this cannot be accomplished if the EMT allows himself or herself to become injured.

6. **(C)** Objective 6

   EMTs often work closely with paramedics and follow their guidance, but medical direction can only be provided by a physician, either in advance in the form of protocols or standing orders, or verbally at the time of the call.

7. **(D)** Objective 3

   BSI is primarily used to protect the EMT from potentially infectious blood or body fluids. BSI is used whenever there is a risk of exposure to blood or body fluids, because it is not always possible to tell whether a patient has an infectious disease.

8. **(A)** Objective 1

   Communication, including communication from the public to the dispatch center, is a critical part of EMS systems. The EMT has an essential role to play in ensuring that this part of the EMS system works by providing the public with information about how to request EMS.

9. **(D)** Objective 4

   The EMT can best carry out his or her responsibilities to the patient and the public by keeping informed, maintaining a professional image, and placing the patient's needs above all else except personal safety.

10. **(B)** Objective 7

    Federal laws cannot account for the individual needs of each state, therefore, in most states, laws governing EMS are at the state level of government, although in some areas, state laws may be modified in particular municipalities.

Well-Being of the EMT

 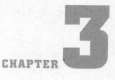

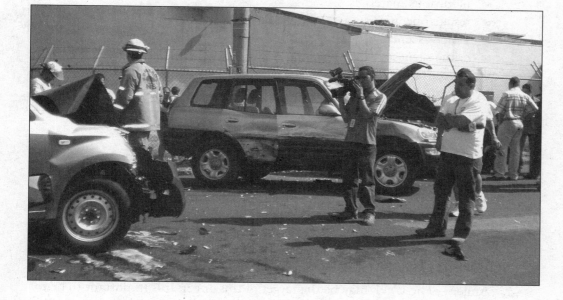

CHAPTER 3

OBJECTIVES

This chapter and the review questions will help readers determine if they are able to

1. list possible emotional reactions that the EMT may experience when faced with trauma, illness, death, and dying;

2. discuss the possible reactions that a family member may exhibit when confronted with death and dying;

3. state the steps in the EMT's approach to the family confronted with death and dying;

4. state the possible reactions that the family of the EMT may exhibit due to their outside involvement in EMS;

5. recognize the signs and symptoms of critical incident stress;

6. state the possible steps that the EMT should take for protection from blood-borne pathogens;

7. explain the need to determine scene safety;

8. discuss the importance of body substance isolation;

9. describe the steps the EMT should take for personal protection from airborne and blood-borne pathogens;

10. list the personal protective equipment necessary for each of the following situations:

   ✔ hazardous materials
   ✔ rescue operations
   ✔ violent scenes
   ✔ crime scenes
   ✔ exposure to blood-borne pathogens
   ✔ exposure to airborne pathogens

EMOTIONAL ASPECTS OF EMERGENCY CARE

The EMT must be prepared for the emotional aspects of our work. This includes dealing with death and dying. People faced with death, either their own or someone close to them, go through five stages toward acceptance. These stages are

1. **Denial**—"No, not me."

2. **Anger**—The EMT may be the target of this anger. It is important to be tolerant and not become defensive. Good listening skills and empathy will be key to helping them though this.

3. **Bargaining**—This is an attempt to postpone the death for a time, to make a deal. "I'll be a better person if you just bring him or her back."

4. **Depression**—Characterized by sadness and/or despair with the patient becoming quiet and withdrawing.

5. **Acceptance**—While the patient may have accepted dying at this time, he or she may still be very sad and unhappy. The family will require a great deal of support at this point.

In dealing with dying patients and their family the EMT needs to address the patient's needs by treating him or her with dignity and respect. The patient will also want to share in decisions about his or her care, so communication is key. The patient also has a need and right to privacy, which should be given as much as possible.

The family of the dying patient may express rage, anger, and/or despair. The EMT should listen empathetically and speak using a gentle tone of voice while being careful not to falsely reassure. Holding the patient's hand or a gentle touch on the arm may also serve to show genuine concern and attention to his or her needs. Let the patient and family know that everything that can be done will be done and give as much comfort as possible.

STRESSFUL SITUATIONS

Examples of situations that may cause stress to the EMT may include

- ✔ mass casualty situations;
- ✔ infant and child trauma;
- ✔ amputations;
- ✔ infant, child, elder, or spousal abuse;
- ✔ death or injury of coworker or other public safety personnel.

The EMT may experience personal stress as well as having to deal with patients, bystanders, and family members who are experiencing stress.

STRESS MANAGEMENT

The EMT must be able to recognize the warning signs of stress in themselves and their coworkers:

- ✔ irritability toward coworkers, family, and friends
- ✔ inability to concentrate
- ✔ difficulty sleeping and/or nightmares
- ✔ anxiety
- ✔ indecisiveness
- ✔ guilt
- ✔ loss of appetite
- ✔ loss of interest in sexual activitiy
- ✔ isolation
- ✔ loss of interest in work

Lifestyle changes can be helpful in dealing with job stress and "burn-out." Changing your diet by reducing sugar, caffeine, and alcohol intake, avoiding fatty foods, and increasing carbohydrates will help. Exercise and practicing relaxation techniques, meditation, or visual imagery can also help reduce or regulate stress. In any case, balancing work, recreation, family, and personal well-being promotes health and career longevity.

FRIENDS AND FAMILY

Friends and family of the EMT can either help the EMT to deal with stress or they can contribute to the stress. They may have a lack of understanding for your work. This can contribute to a fear of separation and being ignored. Irregular work schedules and the complications to family life of being on-call make it difficult to plan activities and may cause those close to us to feel they cannot count on us. Wanting to share and not feeling understood can be frustrating and hurtful.

You can address this by requesting shifts that allow more time with friends and family. Make an effort to express the things you need to share with your family while making sure to hear their concerns as well. If you cannot get a handle on this, seek professional help before things get too far out of hand.

CRITICAL INCIDENT STRESS DEBRIEFING (CISD)

Critical incident stress debriefing teams are teams of peer counselors and mental health professionals who can be called together to help emergency care workers deal with critical incident stress. The meeting must be held within 24 to 72 hours of the incident to be effective and consists of open discussions of feelings, fears, and reactions. It is not a critique or an investigation and all of the information and discussions are confidential. The team makes recommendations or suggestions to help the care workers overcome the stress of the incident. Sessions are designed to accelerate the normal recovery process after a critical incident and succeed through venting feelings in a nonthreatening environment.

Comprehensive critical incident stress management includes

✔ pre-incident stress education;
✔ on-scene peer support;
✔ one-on-one support;
✔ disaster support services;
✔ defusing;
✔ debriefing;
✔ follow-up services;
✔ spouse/family support;
✔ community outreach programs;
✔ other health and welfare programs, such as wellness programs.

Check with your EMS system on how to access CISDs in your area. While there has been some controversy as to the effectiveness of CISD in recent years it continues to be in wide use in EMS.

SCENE SAFETY

The first part of scene safety is BSI. For the protection of yourself and your patients you should

✔ wash hands before and after patient contacts.
✔ use eye protection (glasses or goggles).
✔ wear vinyl or latex gloves.
✔ use heavier gloves for cleaning the vehicle and equipment.
✔ wear a gown when there is body fluid splash potential and change uniforms when exposed.
✔ wear a mask to protect against inhaled hazards.
✔ use a special High Efficiency Particulate Air (HEPA) mask for treating patients with tuberculosis.
✔ have patients with respiratory disease wear surgical masks as long as it does not interfere with breathing or oxygen delivery.

You should also familiarize yourself with Occupational Safety and Health Administration (OSHA) and state regulations regarding BSI and rules on notification of exposure.

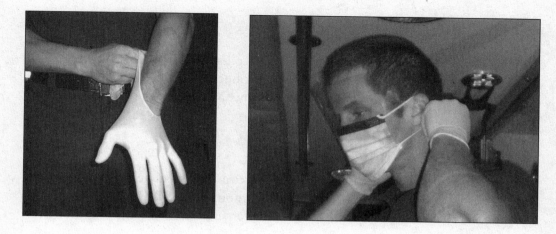

Personal Protection

In dealing with hazardous materials, your most important equipment will be binoculars and the *Hazardous Materials, The Emergency Response Handbook*, published by the U.S. DOT. Use the binoculars to find the placard on container(s) and use the guidebook to determine the hazards. Unless you are specially trained to deal with hazardous environments, do not enter a hazardous scene. Even if you are trained, you cannot approach the hazards without HAZMAT suits and self-contained breathing apparatus. Specially trained hazardous materials teams are in control of these scenes and you should do as instructed by the team. Should there be patients for you to treat, the team will decontaminate them and deliver them to you.

Rescue

Safe rescue depends on first identifying and securing hazards. These hazards might include

- ✔ electricity;
- ✔ fire;
- ✔ explosions;
- ✔ hazardous materials.

These hazards must be secured before rescue can be accomplished. To effect rescue safely, the EMT should wear full protective clothing, including

- ✔ turnout gear;
- ✔ puncture-proof gloves;
- ✔ helmet;
- ✔ eye protection.

In confined space or entrapment situations, special rescue teams need to be used. In the case of violence at the scene, police should secure the scene before the EMT enters. If you know that the scene is a violent one, ask dispatch if police are on the scene before you get there. If not, inform them that you will be staging a safe distance away until police secure the scene. Violent scenes can present hazards from the perpetrator of a crime, family, or bystanders. If you find yourself at a crime scene, do not disturb the scene any more than necessary for patient care.

Scenario 1

You are called to the scene of a motor vehicle collision; the victim is entrapped in the car. The extrication team has gained access but you are being called to remove the victim from the vehicle. What do you as an EMT have to do in order to work on this scene?

SOLUTION

The EMT needs to take personal protection precautions that are appropriate to the scene. In this case besides BSI precautions, turnout gear including helmet, gloves, coat, boots, and eye protection must be worn to participate in removing the victim from the car.

Scenario 2

You arrive on the scene where a child has died. The mother is sitting quietly in the corner by herself and the father is shouting that the rescuers are all idiots and do not know what they are doing. What is happening here and what should you do?

SOLUTION

The mother appears to be slipping into the depression stage of acceptance while the father is in the anger phase. Have the child quickly packaged for transport and try to make time or have someone else make time to listen to and be empathetic toward the family.

Scenario 3

You have arrived at the scene of a hazardous materials incident. Should you go to the patients?

SOLUTION

In hazardous materials incidents special training and equipment are needed. The patients will be decontaminated and brought to you.

Review Questions

EXERCISES

The exercises in this review are designed to help reinforce your knowledge of the objectives for this chapter. If you find it difficult to meet any of the objectives stated, go back and review those materials again.

1. List 10 emotional reactions that EMTs may experience in response to stressful situations. (Objective 1)

_____

_____

_____

_____

2. List and describe each of the five stages of loss associated with one's own death or that of a loved one. (Objective 2)

Stage of Loss	Description

3. You and your partner have been dispatched to respond to "an unresponsive person." On your arrival, you find that the patient is a 57-year-old female with a history of ovarian cancer. She is not breathing and does not have a pulse. The family produces a valid, signed "Do not resuscitate" (DNR) order from the patient's physician. Therefore, you are obligated to withhold resuscitative efforts. Discuss below how you will interact with the patient's family in this situation. (Objective 3)

_____

_____

_____

_____

4. You have just begun volunteering for a rescue squad in your community. Discuss below how family members may respond to an EMT's involvement in EMS. (Objective 4)

_____

_____

_____

_____

5. Last week, on your day off, your partner responded to the scene of a house fire in which four small children were killed. Explain how you will recognize whether your partner begins to experience critical incident stress. (Objective 5)

_____

_____

_____

_____

6. You just responded to a motor vehicle collision (MVC) in which your patient, the driver of a vehicle that rolled over down an embankment, was ejected through the windshield. The patient has numerous lacerations and is vomiting. Explain how you will protect yourself from exposure to the patient's body fluids. (Objective 6)

   _____

   _____

   _____

   _____

7. Explain the importance of establishing scene safety by listing hazards you should anticipate at each of the scenes below. (Objective 7)
   (A) A vehicle that crashed into a utility pole, downing electrical lines, is leaking fluids.

   _____

   _____

   (B) You have been called to an apartment to treat a woman reporting that her boyfriend "tried to choke her to death."

   _____

   _____

   (C) You have been called to a college dorm where a party got out of hand and a 19-year-old male student fell from a second-story balcony.

   _____

   _____

8. What are some of the infectious diseases to which the EMT can minimize exposure by using appropriate BSI? (Objective 8)

   _____

   _____

9. Your patient is a resident of an extended care facility in which there is a high prevalence of tuberculosis. The patient, a 75-year-old male, is complaining of a fever and cough. What will you do to minimize your risk of exposure to airborne pathogens? (Objective 9)

_____

_____

10. Fill in the matrix below to describe the PPE necessary for the situations listed. (Objective 10)

Situation	PPE Required
Hazardous Materials	
Rescue Operations	
Violent Scenes	
Crime Scenes	

MULTIPLE-CHOICE QUESTIONS

1. You are treating a critically injured child. The child's mother is crying and saying, "Please, God, let him live. I swear I will never ask for anything again." The mother's reaction is best described as
   (A) bargaining.
   (B) anger.
   (C) denial.
   (D) depression.

2. You just informed a family that their loved one is dead and that there is nothing you can do for her. The patient's son screams at you and punches the wall. This is best described as _____ , which is an _____ response to the death of a loved one.
   (A) anguish; expected
   (B) anguish; unexpected
   (C) anger; expected
   (D) anger; unexpected

3. Which of the following situations would most predictably produce critical incident stress in EMS personnel?
   (A) repeatedly responding to the same address for a patient who does not really seem to be sick
   (B) delivering a baby
   (C) responding to an elderly female who was forced by her caregiver to sit in a bathtub of hot water until she received full-thickness (third-degree) burns
   (D) inability to successfully resuscitate an 80-year-old male who was found in cardiac arrest in his bed

4. You respond to a home where an 85-year-old male apparently died in his sleep during the night. The body is cool to the touch, mottled, and rigored. The patient's wife is looking at you anxiously, asking, "Isn't there anything you can do?" What is the best way to handle this situation?
   (A) State, "I am sorry ma'am. Your husband is dead."
   (B) State, "Yes ma'am. We will do our best." Then, initiate resuscitation attempts and transport the patient.
   (C) State, "No, I'm afraid he has passed."
   (D) Initiate resuscitation attempts, but stop as soon as you are in the back of the ambulance, where the wife cannot see you.

5. Your patient has signs and symptoms suggestive of tuberculosis. He is coughing and needs oxygen. Which action is most appropriate in protecting yourself from exposure to tuberculosis?
   (A) wear a HEPA mask or N-95 respirator and gloves
   (B) place a HEPA mask or N-95 respirator on your patient
   (C) place a non-rebreather oxygen mask on the patient and sit as far away as possible during transportation
   (D) place surgical masks on yourself and your patient, and wear gloves, goggles, and a gown

6. Your partner's spouse is placing a lot of pressure on her because of the time she spends away from him doing her job. She says she does not know what to do about it, but it is really "stressing her out." Which response would be most appropriate?
   (A) "Don't worry about it. He'll get used to it in time."
   (B) "What a jerk! Don't let him lay this on you."
   (C) "Have you thought about requesting a shift that might allow you to spend more time together?"
   (D) "It seldom works out when a person in EMS is married to someone who isn't in the medical field."

7. Critical incident stress debriefing is effective when it is conducted within _____ of the event.
   (A) 1 hour
   (B) 24 to 72 hours
   (C) 4 days
   (D) 1 week

8. Which of the following dietary habits is helpful in minimizing the effects of stress?
   (A) using caffeine to stay awake when working the night shift
   (B) having three to four alcoholic drinks each day
   (C) eating a variety foods, limiting fat and sugar intake
   (D) all of the above

9. You recently notice that you are irritated with your spouse, children, and just about everyone. You are not sleeping well, and find it difficult to sit through a movie, which is usually an enjoyable activity for you. Which of the following is most likely to be helpful?
   (A) request a couple of overtime shifts to avoid conflict with your family
   (B) walk a mile or so before or after your shift and on your days off
   (C) have a beer or glass of wine before bed to help you relax and fall asleep
   (D) call in sick for your next shift

10. Personal protective equipment for rescue situations includes all of the following EXCEPT
    (A) turnout gear.
    (B) helmet.
    (C) eye protection.
    (D) latex or vinyl gloves.

ANSWERS TO REVIEW QUESTIONS

Exercises

1. Irritability toward coworkers, family, and friends; inability to concentrate; difficulty sleeping and/or nightmares; anxiety; indecisiveness; guilt; loss of appetite; loss of interest in sex; isolation; and loss of interest in work.

2.

Stage of Loss	Description
Denial	"No, not me."
Anger	The patient or family may direct this anger toward the EMT, making the EMT's ability to listen and demonstrate empathy critical
Bargaining	Attempting to make a deal to forestall death
Depression	Sadness and despair, which may manifest as withdrawal
Acceptance	Coming to terms with the situation

3. The family requires the EMT's support at this time. The EMT must treat them with dignity and respect, and must not provide false reassurance. Showing empathy and concern is critical.

4. Some family members may be supportive, but in other situations, the family's feelings may cause additional stress for the EMT. The family may be upset by separation and time apart, feel ignored, and find it difficult to plan activities due to the EMT's schedule and obligations.

5. Signs of critical incident stress include irritability toward coworkers, family, and friends; inability to concentrate; difficulty sleeping and/or nightmares; anxiety; indecisiveness; guilt; loss of appetite; loss of interest in sex; isolation; and loss of interest in work.

6. At a minimum, this situation requires gloves and protective eyewear. Depending on the amount of blood and whether the patient is actively bleeding or vomiting, a mask and gown may be required, as well.

7. (A) The vehicle may be unstable, air bags may not have deployed and may deploy during extrication, the utility pole may be unstable, the power company must be notified to shut off power to the downed lines, and the fluids leaking may be flammable, or may cause a slip hazard.

   (B) The assailant may still be on the scene, and EMTs should not approach until law enforcement has secured the scene.

(C) Potential hazards in this situation include a crowd of bystanders in a situation where alcohol, and perhaps other drugs, have likely been consumed, altering judgment. Additionally, it is not known if the balcony is unstable, and perhaps shifted, contributing to the fall.

8. Exposure to hepatitis B and C, HIV, tuberculosis, as well as other less concerning diseases, such as childhood illness, can be minimized by BSI.

9. The EMT must wear a HEPA or N-95 respirator in addition to BSI worn for other patients. Disinfection of equipment and the ambulance, and good hand-washing are also critical.

10.

Situation	PPE Required
Hazardous Materials	Special training and equipment are required. The EMT caring for patients who have been exposed to hazardous materials includes binoculars, and depending upon other training the EMT may have received, HAZMAT suits and SCBA.
Rescue Operations	Turnout gear, puncture-proof gloves, helmet, and eye protection.
Violent Scenes	The EMT should not enter violent scenes until the scene has been secured by law enforcement.
Crime Scenes	The EMT's primary responsibility is patient care, but he or she should be cautious not to unnecessarily touch anything or otherwise disturb the scene.

Multiple-Choice Answers

1. (A) Objective 2
   Bargaining is the stage of grief or loss in which the patient or loved one tries to make a deal in order to avert death.

2. (C) Objective 2
   Anger is an expected reaction to the death of a loved one. The EMT must be willing to listen and demonstrate empathy to defuse this anger, when necessary.

3. **(C)** Objective 5

   Some of the situations that commonly produce stress reactions in EMS personnel include: mass casualty situations; trauma to infants and children; amputations; infant, child, elder, or spousal abuse; and death or injury of a coworker or other public safety personnel.

4. **(A)** Objective 3

   It is important that the EMT be honest, clear, and empathetic when dealing with situations like this. Clear language, such as the term "dead" may seem harsh, but it is not likely to be mistaken for another meaning, as less direct terms may be. The EMT must not give false reassurance that the patient can be resuscitated.

5. **(A)** Objective 9

   Exposure to airborne pathogens is best prevented with a high-efficiency mask that eliminates small particulates in inspired air. While surgical masks on the patient may sometimes be acceptable, this patient requires oxygen.

6. **(C)** Objective 4

   Neither ignoring the problem, putting blame on the spouse, nor expressing hopelessness about the situation is likely to make the situation better. The most productive response is to suggest requesting a shift that might allow the couple to spend more time together.

7. **(B)** Objective 5

   CISD is effective within 72 hours.

8. **(C)** Objective 1

   Using caffeine and alcohol are not effective or healthy strategies to cope with stress. A healthy diet, low in fat and sugar, is helpful in maintaining overall health and assisting in coping with stress.

9. **(B)** Objective 1

   Regular exercise is a positive step in coping with stress, while the other responses avoid dealing with stress.

10. **(D)** Objective 10

    When performing rescue operations, latex or vinyl gloves will not provide adequate protection. The EMT must wear puncture-resistant gloves.

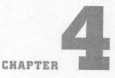
Medical, Legal, and Ethical Issues

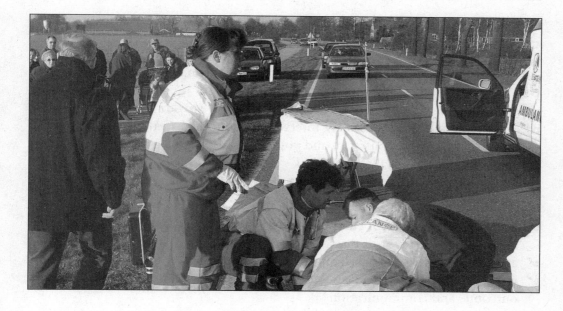

OBJECTIVES

This chapter and the review questions will help readers determine if they are able to

1. define the EMT's scope of practice;

2. discuss the importance of do not resuscitate (DNR), advance directives, and local or state provisions regarding EMS application;

3. define consent and discuss the methods of obtaining consent;

4. differentiate between expressed and implied consent;

5. explain the role of consent of minors in providing care;

6. discuss the implications for the EMT in patient refusal of transport;

7. discuss the issues of abandonment, negligence, and battery and their implications to the EMT;

8. state the conditions necessary for the EMT to have a duty to act;

9. explain the importance, necessity, and legality of patient confidentiality;

10. discuss the considerations of the EMT in issues of organ retrieval;

11. differentiate the actions that the EMT should take to assist in the preservation of a crime scene;

12. State the conditions that require the EMT to notify local law enforcement officials keep.

SCOPE OF PRACTICE

The EMT's scope of practice is to render basic life support (BLS) to the sick and injured. The EMTs scope of practice also includes legal duties to the patient, the medical director, and the public. The EMT must provide for the well-being of the patient by rendering necessary interventions outlined in the scope of practice dictated by the laws in your state and your medical director and referenced to the National Standard curricula. The EMT's legal right to function may also be contingent on medical direction by radio or phone communications or protocols.

The EMT's ethical responsibilities are:

✔ to meet the physical and emotional needs of the patient, and practice and maintain skills to the point of mastery
✔ attend continuing education and refresher programs
✔ critically review performances and seek ways to improve response time, patient outcome, and communication
✔ honesty in reporting

DO NOT RESUSCITATE ORDERS AND ADVANCE DIRECTIVES

A DNR is a document expressing a patient's wish to not be resuscitated if found pulseless and nonbreathing. Patients have a right to refuse resuscitation and you should know your state, local, and EMS system rules on what constitutes a legal "Do Not Resuscitate" order. In general, a written order from a physician is the model used. If there is any doubt, the EMT should begin resuscitation efforts. Advance directives can include DNRs but may also be statements limiting the care a patient may wish to receive. Examples may include "comfort measures only" or "do not place on ventilator."

CONSENT

The EMT must have consent to treat a patient; there are three different types of consent to be familiar with.

1. **Expressed consent** is verbal consent given by a patient of legal age to give it. The patient must be informed of the steps of the procedure and the risks of treating or not treating. All conscious, mentally competent adults must give this type of consent.
2. **Implied consent** is assumed in unconscious patients requiring emergency care. It is based on the assumption that the patient would give consent to life-saving care were they able to do so.
3. **Children and mentally incompetent adults** must have consent given by a parent or legal guardian. Review your state laws regarding emancipation and the age of minors in your state. In life-threatening situations where there is no guardian present, treat the patient using the rule of implied consent.

ASSAULT AND/OR BATTERY

Assault and battery are charges that can be brought against an EMT for violating a patient's rights or creating a threat of harm. A charge of battery can be brought for touching a patient without permission and assault may be charged if the EMT caused the patient to be in fear of injury.

REFUSALS

Patients have a right to refuse care. They may withdraw from care at any time, even if they regain consciousness and want you to discontinue care. Refusals may be given by mentally competent adults following the rules of expressed consent. This means you must explain the possible complications should they refuse or discontinue care. Again, when in doubt, treat. Documentation is important in protecting the EMT in refusals. Before leaving the scene, try again to persuade the patient and make sure the patient is able to make a rational, informed decision. This means that the patient must not be under the influence of drugs, alcohol, or illness or injury. Consult medical direction as your protocols dictate and consider assistance from the police if needed. Document any findings and care given and have the patient sign a refusal-of-care form.

ABANDONMENT

Abandonment is terminating care without assuring the continuation of care at the same level or higher.

NEGLIGENCE

Negligence is deviation from the accepted standard of care resulting in further injury to the patient. In order for negligence to be found, all of these components must be present:

- ✔ duty to act
- ✔ breach of duty
- ✔ injury or damages inflicted
    - physical
    - psychological
- ✔ actions of the EMT caused the injury or damage

DUTY TO ACT

For duty to act to be present, a contractual or legal obligation must exist. It is implied if a patient calls for an ambulance and it is confirmed that the ambulance will be sent. It is also implied once treatment on the patient begins.

Formal obligation occurs when an ambulance service has a written contract with a municipality or an individual.

Legal duty to act may not apply but there still may be moral or ethical considerations. In some states, duty to act is established when an EMT sees that someone is is need of care. Documentation again is important in determining when duty to act is established. Know the rules regarding this in your state.

CONFIDENTIALITY

Your patient's history, your assessment, and treatments provided are confidential information and cannot be shared with anyone not involved in the patient's care unless released in writing by the patient. Release is not required if state law requires reporting, such as in criminal assaults (rape or gunshots), or if a legal subpoena is produced.

SPECIAL SITUATIONS

Organ Donors

One example of a special situation the EMT will face is the organ donor. Organ donors may have a card expressing their wishes or they will have signed a space on their driver's license. First and foremost, you should not treat the organ donor any differently than you would any other patient. Your role in these situations is to identify the patient as a potential donor in your communication with the hospital and then to the team that receives your patient. You can also reassure the family that you will do you best to honor their wishes.

Medical Identification Insignia

EMTs should also be on the lookout for medical identification insignia. Bracelets, necklaces, or cards can identify the patient as a diabetic, heart patient, or having any significant medical condition. They may also list medications the patient may be taking or allergies.

Crime Scene Evidence

At a crime scene the patient's needs are the EMT's first priority. Dispatch should be notified that you have happened upon the scene of a crime if they are not aware. Do not disturb anything at the scene unless patient care makes it necessary. Document any observations you may have about the scene. Your patient care may involve removing the patient's clothing; if so, avoid cutting through rips, tears, bullet, or knife holes that may have been made in commission of the crime.

Special Reporting Situations

While it differs by state, each state has situations or events that must be reported. Infant, child, elder, and/or spousal abuse, wounds resulting from a crime, and sexual assault are examples of required reporting situations. Familiarize yourself with the laws in your state.

Scenario 1

You are treating an unconscious male patient on the street. You determine that the man is in critical condition and should be transported immediately. The police have been unable to locate family to give consent for treatment and transport. What should the EMT do in this case?

SOLUTION

The EMT should treat and transport this critical patient. An EMT can treat an unconscious patient under implied consent.

Scenario 2

An off-duty EMT drives by the scene of a motor vehicle collision with injuries. Has this EMT violated any law by not stopping to help?

SOLUTION

In most states, "duty to act" must be established in order for the EMT to be required to render aid. In most states this EMT would not be in violation. It is important that all EMTs examine their own state laws, as there are laws in some states that require medically trained individuals to stop and render aid.

Scenario 3

An alert adult male who was struck in the head with a rock allowed you to bandage his head but is refusing transport. What should the EMT do in this situation?

SOLUTION

Alert adult patients have the right to refuse treatment and/or transport at any time during their care, so even though you have begun treatment he has the right to tell you that is all he wants. You should encourage him to go to the hospital and advise him of the possible complications that not going to the hospital could cause. Once you inform him of the dangers of not going to the hospital, have him sign a release and have family and/or police officers sign as witnesses.

Review Questions

EXERCISES

The exercises in this review are designed to help reinforce your knowledge of the objectives for this chapter. If you find it difficult to meet any of the objectives stated, go back and review those materials again.

1. What is an EMT's scope of practice? Who determines an EMT's scope of practice? (Objective 1)

   _____

   _____

   _____

   _____

2. How do DNR orders differ from advance directives? How do local or state provisions affect how EMTs follow DNRs and advanced directives? (Objective 2)

   _____

   _____

   _____

   _____

3. You respond to the home of a woman whose husband called for EMS because the woman has slurred speech. Is it necessary to obtain consent? If so, explain how you will obtain consent. (Objective 3)

_____

_____

_____

_____

4. Describe two scenarios: one in which you must obtain expressed consent, and one in which implied consent applies. (Objective 4)

_____

_____

_____

_____

5. You respond to a high school where a 15-year-old pregnant female appears to be in labor. Describe the considerations in obtaining consent to treat and transport this patient. (Objective 5)

_____

_____

_____

6. Your patient is a 35-year-old male kitchen worker who cut his thumb while slicing vegetables. The laceration appears to need sutures, but the patient refuses your treatment or transport. What should you do? (Objective 6)

_____

_____

_____

_____

7. Describe a scenario for each of the following. (Objective 7)
   Abandonment:

   _____

   _____

   Negligence:

   _____

   _____

   Battery:

   _____

   _____

8. You are in the ambulance on your way to a call for an injured football player. En route, a man on the sidewalk flags you down and states that there is an unresponsive man in the alley behind his house. What should you do? Explain your decision. (Objective 8)

   _____

   _____

   _____

   _____

9. As you are loading a patient injured in a motor vehicle collision into your ambulance, a man approaches the back of the ambulance and states he is a personal injury attorney. He offers you $200 for a copy of the patient care report. Explain your rationale for denying this request. (Objective 9)

   _____

   _____

   _____

   _____

10. Your patient is a 25-year-old female cyclist who was struck by a vehicle and was not wearing a helmet. She is alive, but is unresponsive and has significant injuries to her head. You feel that there is a good chance the patient may not survive. Do you have any obligations concerning potential organ donation? If so, what are they? (Objective 10)

_____

_____

_____

_____

11. Law enforcement has just secured the scene of a shooting and indicates to you that you have a single victim at the top of the stairs. You notice that there are shell casings present on the staircase. What significance does this have to you? (Objective 11)

_____

_____

_____

_____

12. In your state, in what situations are you required to notify local law enforcement? (Objective 12)

_____

_____

_____

_____

MULTIPLE-CHOICE QUESTIONS

1. You have responded to the home of an 80-year-old female in cardiac arrest. The patient's husband states, "She doesn't want to be kept alive by machines." The husband is not able to produce a written document from the patient's physician verifying these wishes. What should you do?
   (A) withhold resuscitation because the husband has not given consent
   (B) call the physician before attempting resuscitation
   (C) begin resuscitation
   (D) ask the husband to put his wishes in writing

2. Your patient is a 45-year-old male who is complaining of chest pain. He is diaphoretic and pale. He refuses your treatment and transport. Which of the following is most appropriate?
   (A) call law enforcement to place the patient under immediate detention so you can treat him
   (B) tell the patient he is having a heart attack and there is a high likelihood he will die within the next few hours
   (C) have the patient sign a release and leave the scene
   (D) contact medical direction and have the patient speak to the physician

3. Your patient is a 70-year-old female who does not want you to take her blood pressure. You apply the blood pressure cuff, causing the patient to become very upset. Your action is best described as
   (A) battery.
   (B) assault.
   (C) negligence.
   (D) duty to act.

4. You just transported a patient with an injured ankle to the emergency department and placed her in a wheelchair in the waiting room, without talking to a nurse or leaving a report. This is best described as
   (A) breach of contract.
   (B) negligence.
   (C) abandonment.
   (D) assault.

5. True or False: Any patient who has been drinking alcohol is incompetent to consent to or refuse medical care.
   (A) True
   (B) False

6. An EMT responds to the scene of a patient who was injured when she was thrown from a horse. The patient is complaining of neck pain, but refuses to be immobilized. The EMT explains the risks to the patient, but she still refuses. At the emergency department, a nurse threatens to report the EMT for negligence. Fortunately, the patient does not have a serious injury. Which of the following components to prove negligence is missing?
   (A) breach of duty
   (B) infliction of injury
   (C) a causal link between the EMT's actions and the patient's injury
   (D) all of the above

7. Under what conditions can confidential patient information be released to someone not directly involved in the patient's care?
   (A) under state law, the case involves a reportable situation such as a gunshot wound
   (B) a subpoena has been issued for the information
   (C) the patient signs a written release requesting the release of information
   (D) all of the above

8. Which of the following applies to expressed consent to or refusal of medical care?
   (A) The patient must be informed of the risks, benefits, and alternatives available to the proposed treatment.
   (B) The patient's family must also agree to treatment or refusal of treatment.
   (C) If the patient agrees to treatment, his or her understanding of the treatment offered is implied.
   (D) Once the patient consents to treatment, he or she is obligated to complete the treatment offered.

9. The EMT's scope of practice is usually determined by
   (A) the National Registry of EMTs.
   (B) the state in which the EMT practices.
   (C) the National Highway Traffic Safety Administration.
   (D) the EMT's employer.

10. Which of the following creates a duty to act?
    (A) being dispatched to a call while on duty
    (B) seeing someone who is injured while you are off duty
    (C) receiving a card from the National Registry of EMTs
    (D) all of the above

ANSWERS TO REVIEW QUESTIONS

Exercises

1. Scope of practice refers to the treatment EMTs can, and are expected to, perform in the care of their patients. A general scope of practice is determined at the federal level and published by NHTSA, but each state is responsible for declaring its scope of practice. In most cases, the state scope of practice is similar to the NHTSA document, but individual states may expand or restrict the scope of practice.

2. DNRs and advance directives are both documents that communicate a patient's wishes regarding end-of-life care. A DNR is a physician's order and must be signed by the physician. Most states require that the DNR be dated within a specific period of time prior to the need for resuscitation. States and EMS services vary in the degree of autonomy an EMT may use in honoring a DNR. In most cases, the EMT must at least contact medical control (an advising physician) to advise them of the DNR. An advance directive is typically signed by the patient and may contain more details about what and how actions should be carried out at the time of death. Usually, EMTs cannot honor advance directives. All EMTs must be familiar with state and service regulations regarding DNRs and advance directives.

3. Consent is the patient's legal acceptance of medical care. Expressed consent is verbal consent given by a patient of legal age. The patient must be informed about procedure, risks, and benefits. Implied consent is assumed in patients who, for medical reasons, cannot give expressed consent. Minors and mentally incompetent adults must have consent given by a parent or legal guardian. In this scenario, it is essential to obtain the patient's consent. Even though the patient's speech is slurred, she may be understandable, or may nod her head or otherwise indicate that she agrees to treatment.

4. **Scenario 1:** You arrive on the scene of a motor vehicle collision where a patient is awake and complaining of neck pain. The patient is alert and oriented to person, time, and place. You must obtain expressed consent.
   Scenario 2: You arrive at an office where an adult male, who is known to be a diabetic, is unconscious. The patient is in need of immediate treatment but unable to consent; therefore implied consent applies.

5. Laws may vary from state to state, but a pregnant teenager is often considered to be emancipated and capable of consenting to medical care, despite being under the age of 18.

6. All competent patients have the right to refuse care. However, the EMT is obligated to explain the potential consequences of refusing medical care. In this case, it is reasonable that the patient would rather go to the emergency department on his own, rather than by ambulance.

7. **Abandonment:** An EMT who leaves a patient in the emergency department waiting room without giving a report to a nurse at the emergency department may be accused of abandonment. He or she has terminated the patient–provider relationship without ensuring ongoing care by a provider at an equal or higher level.

   Negligence: An EMT fails to suction the airway of an unconscious patient who vomits, and leaves the patient in a supine position. The patient aspirates her stomach contents and subsequently develops pneumonia and dies. This EMT has most likely met all three conditions required to prove negligence: 1) Failure to act as a reasonable person with similar training would act; 2) An injury occurred to the patient; and 3) The EMT's failure to act is likely to have caused or substantially contributed to the patient's pneumonia and subsequent death.

   Battery: An EMT is annoyed with a patient whom she thinks is "faking" unconsciousness. She uses unnecessary force to apply a sternal rub, and leaves a contusion on the patient's chest.

8. The duty to respond is to the patient for whom you have already been dispatched. The reasonable thing to do is to contact dispatch and advise them of the situation. Depending on the nature of the original call, the dispatcher may either have you continue on and dispatch a second ambulance to the unresponsive person; or may have you stay on the scene of the unresponsive person and dispatch a second ambulance to the original call.

9. Complying with the request is an obvious breech of patient confidentiality.

10. Organ donation laws and the obligations of EMS providers may vary from state to state, and the EMT must be aware of the legal obligations in his or her state of employment. However, there is an ethical obligation, regardless of legal obligation, to ensure the patient receives optimal prehospital care and is delivered to an appropriate facility in the event the patient is an organ donor, or her family decides to donate her organs if her injuries are unsurvivable.

11. The greatest significance in this case is that you should avoid touching or moving the casings, and should point out their presence to law enforcement if they have not already been identified and marked. The presence of casings should not cause the EMT to make assumptions about the nature or number of injuries to the patient.

12. Reportable situations can vary from state to state. Some common situations that are reportable include child, elder, and dependent adult abuse, gunshot wounds, and animal bites.

Multiple-Choice Answers

1. **(C)** Objective 2
   In this case, the EMT should err on the side of resuscitation by beginning resuscitation and then contacting medical direction. The EMT cannot risk delaying resuscitation in the absence of a valid DNR.

2. **(D)** Objective 4
   Even though competent adults may refuse medical care, the EMT has an ethical obligation to ensure everything possible is done to convince this very sick patient to receive the care he needs. The EMT cannot diagnose a heart attack, and little is to be gained by telling the patient he is going to die.

3. **(A)** Objective 7
   Assault and battery are closely related. Most often, battery is defined as touching another person without consent. This usually does not apply to situations where one can reasonably expect inadvertent contact with others, such as crowded public places.

4. **(C)** Objective 7
   Abandonment refers to leaving a patient in need of care without transferring care of the patient to a provider of equal or higher training.

5. **(B)** Objective 4
   The mere ingestion of alcohol does not mean that a patient is not competent to consent to medical care.

6. **(D)** Objective 7
   The EMT was prevented from providing the indicated care by the patient's refusal. To have provided the care against the patient's wishes could amount to battery or false imprisonment. The EMT took the reasonable actions of explaining risks to the patient; therefore, there was no breach of duty. No injury occurred as a result of the nontreatment, and there was no link between the EMT's actions and the patient's injury.

7. **(D)** Objective 9
   Patient information can be released in each of the situations described.

8. **(A)** Objective 4
   It is not enough to simply obtain the patient's agreement to medical treatment. He or she must understand to what he or she is consenting. The family of a competent adult need not agree with the treatment, and a patient can withdraw consent at any time.

9. **(B)** Objective 1
   Legally, scope of practice is typically defined by states, although medical directors may restrict or ask for legal exceptions to the scope of practice for a particular service.

10. **(A)** Objective 8
    Only being on duty and being dispatched to a call constitute a duty to act.

The Human Body

 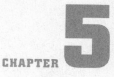

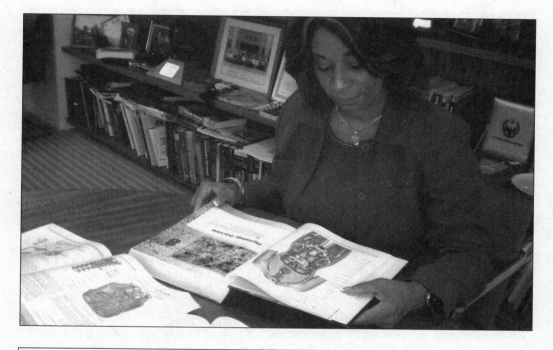

OBJECTIVES

This chapter and the review questions will help readers determine if they are able to

1. Identify the following topographic terms:

   medial
   lateral
   proximal
   distal
   superior
   inferior
   anterior
   posterior
   midline
   right and left
   mid-clavicular
   bilateral
   mid-axillary

> **2.** Describe the anatomy and function of the following major body systems:
>
> respiratory
> circulatory
> musculoskeletal
> nervous
> endocrine

ANATOMICAL TERMS

In order to review the anatomical terms you need to know, we start with normal anatomical position, or the position the body is in when these terms and landmarks are identified. **Correct anatomical position** is a person standing facing forward with palms facing forward. **Midline** is an imaginary line drawn down the center of the body, through the nose and umbilicus (belly button), dividing the body into right and left halves. **Mid-axillary lines** are imaginary lines on both sides of the body drawn from the armpit to the ankle, dividing the body into **anterior** (front) and **posterior** (back).

The word **torso** refers to the chest. **Medial** means toward midline and **lateral** means away from midline. A cut on the inside of your thigh is medial, while one on the outside of your thigh is **lateral**. **Proximal** and **distal** are words that are used to describe where something lies on an extremity. Toward the fingers or toes is distal, while something near where the extremity attaches to the body is proximal.

Superior and **inferior** refers to where something is in relation to the whole body. Superior is toward the head and inferior is toward the feet.

When using the words **right** and **left**, remember that this means the patient's right and left. So in order to grab the patient's right and left hands with your right and left hands with the patient facing you, you have to cross your hands.

Unilateral refers to one-sided and **bilateral** refers to both sides. **Dorsal** is another term for the back of something like your hand, while **ventral** is the front side (your palm). **Plantar** is another term that refers to the feet, while **palmar** refers to the hand.

If you are lying on your stomach you are in a **prone** position, while on your back you are **supine**. **Fowler's position** is a sitting position and **Trendelenburg** is sitting with your knees elevated. The **shock position** is supine with the legs higher than the heart (elevating the legs or tilting the bed).

THE SKELETAL SYSTEM

The skeletal system gives the body shape, protects vital organs, and provides the support needed for us to be able to move. The skeletal system is made up of sections.

The **skull** houses and protects the brain.

The **face** is made up of the orbits (around the eyes), nasal bone, maxilla (upper jaw), mandible (jawbone), and zygoma (cheekbones).

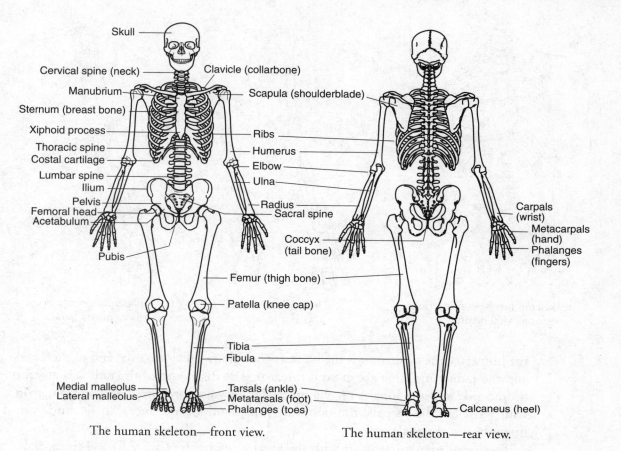

The human skeleton—front view. The human skeleton—rear view.

The **spinal column** is made up of 5 sections containing 33 vertebrae in all. The division is as follows:

- cervical   7
- thoracic   12 (one for each rib)
- lumbar   5
- sacral   5
- coccyx   4

All of these vertebrae are separated by flexible disks with the exception of the sacrum and coccyx (sometimes called the **sacrococcygeal spine**), which is a single fused bony mass.

The **thorax** or **chest** is made up of 12 ribs, which come out of each side of the 12 thoracic vertebrae. Ten of these come together at the sternum in the center of the anterior chest. The last two float freely. The sternum is divided into three parts: the manubrium (top), body (middle), and xiphoid (inferior portion).

The **pelvis** consists of the iliac crests (pelvic wings), pubis (the anterior portion you can palpate, and the ichium, which is inferior and posterior. This is the bone you hurt when you fall on your rear end.

The **upper extremities** consist of the clavicles or collarbones, the scapula (shoulder blade), and the acromion process or the tip of your shoulder. Your upper arm is

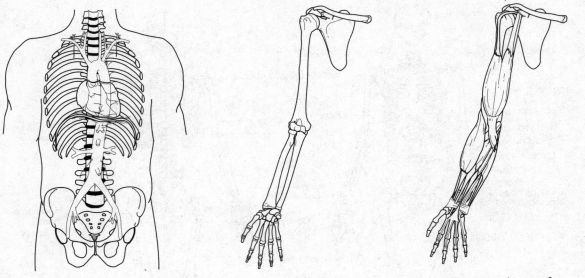

The skeleton furnishes protection for all vital organs.

The bones of the arm and hand.

The musculature of the arm and hand.

the humerus, the olecrenon is the bone at your elbow (the proximal end of the ulna) and the radius and ulna are in your forearm. The distal end of the radius is at your thumb side and the ulna is on the other side of your forearm. The small bones in your wrist are the carpals, the bones in your hand are the metacarpals, and your finger bones are phalanges.

The **lower extremities** start with the greater trochanter (the ball) and the acetabulum (socket) that form the hip joint. The trochanter is the proximal end of the long bone in your thigh, the femur. Your kneecap is the patella and the lower leg is made up of the tibia (shin bone) and the fibula. The distal end of the fibula is the

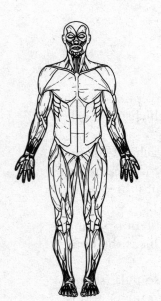

The musculature of the body.

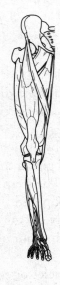

The musculature of the leg and foot.

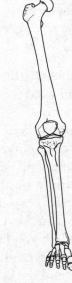

The bones of the leg and foot.

knob on the outside of your ankle and the distal end of the tibia is the knob on the inside of your ankle.

The **tarsals** are the small bones in your ankle and the metatarsals are the bones in your foot. The toe bones are called phalanges, like the fingers.

Where two bones come together is called a *joint*. The two types that we are concerned with are the ball-and-socket and hinge type. Your hip and shoulder joints are ball-and-socket; the knee is a hinge joint.

THE RESPIRATORY SYSTEM

The respiratory system starts with the nose and mouth, which house the **oropharynx** (mouth) and **nasopharynx** (nose). There are two tubes in your neck leading into the chest cavity. The anterior tube is the **trachea**, which carries air to the lungs. The posterior tube is the **esophagus**, which is part of the digestive system. A leaf-shaped valve called the **epiglottis** moves back and forth above these tubes to keep food out of the trachea and air out of the esophagus. Near the "Adam's apple" in the center of your anterior neck is the **cricoid cartilage larynx.**

Past the larynx your trachea splits into two **bronchi**, right and left, which bring the air into the lungs. In the lungs the bronchi divide into small bronchi called **bronchioles**. These bronchioles lead to **alveoli**, which are surrounded by **capillary beds**. The capillary beds bring blood into the lungs to exchange carbon dioxide for oxygen with the alveoli.

Breathing is brought about by the action of the intercostals (chest wall muscles) and the **diaphragm** (muscle separating the chest and abdominal cavities). The active part of breathing is **inspiration**, which is brought about by the contraction of these respiratory muscles, which increase the size of the chest cavity, bringing air into the lungs. The passive part of breathing is brought about by the relaxation of these muscles decreasing the size of the chest cavity forcing the air out of the lungs.

During each breath, oxygen-rich air enters the alveoli, while oxygen-poor blood arrives in the lungs at the **capillaries** surrounding the alveoli. The oxygen in the alveoli is then exchanged with the carbon dioxide in the capillaries and the oxygen is carried by the blood out to the body, where the opposite exchange takes place in the capillaries in all of the body's tissues.

Normal breathing rates are: adult: 12–20 breaths per minute
children: 15–30 breaths per minute
infants: 25–50 breaths per minute

Breathing should be effortless. Any sign of effort is an indication of respiratory distress. Breathing should have a regular rhythm with adequate and equal chest wall expansion. Breath sounds can confirm the presence and quality of respirations.

Inadequate respirations can be indicated by irregular rhythm or rates outside the normal range. Cyanosis, cold and clammy skin, diminished or absent breath sounds, unequal or inadequate chest wall expansion, or increased effort to breathe also indicate respiratory distress. Use of accessory muscles, particularly in children, is also a sign of respiratory distress. Agonal, or occasional gasping breaths, are usually the type of breathing seen just before a patient dies.

Special considerations for infants and children include smaller airways in which the tongue takes up proportionally more space. The trachea is narrower and softer making it more easily obstructed by foreign bodies or positioning. The cricoid cartilage is less rigid in infants. The chest wall is also softer, making infants rely more on their diaphragm to breath.

THE CIRCULATORY SYSTEM

The circulatory system is made up of the heart (the pump), the blood vessels that carry the blood, and the blood itself.

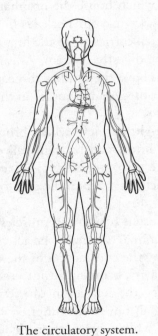

The circulatory system.

The Heart

The **heart** is a four-chambered muscle. The top two chambers are called the **atria**. The bottom two are called the **ventricles**. The right atrium receives oxygen-poor blood from the veins and the left atrium receives oxygen-poor blood from the lungs. The atria contract, forcing the blood into the ventricles; then the ventricles contract. The right ventricle pumps blood to the lungs to exchange carbon dioxide for oxygen; the left ventricle sends the blood into the arteries to carry the blood out to the body, where oxygen will be exchanged for carbon dioxide at capillaries in the body's tissues.

Blood Vessels

Arteries are double-walled tubular muscles that carry blood from the heart to the body's tissues. The largest is the **aorta**, which comes from the left ventricle and divides into the ascending and descending aorta in the chest. The **coronary arteries** run from the aorta to the heart muscle, supplying the heart with blood. The **pulmonary arteries** are the only arteries that carry oxygen-poor blood. They carry blood from the right ventricle to the lungs. The **carotid arteries** branch off from the ascending aorta and carry blood to the brain. The **femoral arteries** branch off from the descending aorta and carry blood into the lower extremities. The **brachial arteries** run from the ascending aorta into the upper extremities. The **radial arteries** run from the brachial arteries along the radial bones toward the hands. Wherever an artery runs over a bone or muscle and comes close to the surface of the skin, a pulse can be palpated. Smaller extensions of arteries are called **arterioles**. Examples are:

carotid: either side of the neck
brachial: inside the elbows
radial: anterior, thumb side of wrist
posterior tibial: medial aspect of ankle, posterior to distal tibia
dorsalis pedis: top of the foot

Veins are single-walled tubular muscles that carry oxygen-poor blood back to the heart. Smaller veins are called **venules**. Between the venules and the arterioles are the **capillaries**. The capillaries are where the exchange of oxygen and carbon dioxide takes place. At the tissue levels, nutrients and waste are also exchanged. The pulmonary vein is the only vein that carries oxygen-rich blood from the lungs to the left atrium. The largest veins are the **inferior** and **superior vena cava**, which bring the blood back to the heart from the body.

Blood

Blood is made up of **red blood cells**, **white blood cells**, and **platelets**. Red blood cells give blood its color and carry oxygen and/or carbon dioxide. White blood cells are part of the body's defense against infection. The platelets are part of the body's clot-forming capability.

Blood pressure consists of **systolic** and **diastolic pressures**. The systolic pressure represents the pressure within the arteries during the contraction of the heart and the arteries. The diastolic is the pressure in the arteries between the contractions.

Inadequate circulation is **shock** or **hypoperfusion**. This lack of perfusion can be recognized by changes in the level of consciousness (restlessness, nervousness, agitation, and mental dullness); pale, cool, and clammy skin; rapid weak pulses; nausea and vomiting; and rapid shallow breathing.

THE NERVOUS SYSTEM

The nervous system is divided into the **central** and **peripheral nervous systems**. The central nervous system includes the **spinal cord** and the **brain** and the peripheral nervous system includes **motor** and **sensory nerves**. Sensory nerves bring information about the body's environment back to the central nervous system. The central nervous system then uses motor nerves to act on conscious or automatic instructions from the brain or spinal cord. The peripheral nervous system branches out of the central nervous system from the spinal cord and through the vertebrae. Injury to the spine can cause injury to peripheral nerves, or even worse, damage to the spinal cord. Injury to the cord or any nerve causes dysfunction beyond the site of injury: paralysis and parasthesia (inability to move or feel).

THE ENDOCRINE SYSTEM

The endocrine system is comprised of glands that produce and secrete hormones that are essential to normal body function. The **hypothalamus** affects fluids and temperature and stimulates the release of hormones in the **pituitary gland**. These hormones stimulate the development of adrenal and thyroid glands, pigment-producing skin cells, and the ovaries and testes. The pituitary also secretes growth hormone, antidiuretic hormones, and prolactin. The **thyroid gland** secretes hormones that affect body heat, bone growth, and the body's metabolism. The **pancreas** secretes insulin and glucagons, which enable the body to facilitate the movement of glucose into the cells. The cells consume the glucose, producing energy that allows the cells to do their work. Other endocrine glands include the adrenal cortex of the **adrenal gland**, which secretes adrenalin and norepinephrine along with hyrdrocortisone, affecting metabolism, blood pressure, and the balance of the body's salt levels. **Testes** and **ovaries** (gonads) secrete a variety of hormones that promote maleness or femaleness. The **pineal gland** secretes melatonin, which plays a role in regulating sleep–wake cycles. The **thymus** is the site of maturation of T-lymphocytes, which help the body fight infection.

THE MUSCULAR SYSTEM

Like the skeletal system, the muscular system gives the body shape, protects internal organs, and provides for movement. There are three types of muscle:

1. **Voluntary** or **skeletal muscle** is attached to bones, forms the major muscle mass of the body, and can be instructed by the nervous system and the brain to be contracted or relaxed at command of the individual.
2. **Involuntary** or **smooth muscle** can be found in the walls of tubular structures like the gastrointestinal tract, urinary system, and blood vessels. The individual has no control over these muscles, but the nervous system instructs them to move food, blood, or waste material through them.
3. **Cardiac muscle** is highly specialized muscle. It is found only in the heart and can only tolerate brief interruptions of blood flow. Most importantly, cardiac muscle can function independent of control from the brain or nervous system.

THE SKIN

The skin protects the body from the environment, bacteria, and other organisms. It plays a role in temperature regulation and is a huge sensory organ, collecting information about heat, cold, pressure, and pain and sending it back to the spinal cord and the brain. The skin is made up of three layers:

1. The **epidermis** is the outermost and thinnest layer that is made up of cells that die, flake off, and replace themselves.
2. The **dermis** is the next layer and contains sweat and sebaceous glands, hair follicles, and nerve endings.
3. The deepest layer is the **subcutaneous** layer, which is made up of fat cells that store nutrients and water and is responsible for the curves and appearance of the exterior of our bodies.

Scenario 1

You are giving aid to a patient who was struck by a car. During your exam you notice swelling and deformity to his right thigh. This injury most likely has involved what structure?

SOLUTION

You would suspect that this patient has broken the largest long bone in his body, the femur. You should check for pulses and sensation below the injury (ankle) to make sure nerves and blood vessels have not been disrupted.

Scenario 2

Your patient is complaining of tenderness in the right upper quadrant of his abdomen after being involved in a fistfight. What injuries do you suspect?

SOLUTION

The liver is the largest solid organ and takes up most of the right upper quadrant and part of the left upper quadrant. You might also suspect injury to the ribs, gallbladder, kidneys, and colon.

Review Questions

EXERCISES

The exercises in this review are designed to help reinforce your knowledge of the objectives for this chapter. If you find it difficult to meet any of the objectives stated, go back and review those materials again.

1. Complete the following sentences. (Objective 1)

    (a) The anatomical position is described when the person is facing

    _____ with his palms facing _____ .

    (b) An imaginary line that divides the body into equal right and left halves

    is the _____ .

    (c) An imaginary line on the lateral aspect of the body that starts in the center of the armpit and runs to the ankle is called the right or left

    _____ .

    (d) The inner aspect of the arm is known as the _____ aspect, while the outer aspect of the arm is known as the _____ aspect.

    (e) In terms of anatomical direction, the hand is _____ to the elbow, while the knee is _____ to the foot.

(f) When assessing a patient we begin at the head and move in a(n) _____ direction. The opposite of this direction is

_____ .

(g) The front of the body is called the _____ aspect, while the back of the body is the _____ aspect.

(h) Something that is present on both sides of the body is said to be

_____ .

2. Label the parts of the lower respiratory system. (Objective 2)

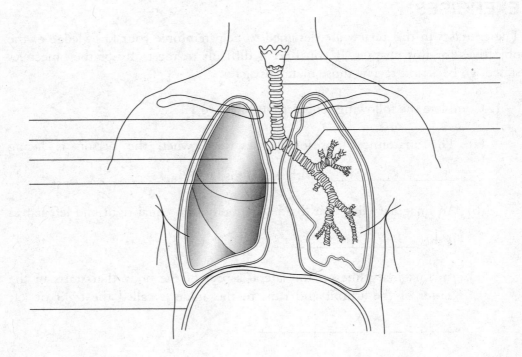

3. Label the parts of the skeletal system. (Objective 2)

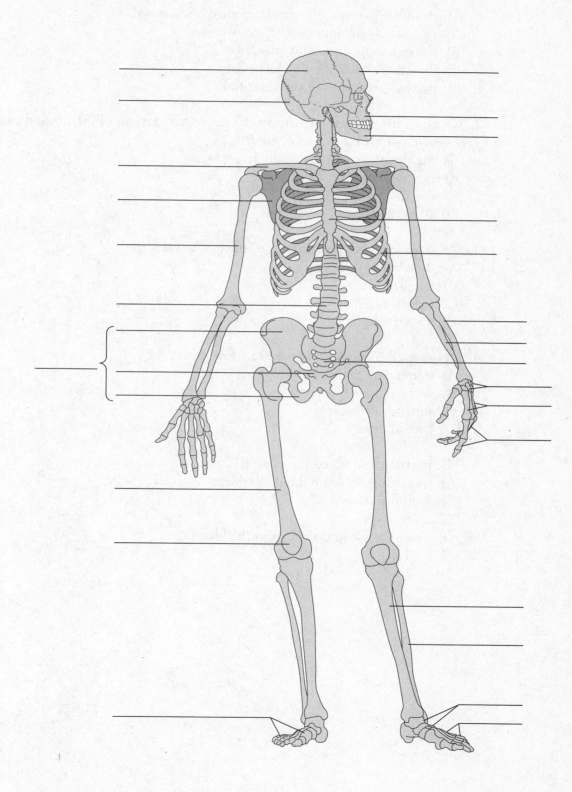

MULTIPLE-CHOICE QUESTIONS

1. Which of the following is associated with inspiration?
   (A) relaxation of diaphragm
   (B) relaxation of intercostal muscles
   (C) increased size of the thoracic cavity
   (D) passive movement of the chest wall

2. Which of the following is true of the respiratory system of infants and small children, compared to that of adults?
   (A) the tongue is proportionally larger
   (B) the trachea is soft and flexible
   (C) the airways are smaller
   (D) all of the above

3. Blood returning to the heart from the lungs enters the
   (A) right atrium.
   (B) left atrium.
   (C) right ventricle.
   (D) left ventricle.

4. Oxygenated blood leaving the heart first enters the
   (A) pulmonary artery.
   (B) aorta.
   (C) superior vena cava.
   (D) carotid artery.

5. The primary role of red blood cells is to
   (A) form plugs in injured blood vessels.
   (B) fight infection.
   (C) carry oxygen.
   (D) recognize foreign material in the blood.

6. Smooth muscle is found
    (A) in the heart.
    (B) in the nervous system.
    (C) attached to bones.
    (D) in organs and blood vessels.

7. The outermost layer of the skin is the
    (A) dermis.
    (B) subcutaneous layer.
    (C) epidermis.
    (D) fascia.

8. Insulin is secreted from the
    (A) adrenal glands.
    (B) liver.
    (C) thyroid gland.
    (D) pancreas.

9. The part of the brain that is most responsible for regulation of normal breathing is the
    (A) medulla oblongata.
    (B) cerebellum.
    (C) pons.
    (D) cerebral cortex.

10. A patient described as prone would be positioned:
    (A) lying on either side
    (B) lying face-down
    (C) lying face-up
    (D) semi-reclined, face-up

ANSWERS TO REVIEW QUESTIONS

Exercises

1. (a) The anatomical position is described when the person is facing **forward** with his palms facing **forward**.

   (b) An imaginary line that divides the body into equal right and left halves is the **midline**.

   (c) An imaginary line on the lateral aspect of the body that starts in the center of the armpit and runs to the ankle is called the right or left **midaxillary line**.

   (d) The inner aspect of the arm is also known as the **medial** aspect, while the outer aspect of the arm is also known as the **lateral** aspect.

   (e) In terms of anatomical direction, the hand is **distal** to the elbow, while the knee is **proximal** to the foot.

   (f) When assessing a patient we begin at the head and move in a(n) **inferior** direction. The opposite of this direction is **superior**.

   (g) The front of the body is called the **anterior** aspect, while the back of the body is the **posterior** aspect.

   (h) Something that is present on both sides of the body is said to be **bilateral**.

2.

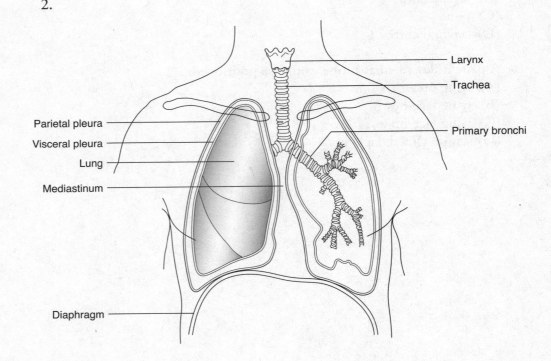

3.

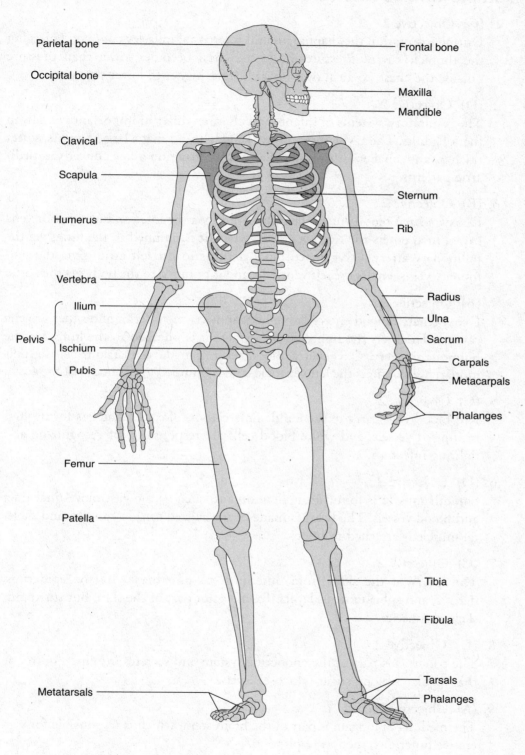

Parietal bone

Occipital bone

Frontal bone

Maxilla

Mandible

Clavical

Scapula

Sternum

Humerus

Rib

Vertebra

Radius

Ilium

Ulna

Pelvis

Sacrum

Ischium

Carpals

Pubis

Metacarpals

Phalanges

Femur

Patella

Tibia

Fibula

Tarsals

Metatarsals

Phalanges

Multiple-Choice Answers

1. **(C)** Objective 2
   During inspiration the diaphragm and intercostal muscles contract, enlarging the thoracic cavity. Pressure inside the chest becomes lower than pressure outside the chest, so air moves inward, from higher to lower pressure.

2. **(D)** Objective 2
   The respiratory systems of infants and children differ in important ways from that of adults. The EMT must always keep in mind that a larger tongue, softer trachea, and smaller airways make airway obstruction a key concern in pediatric patients.

3. **(B)** Objective 2
   Deoxygenated blood enters the right atrium via the inferior and superior vena cavae, then enters the right ventricle, where it is pumped to the lungs via the pulmonary artery. Oxygenated blood returns to the left atrium via the pulmonary veins, enters the left ventricle, and is pumped to the body via the aorta.

4. **(B)** Objective 2
   Deoxygenated blood enters the right atrium via the inferior and superior vena cavae, then enters the right ventricle where it is pumped to the lungs via the pulmonary artery. Oxygenated blood returns to the left atrium via the pulmonary veins, enters the left ventricle, and is pumped to the body via the aorta.

5. **(C)** Objective 2
   Red blood cells carry oxygen and some carbon dioxide. Platelets form plugs in injured vessels, and white blood cells are responsible for recognizing and fighting infection.

6. **(D)** Objective 2
   Smooth muscle is found in hollow organs, such as the gastrointestinal tract and blood vessels. The heart is made of specialized cardiac muscle, and skeletal muscle is attached to bones.

7. **(C)** Objective 2
   The layers of the skin, from outermost to innermost, are the epidermis, dermis, and subcutaneous layers. Fascia is not part of the skin, but surrounds skeletal muscle.

8. **(D)** Objective 2
   The pancreas is part of the endocrine system and secretes insulin, a hormone that regulates blood sugar (glucose) levels.

9. **(A)** Objective 2
   The medulla oblongata is part of the brain stem, which is responsible for vegetative functions, such as respiration.

10. **(B)** Objective 2
    If you are lying on your stomach you are in the prone position; while on your back you are supine.

Baseline Vital Signs and SAMPLE History

 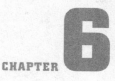

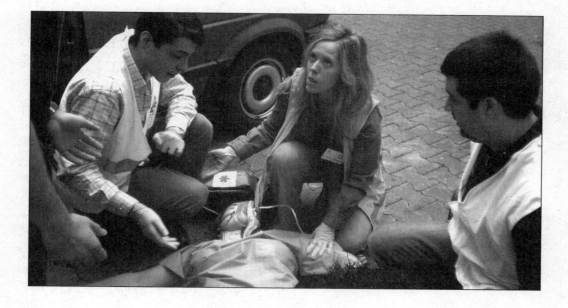

OBJECTIVES

This chapter and the review questions will help readers determine if they are able to

1. identify the components of vital signs;

2. describe the methods to obtain a breathing rate;

3. identify the attributes that should be obtained when assessing breathing;

4. differentiate between shallow, labored, and noisy breathing;

5. describe the methods to obtain a pulse rate;

6. identify the information obtained when assessing the patient's pulse;

7. differentiate between a strong, weak, regular, and irregular pulse;

8. describe the methods to assess skin color, temperature, and condition (capillary refill in infants and children);

9. identify normal and abnormal skin colors;

10. differentiate between pale, blue, red, and yellow skin colors;

11. identify normal and abnormal skin temperature;

12. differentiate between hot, cool, and cold skin temperatures;

13. identify normal and abnormal skin conditions;

14. identify normal and abnormal capillary refill in infants and children;

15. describe the methods to assess the pupils;

16. identify normal and abnormal pupil size;

17. differentiate between dilated (big) and constricted (small) pupil size;

18. differentiate between reactive and nonreactive pupils and equal and unequal pupils;

19. describe the methods to assess blood pressure;

20. define systolic pressure;

21. define diastolic pressure;

22. explain the difference between auscultation and palpation for obtaining a blood pressure;

23. identify the components of the SAMPLE history;

24. differentiate between a sign and a symptom;

25. state the importance of accurately reporting and recording the baseline vital signs;

26. discuss the need to search for additional medical identification.

GENERAL INFORMATION

You will need to collect general information on your patient. This information includes the chief complaint, or why EMS was called. This information also includes age, sex, and race.

VITAL SIGNS

Baseline vital signs include assessing breathing, pulse, skin, pupils, blood pressure, and a reassessment of these vital signs.

In obtaining a breathing rate, it is important that the patient not know you are counting his or her breaths as it may influence the rate of breathing. Count the breaths for 30 seconds and double that to obtain the rate of breaths per minute. You should also note the quality of breathing.

- **Normal breathing** is the average chest wall movement without use of accessory muscles.
- **Shallow breathing** has slight movement of the chest wall.
- **Labored breathing** is evidenced by an obvious increased effort to breathe. Sounds like grunting or stridor may be heard and the use of accessory muscles can be seen. In infants and children, nasal flaring and supraclavicular and intercostal retractions are common. Patients may also gasp for breath. Noisy respirations can include snoring, wheezing, gurgling, and crowing sounds.

Pulse

In all patients over one year old, the pulse you obtain initially is the **radial pulse**. Once you obtain the radial pulse, assess its rate and quality. As with breathing, count the pulse for 30 seconds and double it to get the rate per minute. The quality of the pulse should be described as weak or strong. You should also determine whether the rhythm is regular or irregular. If you are unable to get the radial pulse, check for a **carotid pulse**. When assessing the carotid it is important to check only one at a time and not use excessive pressure, particularly in geriatric patients.

Skin

Skin color is assessed to determine **tissue perfusion**. You can examine nail beds, oral mucosa, and/or conjunctiva. In infants and children, you can check the palms of the hands and soles of the feet. Normally, skin color should be pink. Pale skin indicates poor perfusion. Bluish or cyanotic skin indicates poor tissue perfusion and/or inadequate oxygenation. Red or flushed skin can occur because of exposure to heat or carbon monoxide poisoning. Yellow or jaundiced skin indicates illness involving the liver.

Skin temperature should be assessed by placing the back of your hand on the patient's skin. **Normal skin** feels warm. **Abnormal skin** temperatures include: **hot**, which indicates fever or exposure to heat; **cool**, which indicates poor perfusion or cold exposure; and **cold**, which indicates exposure to extreme cold.

Normal skin condition should be dry. Wet, moist, or extremely dry skin is abnormal.

In infants and children less than 6 years old, you should assess **capillary refill** to evaluate tissue perfusion. This is done by pressing on the skin or nail beds and counting the seconds it takes for the initial color to return. In infants, this should take 2 seconds or less. More time than this is abnormal.

Briefly shine a light into your patient's eyes and evaluate the size and reactivity of the pupils. A large pupil is described as **dilated**, while small is described as **constricted**. The pupils should be described as equal or unequal and reactive or nonreactive to the light.

Blood Pressure

The blood pressure reading includes the **systolic** and **diastolic** values. When auscultating the blood pressure, the first sound heard is the systolic pressure, which represents the pressure in the arteries during heart contraction. The second sound heard is the diastolic, which represents the pressure in the arteries between the heart contractions. When palpating the pressure the EMT will only get the systolic pressure. Blood pressures should be obtained in all patients over the age of three.

It is important to remember that general physical condition may be more important than the vital signs, particularly in children. Noting that the patient is unresponsive or in respiratory distress is more descriptive of the patient's condition than the numbers.

Also of importance is reassessing the patient's vital signs. This should be done at least every 15 minutes and every 5 minutes if the patient is unstable. You should also recheck vitals after every treatment, intervention, or change in patient condition.

SAMPLE

SAMPLE is an acronym that helps to remember the parts of the patient history you need to obtain.

S	=	Signs and symptoms
A	=	Allergies
M	=	Medications
P	=	Pertinent past history
L	=	Last oral intake
E	=	Events leading to the injury or illness

A **sign** is measurable, like a pulse or the color of the skin. **Symptoms** are descriptions by the patient of how he or she feels: discomfort or disability. Examples of symptoms are nausea, chest pain, or light-headedness.

Baseline Vital Signs

It is important to get baseline vital signs on your patient. This enables you to determine whether the patient's condition is worsening or improving and measure the effectiveness of your treatments.

MEDICAL IDENTIFICATION

Many patients who want others to be aware of their medical history wear or carry medical identification. These bracelets, necklaces, cards, or other form of identification alert EMTs to conditions like diabetes, heart disease, or allergies. They also let us know that patients may have other special needs or disabilities. EMTs should be on the lookout for medical IDs, particularly if the patient is unconscious and/or unable to give history.

Scenario 1

Your partner has asked you to obtain a blood pressure on your patient. How will you do that?

SOLUTION

After confirming the location of the brachial pulse in the arm you have selected, place the cuff around the arm so the bladder is centered over the anterior surface of the forearm. (Many cuffs have arrows showing how to line it up.) Once done, put the bell of your stethoscope over the place you felt the pulse and pump up the cuff to about 150 mmhg. Place the earpieces of the stethoscope in your ears and listen as you slowly let the air out of the cuff. The first sound you hear is the systolic pressure and the last you hear is the diastolic.

Scenario 2

Next your partner asks you to check the patient's pupils. How will you do that and what are you looking for?

SOLUTION

You are looking to determine PERL. That is, pupils equal and reactive to light. In order to do this, hold open one eye at a time and move the light across the eye from the outside (lateral) to the inside (medial). Check the pupil size before the light is shone into it and how it responds. Then compare the eyes.

Scenario 3

It appears your patient has an injury to his knee. You are asked to check circulation and sensation below the injury. How will you do that?

SOLUTION

You need to check for distal pulses, below the injury, to check for the posterior tibial or dorsalis pedis pulses. Also check if the nerves are intact by asking the patient to wiggle his toes to see if he feels you touching the inside and outside of his toes.

Review Questions

EXERCISES

The exercises in this review are designed to help reinforce your knowledge of the objectives for this chapter. If you find it difficult to meet any of the objectives stated, go back and review those materials again.

1. What are the components of vital signs? (Objective 1)

   _____

   _____

2. How would you assess a patient's respiratory rate? (Objective 2)

   _____

   _____

3. When assessing a patient's respirations, you should determine the rate and _____ of respirations. (Objective 3)

4. The depth of breathing can be assessed by looking for movement of the _____ .

   Compared to normal breathing, shallow breathing involves _____ movement.

   Normal breathing is effortless. Labored breathing can be recognized by

   _____

   _____

   Normal breathing is quiet. Abnormal breathing sounds include

   _____

   _____

   (Objective 4)

5. How would you assess a patient's pulse? (Objective 5)

_____

_____

6. When assessing the pulse, in addition to rate, you also check the

_____ and _____ of the pulse, which includes the

_____ and _____ of the pulse. (Objectives 6 and 7)

7. How would you assess a patient's skin during the baseline vital signs?
   (Objective 8)

_____

_____

8. What is the possible significance of each of the following skin colors?
   (Objectives 9 and 10)
   Pale:

_____

   Blue:

_____

   Red:

_____

   Yellow:

_____

9. What is the possible significance of each of the following skin temperatures?
   (Objectives 11–13)
   Hot:

_____

   Cool:

_____

   Cold:

_____

10. Capillary refill time is usually _____ .
    (Objective 14)

11. How would you assess a patient's pupils? (Objective 15)

    _____

    _____

12. What is the normal appearance and reaction to light of the pupils?
    (Objectives 16–18)

    _____

    _____

13. What does the equipment needed to assess blood pressure include?
    (Objective 19)

    _____

    _____

14. The systolic blood pressure represents the pressure in the arteries during

    _____ , while diastolic blood pressure represents

    the pressure in the arteries _____ .
    When auscultating the blood pressure the first sound heard represents the

    _____ blood pressure and the disappearance of sounds

    represents the _____ blood pressure. (Objectives 20 and 21)

15. When palpating the blood pressure only the _____ blood
    pressure can be detected. (Objective 22)

16. Write the component of the history indicated by each letter below. (Objective 23)

    S _____

    A _____

    M _____

    P _____

    L _____

    E _____

17. For each item below, indicate whether it is a sign or a symptom. (Objective 24)

    Headache: _____

    Scraped knee: _____

    Blue skin color: _____

    Dizziness: _____

18. The baseline vital signs provide a basis of _____ for later

    vital signs so that providers can detect _____ in the patient's condition. (Objective 25)

19. Searching for additional information is especially important when the patient

    _____ . (Objective 26)

MULTIPLE-CHOICE QUESTIONS

1. You have observed your patient's chest rise and fall three times in 15 seconds. Therefore, the patient's respiratory rate is _____ per minute, which is considered _____ for an adult patient.
   - (A) 12; normal
   - (B) 12; abnormal
   - (C) 15; normal
   - (D) 15; abnormal

2. The first place the EMT should check for the pulse of most adult patients is at the _____ artery.
   - (A) carotid
   - (B) brachial
   - (C) radial
   - (D) femoral

3. Your patient's right pupil is much larger than the left and does not get smaller in response to light. The right pupil is best described as
   - (A) equal and reactive.
   - (B) constricted and nonreactive.
   - (C) dilated and nonreactive.
   - (D) unequal and reactive.

4. The EMT should check the vital signs of an unstable patient at least every _____ minutes.
   - (A) 2
   - (B) 5
   - (C) 10
   - (D) 15

5. In a patient with poor perfusion, the most likely skin findings would be
   - (A) warm, moist, and pink.
   - (B) warm, dry, and pale.
   - (C) cool, moist, and pale.
   - (D) cool, dry, and pink.

6. Capillary refill time is a useful indication of perfusion in patients _____ years of age.
   - (A) under 6
   - (B) 6 or more
   - (C) under 12
   - (D) 12 or more

7. If you are unable to obtain a patient's radial pulse, you should immediately
   (A) start CPR.
   (B) apply an AED.
   (C) presume the patient is dead.
   (D) check the carotid pulse.

8. Your patient's skin appears blue. You should presume this to be an indication of
   (A) liver disease.
   (B) carbon monoxide poisoning.
   (C) poor oxygenation.
   (D) high fever.

9. Your patient's skin feels hot to the touch. The most likely cause is
   (A) carbon monoxide poisoning.
   (B) poor perfusion.
   (C) fever.
   (D) inadequate oxygenation.

10. It is generally not necessary for the EMT to assess blood pressure in patients who are under _____ years of age.
    (A) 3
    (B) 5
    (C) 8
    (D) 12

ANSWERS TO REVIEW QUESTIONS

Exercises

1. Breathing, pulse, skin, pupils, and blood pressure.

2. Observe the number of times the patient's chest wall rises and falls (1 rise + 1 fall = 1 respiration) in 30 seconds and multiply the number by two.

3. When assessing a patient's respirations, you should determine the rate and **quality** of respirations.

4. The depth of breathing can be assessed by looking for movement of the **chest wall**. Compared to normal breathing, shallow breathing involves **less** movement. Normal breathing is effortless. Labored breathing can be recognized by **increased effort, abnormal noises, use of accessory muscles, nasal flaring, and supraclavicular and intercostal retractions.** Normal breathing is quiet. Abnormal breathing sounds include **snoring, wheezing, gurgling, and crowing.**

5. For patients over 1 year old, the radial pulse is usually checked by locating the pulsation of the radial artery on the wrist at the base of the thumb. The number of pulsations is counted for 30 seconds and multiplied by 2 (or counted for 15 seconds and multiplied by 4) to obtain the pulse rate.

6. When assessing the pulse, in addition to rate, you also check the **quality** and **rhythm** of the pulse, which includes the **strength** and **regularity** of the pulse.

7. Observe the skin color, which may also be noted in the nail beds, oral mucosa, and conjunctiva. The temperature and condition of the skin can be checked by placing the back of the hand on the patient's skin.

8. **Pale:** poor perfusion
   Blue: poor oxygenation
   Red: fever, exposure to heat
   Yellow: liver disease

9. **Hot:** fever, exposure to heat
   Cool: poor perfusion
   Cold: exposure to cold

10. Capillary refill time is usually **less than 2 seconds**.

11. The pupils are visualized for size, equality, and symmetry and reaction to a penlight shone into the eye.

12. Pupils are normally equal in size, round, larger in dim light, and smaller in bright light and both pupils should become smaller when a light is shone into each eye.

13. A blood pressure cuff (sphygmomanometer) and stethoscope is used to assess blood pressure.

14. The systolic blood pressure represents the pressure in the arteries during **contraction of the ventricles**, while diastolic blood pressure represents the pressure in the arteries **during relaxation of the ventricles**. When auscultating the blood pressure the first sound heard represents the **systolic** blood pressure and the disappearance of sounds represents the **diastolic** blood pressure.

15. When palpating the blood pressure only the *systolic* blood pressure can be detected.

16. S = signs and symptoms
    A = allergies
    M = medications
    P = pertinent past medical history
    L = last oral intake
    E = events leading up to the illness or injury

17. **Headache:** symptom
    Scraped knee: sign
    Blue skin color: sign
    Dizziness: symptom

18. The baseline vital signs provide a basis of **comparison** for later vital signs so that providers can detect **trends (changes)** in the patient's condition.

19. Searching for additional information is especially important when the patient **is unconscious or otherwise unable to give a history**.

Multiple-Choice Answers

1. **(A)** Objective 2
   The respiratory rate is obtained by counting the rise and fall of the chest for 15 seconds and multiplying by 4. The normal adult respiratory rate is 12 to 20 breaths per minute.

2. **(C)** Objective 5
   The radial pulse is the most convenient, accessible, and nonintrusive site for routine patient care. However, in unresponsive patients the carotid pulse is checked first.

3. **(C)** Objective 18
   The pupils should be equal in size and should respond (react) to light by getting smaller (constricting).

4. **(B)** Objective 25
   Vital signs must be rechecked frequently in the critically ill or injured patient to detect deterioration and monitor the effects of treatment.

5. **(C)** Objective 13
   Cool, moist, and pale skin is most indicative of poor perfusion. Warmth and good color indicate adequate perfusion and skin is normally dry to the touch.

6. **(A)** Objective 14
   In older children and adults capillary refill time can be affected by a number of factors and is not as reliable.

7. **(D)** Objective 5
   Patients with poor perfusion may not have a radial pulse, but may have a carotid pulse. Neither further interventions nor presumption that the patient is dead are based on the absence of a radial pulse.

8. **(C)** Objective 9
   Patients with cyanosis, a blue discoloration of the skin, are presumed to have poor tissue oxygenation.

9. **(C)** Objective 12
   Of these answer choices, only fever—an increase in the production of body heat—would cause hot skin.

10. **(A)** Objective 19
    The blood pressure is generally difficult to obtain and gives little additional information about perfusion beyond the pulse and capillary refill in small children.

Lifting and Moving Patients

 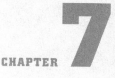

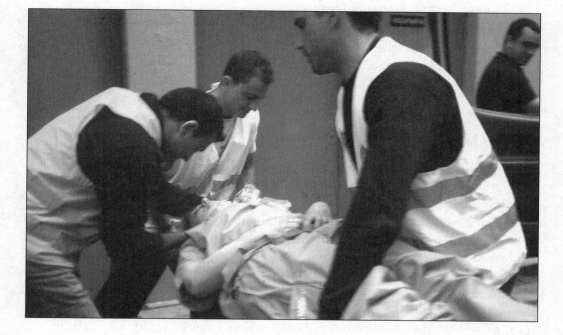

OBJECTIVES

This chapter and the review questions will help readers determine if they are able to

1. define body mechanics;

2. discuss the guidelines and safety precautions that need to be followed when lifting the patient;

3. describe the safe lifting of cots and stretchers;

4. describe the guidelines and safety precautions for carrying patients and/or equipment;

5. discuss one-handed carrying techniques;

6. describe correct and safe carrying procedures on stairs;

7. state the guidelines for reaching and their application;

8. describe the correct reaching technique for logrolls;

9. state the guidelines for pushing and pulling;

10. discuss the general considerations of moving patients;

11. state three situations that may require the use of an emergency move;

12. identify the following patient carrying devices:

✔ wheeled ambulance stretcher
✔ portable ambulance stretcher
✔ long spine board
✔ basket stretcher
✔ flexible stretcher

BODY MECHANICS

Proper lifting techniques include the basic safety precautions of using your legs and not your back to lift, and keeping the weight as close to your body as possible. Guidelines for lifting include taking the patient's weight into consideration and whether you need additional help. You should always lift without twisting, with your feet properly positioned, while communicating clearly and frequently with your team members.

Lifting cots and stretchers calls for using the proper number of people. When possible, consider a stair chair when traversing stairs for safety and patient comfort. Before placing the patient on the device try to determine the patient's weight. The team should consist of an even number of people to provide balance when lifting. You should also make sure you know the weight limitations of your equipment and what to do when patient weight exceeds the limits of your gear. When lifting, use the power-lift or squat-lift position, maintaining your back locked in normal curvature and position. Even with weak knees or thighs the power lift can be helpful. Feet should be flat and evenly spaced to distribute the weight. When you lift it is important that the upper body come up before your hips.

The power grip maintains the maximum surface of your hands in contact with what you are lifting. Always avoid bending at the waist.

When carrying it is important to use devices that can be rolled whenever possible. Know the weight that your device and team are capable of lifting. Weight close to your body, good communication with your team members, back in proper position, refraining from twisting when lifting, bending at the knees and not the back, while avoiding hyperextension of the back, are all essential. Use correct lifting techniques and choose teammates of similar strength and height for best results.

The one-handed technique calls for picking up and carrying with the back in the locked-in position, while avoiding leaning to either side to compensate for the imbalance.

As mentioned, correct procedure on stairs should include the use of a stair chair when possible with the back in locked-in position, flexing at the hips, not the waist, while bending at the knees. As with all lifts and carries, keep weight and arms as close to the body as possible.

When reaching, avoid reaching overhead and a hyperextended position. Do not twist while reaching and keep the back in a locked-in position. You should avoid reaching more than 15 to 20 inches in front of your body; situations where strenuous effort must be maintained for longer than a minute should be avoided.

When reaching to logroll patients, lean from the hips with your back straight, using your shoulder muscles to help with the roll.

You should push whenever possible rather than pull with your back in locked-in position, keeping the line of pull through the center of the body by bending your knees. Keep the weight close to your body while pushing from the area between the waist and shoulder. If the weight is low, use the kneeling position. Avoid pushing or pulling if the weight is in an overhead position. Keep your elbows bent and close to your sides.

TYPES OF MOVES

The EMT must be able to determine the kinds of moves to be undertaken when handling various categories of patients.

Emergency Moves

Emergency moves are used when there is imminent danger to the patient if not moved immediately. Fire or danger of fire or explosion, an inability to protect the patient from hazards, or the need to gain access to another patient in need of life-saving care are reasons for using emergency moves. Urgent moves are used when there is an immediate threat to life. Urgent moves should be used when the patient has an altered mental status, inadequate breathing, or shock. If there is no threat to life, nonurgent moves or moves using normal precautions should be used.

Using emergency moves may aggravate spine injuries; moving the patient by pulling in the direction of the long axis of the spine can limit the hazard. It is not possible to completely protect the spine without immobilization devices, so emergency moves should only be used when there is imminent danger to the patient or the rescuers, or there is another patient in more imminent need that necessitates moving the patient. If the patient is on the ground (or floor), pull on the patient's clothing in the neck and shoulder area, put the patient in a blanket, and drag the blanket or drag the patient with your hands under the patient's armpits while grasping the forearms.

Urgent moves include using rapid extrication (e.g., a motor vehicle collision). This entails getting behind the patient, providing in-line immobilization, while a second EMT applies a cervical collar (c-collar), and a third EMT places a long board under the patient and then moves into the passenger seat. The second EMT supports the thorax as the third frees the patient's legs from the gas and brake pedals. As the EMT at the head and neck directs, the patient is rotated in several short coordinated moves to bring his or her back square to the doorframe. At this point, a fourth EMT must take the head and neck from the EMT in the back seat, as he or she can no longer maintain cervical immobilization while the patient is moved to the board. While the end of the board is supported, the team then lowers the patient from a sitting position to supine. The patient is moved onto the board in short movements that allow the team to maintain in-line immobilization.

Nonurgent Moves

Nonurgent moves are used when there is no suspicion of spinal injury. These moves include the direct ground lift, in which two rescuers, side by side, slide their arms under the patient at the neck, lower back, and just above the buttocks and knees, and lift the patient to their chests. Another nonurgent move is the extremity lift in which a rescuer at the patient's head comes from behind and places his or her hands under the patient's arms and grabs the wrists. A second rescuer grabs the patient under the knees and both rescuers lift the patient together.

Transferring a Supine Patient

Transferring a supine patient from a bed to a stretcher is a variation of the direct ground lift. The stretcher is placed perpendicular to the bed with the head of the stretcher at the foot of the bed. After sliding the patient to the edge of the bed, two rescuers lift the patient in the same manner as the direct ground lift and rotate toward the stretcher. The draw sheet method depends on the strength of the draw sheet and the weight of your patient. It is widely used to transfer patients from a stretcher to a bed or vice versa. In this method, the top sheet is loosened from the bed. Then the cot is pushed up to the bed as the rescuers reach across the stretcher, grasping the sheet firmly at the head, chest, hips, and knees. The patient is then gently slid onto the bed.

Equipment Used in Lifting and Moving

The equipment used in lifting and moving patients includes stretchers or cots, which are commonly used for transport as well as movement to and from the ambulance. The stretchers have collapsible wheel assemblies and are stable only on even terrain. These stretchers can be carried up and down stairs once collapsed by two or four rescuers. Two rescuers would lift from the feet and the head while each of four rescuers would lift at one corner of the stretcher. When loading stretchers into an ambulance, always ensure that there is sufficient lifting power available. It is also important to lift with your legs, maintaining your back in a straight, upright position. Avoid twisting and lifting at the same time. If you are loading an ambulance that includes multiple stretchers, hanging stretchers should be loaded first. All patients and cots should be secured before moving the ambulance.

Other devices for lifting and carrying include portable or collapsible stretchers and stair chairs for bringing patients out of buildings in a sitting position. Long backboards are used to immobilize spine-injured patients and short boards are used for patients that must be extricated from a vehicle or other compartment and brought out onto a long board. Scoop stretchers split at the center and scoop up the patient. Flexible stretchers are just that, flexible enough to assist in moving patients in awkward situations. As with any piece of equipment, all of these should be tested according to manufacturers' recommendations.

PATIENT POSITIONING

Unresponsive patients without spine injury should be placed in the recovery position. This has the patient on his or her side to help keep the airway open. Patients with chest pain or respiratory distress should be placed in a sitting position. Spine-injured patients should be immobilized on a long board in a supine position. Patients in shock may benefit from elevating the foot end of their stretcher. Pregnant patients may suffer from postural hypotension. Placing her left side in the left, lateral recumbent position should relieve this. Uncomfortable, nauseated, or vomiting patients should be placed in a position of comfort or the position they best tolerate with an EMT in position to monitor the airway.

Scenario 1

You are called to assist lifting a patient onto a cot. Is it acceptable to bend at the waist as you lift the cot?

SOLUTION

Proper body mechanics require that you bend at the knees and lift with your back straight. Bending at the waist puts you at risk for serious back injuries.

Scenario 2

You and your partner are confronted with moving a patient in respiratory distress down several flights of stairs. What is the best way to do this?

SOLUTION

When taking patients down stairs, whenever possible it is best to use a stair chair device or at the least, a chair. The patient can be transferred to a sitting position on your cot when you make it to street level.

Scenario 3

You arrive at the scene of a burning vehicle with the victim still inside the vehicle. After donning proper clothing and given the signal to proceed by the fire department, how will you remove the victim from the car?

SOLUTION

Whenever there is an immediate danger to the patient if not moved, emergency moves are to be used. These are manual moves using minimal equipment to move the patient without delay.

Review Questions

EXERCISES

The exercises in this review are designed to help reinforce your knowledge of the objectives for this chapter. If you find it difficult to meet any of the objectives stated, go back and review those materials again.

1. What is meant by body mechanics? (Objective 1)

   _____

   _____

2. List at least six general guidelines for safely lifting a patient. (Objective 2)

   _____

   _____

   _____

   _____

3. List at least four ways to maintain safety while lifting a cot or stretcher. (Objectives 3 and 4)

   _____

   _____

   _____

   _____

4. Describe the technique for a one-handed carry. (Objective 5)

   _____

   _____

5. What piece of equipment should be used for carrying patients on stairs? (Objective 6)

   _____

6. List four guidelines for reaching. (Objective 7)

   _____

   _____

   _____

   _____

7. When reaching to logroll a patient you should lean from the _____

   with the back straight, using your _____ muscles to help with the roll. (Objective 8)

8. Whenever possible you should _____ (push/pull) instead of

   _____ (pushing/pulling). (Objective 9)

9. What are the three classifications of moves used when deciding how to move a patient in a prehospital setting? (Objective 10)

   _____

   _____

   _____

10. Under what conditions should you use an emergency move? (Objective 11)

    _____

    _____

    _____

11. Identify each of the following devices. (Objective 12)

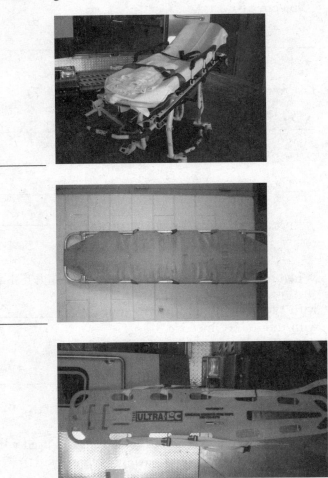

_____

_____

_____

MULTIPLE-CHOICE QUESTIONS

1. Proper body mechanics are best described by bending at the _____ and lifting with the _____.
   (A) waist; back
   (B) knees; back
   (C) waist; legs
   (D) knees; legs

2. When lifting, your feet should be
   (A) turned inward and widely spaced.
   (B) flat and evenly spaced.
   (C) turned inward and evenly spaced.
   (D) flat and widely spaced.

3. In order to accomplish a power lift you must
   (A) wear special arm bands.
   (B) grip with your hands in opposite directions.
   (C) keep the surface of your hands in contact with the stretcher.
   (D) keep your arms straight at a 90-degree angle from your body.

4. When moving a patient, you should try to keep the patient _____ inches from your body.
   (A) 5 to 10
   (B) 10 to 15
   (C) 15 to 20
   (D) 20 to 25

5. The best position for an unresponsive patient who does not require airway management or ventilation and who does not have a spinal injury is
   (A) supine with the head flat.
   (B) prone with the head turned to one side.
   (C) on his or her side.
   (D) supine with the head elevated.

6. You arrive on the scene of a motor vehicle collision. Your patient remains in the vehicle and has a weak, rapid pulse and ineffective respirations. You should use a(n) _____ move to remove the patient from the vehicle.
   (A) standard
   (B) nonurgent
   (C) urgent
   (D) emergency

7. You arrived on the scene of a motor vehicle collision. Your patient is conscious and has normal vital signs, but complains of back pain. You should move this patient using a(n) _____ move.
   (A) standard
   (B) nonurgent
   (C) urgent
   (D) emergency

8. Your patient has a history of asthma and is complaining of difficulty breathing. There is no potential for spinal injury. This patient should be placed in a _____ position.
   (A) supine
   (B) prone
   (C) recovery
   (D) sitting

9. When lifting a patient, it is best if your partner is
    (A) about as strong as you are.
    (B) stronger than you are.
    (C) not as strong as you are.
    (D) any of the above, as long as you both use proper body mechanics.

10. In which of the following situations should an EMT use an emergency move?
    (A) a patient with difficulty breathing who has been involved in a vehicle collision
    (B) a patient who is unresponsive in her home due to possible carbon monoxide poisoning
    (C) a patient with a fever who must be moved from her bed
    (D) a patient who has fallen in her front yard and who is screaming at you to get her inside before her neighbors see her

ANSWERS TO REVIEW QUESTIONS

Exercises

1. The term body mechanics refers to protecting yourself from injury by using proper techniques of walking, standing, bending, lifting, and sitting.

2. Use your legs instead of your back to lift, keeping the weight as close to your body as possible, consider the need for additional help, do not twist while lifting, keep feet properly positioned, and communicate with your team members.

3. Use the proper number of people to help, consider a stair chair if you must go up or down stairs, consider the patient's weight, use an even number of people to balance the weight, and use a power lift or squat lift.

4. Keep your back in the locked-in position and avoid leaning to either side.

5. A stair chair should be used to carry patients on stairs.

6. Do not reach overhead or use a hyperextended position, do not twist, keep the back in a locked-in position, avoid reaching more than 15 to 20 inches, and avoid strenuous effort lasting longer than one minute.

7. When reaching to logroll a patient you should lean from the **hips** with the back straight, using your **shoulder** muscles to help with the roll.

8. Whenever possible you should **push** (push/pull) instead of **pull** (push/pull).

9. Nonurgent, urgent, and/or emergency moves can be used in a prehospital setting.

10. Emergency moves should be used when the patient is in imminent danger if not moved immediately or if the patient must be moved to access another patient in immediate need of lifesaving care.

11.

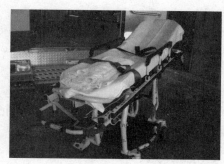

wheeled ambulance stretcher

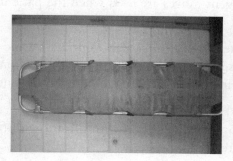

portable ambulance stretcher

long spine board

Multiple-Choice Answers

1. **(D)** Objective 1
   Always bend at the knees with the back straight. Lifting with the legs limits the potential for back injury.

2. **(B)** Objective 2
   Keeping your feet flat and evenly spaced ensures that your legs are in proper lifting position, preventing unnecessary strain to the leg muscles and a solid platform to distribute the weight you are lifting.

3. **(C)** Objective 2
   The intention of the power lift is to position your hands in a way that keeps as much of the anterior surfaces of your palm and fingers on the handle or bar you are lifting.

4. **(A)** Objective 7
Working with the patient 5 to 10 inches from your body allows you to distribute the weight you are lifting without excessive strain on your arms and back.

5. **(C)** Objective 10
The best position for the patient would be on his or her side to protect the airway.

6. **(C)** Objective 11
Urgent moves are used when the patient's condition calls for urgent removal.

7. **(B)** Objective 11
The types of moves appropriate for most patients, taking full precautions to ensure no further harm, are called nonurgent moves. These moves are not time-critical, while urgent and emergency moves are.

8. **(D)** Objective 10
Noninjured patients with breathing difficulty should be kept upright to facilitate breathing.

9. **(A)** Objective 2
It is best if your partner is as strong as you are in order to maintain balance when lifting.

10. **(B)** Objective 11
Emergency moves are used when the environment is hazardous to the patient and/or rescuers.

Airway

 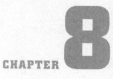

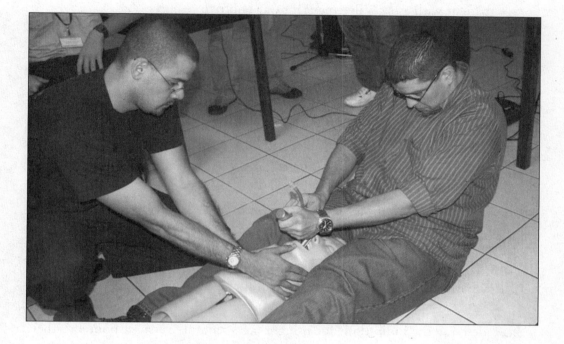

OBJECTIVES

This chapter and the review questions will help readers determine if they are able to

1. name and label the major structures of the respiratory system on a diagram;

2. list the signs of adequate breathing;

3. list the signs of inadequate breathing;

4. describe the steps in performing the head-tilt chin-lift;

5. relate the mechanism of injury to the opening of the airway;

6. describe the steps in performing the jaw thrust;

7. state the importance of having a suction unit ready for immediate use when providing emergency care;

8. describe the techniques of suctioning;

9. describe how to artificially ventilate a patient with a pocket mask;

10. describe the steps in performing the skill of artificially ventilating a patient with a bag-valve mask system while using the jaw thrust;

11. list the parts of the bag-valve mask system;

12. describe the steps in performing the skill of artificially ventilating the patient with a bag-valve mask for one and two rescuers;

13. describe the signs of adequate artificial ventilation using the bag-valve mask;

14. describe the signs of inadequate artificial ventilation using the bag-valve mask;

15. describe the steps in artificially ventilating the patient with a flow-restricted, oxygen-powered ventilation device;

16. list the steps in performing the actions taken when providing mouth-to-mouth and mouth-to-stoma ventilations;

17. describe how to measure and insert an oropharyngeal airway;

18. describe how to measure and insert a nasopharyngeal airway;

19. define the components of an oxygen delivery system;

20. identify a nonrebreather face mask and state the oxygen flow requirements for its use;

21. describe the indications for using a nasal cannula versus a nonrebreather face mask;

22. identify a nasal cannula and state the flow requirements needed for its use.

ANATOMY REVIEW

The respiratory system begins at the mouth and nose and ends with the capillary beds surrounding the alveoli in the lungs. To review, the mouth and nose open into the oropharynx and nasopharynx, joining to form the retropharynx or the back of the throat. The epiglottis covers the esophagus when we breathe to allow the air to enter the trachea and keep it out of the digestive tract. While swallowing, the epiglottis covers the trachea to keep solids and fluids out of the respiratory tract. Further down the trachea is the larynx and cricoid cartilage. Beyond that the trachea divides into the right and left bronchi, one leading into each lung. The bronchi divide into bronchioles, which lead to groups of alveoli, each of which is surrounded by a capillary bed.

Breathing is facilitated by the contraction of the intercostals and diaphragm muscles. As the muscles contract, the lungs expand and air is drawn into the lungs. As the muscles relax, the chest shrinks and the air is forced out.

The cells in every body tissue require oxygen and need to off-load carbon dioxide to function. Blood is circulated to the lungs where the capillaries off-load the carbon dioxide to the alveoli and take oxygen from the alveoli. The carbon dioxide is exhaled and replaced with oxygen with inhalation.

In order for adequate oxygen to reach our body's cells, we need to maintain adequate breathing. Normal rates for adults range from 12 to 20 breaths per minute, while for children it is 15 to 30 and 25 to 50 for infants. Breathing also needs to have a regular rhythm, with clear breath sounds and equal and adequate expansion of both lungs. Breathing should be effortless.

Breathing is inadequate if there is an increased effort to breathe, the rate is outside normal parameters, the rhythm is irregular, or the lungs inflate inadequately or unequally. The patient's skin may become pale, blue, cool, and/or clammy if breathing is inadequate.

Infants and children have some significant differences affecting their airway. All of the structures are smaller and more easily obstructed. Infants' and children's tongues are larger and take up more of the pharynx. Their trachea are narrower and softer, making obstruction more likely. Cartilage and muscles are also less developed and infants and some children may depend more on the diaphragm to breathe.

OPENING THE AIRWAY

When there is no suspicion of spinal injury, the head-tilt chin-lift method of opening the airway should be used. If there is a possibility of injury to the spine, the jaw thrust should be used.

To perform the head-tilt chin-lift maneuver, place your hand on the patient's forehead and tilt the head back. Place your other hand under the bony part of the patient's jaw and lift the jaw upward and outward.

To perform the jaw-thrust maneuver, kneel above the patient's supine head placing your elbows on the surface on which the patient is lying. Place one hand on each side of the patient's head. Grasp the angles of the patient's lower jaw on both sides and move the jaw upward and forward.

SUCTIONING

Gloves and eye protection are a must when providing suction. Suction is done to remove blood, fluids, or other materials from the airway. It is important that you know the operation capabilities and limitations of your equipment, which can be a simple turkey baster or a complex multiple pressure-setting battery-powered unit. When using a commercial battery-powered or mounted suction unit, the preferred suction tip or catheter is the hard or rigid "tonsil tip" suction catheter. This has a large orifice that allows removal of debris from the airway. The soft "French" catheters have a stopcock to apply or release suction, but have a narrow internal diameter and are useful only for light secretions.

Whatever the device, you should premeasure from the corner of the mouth to the earlobe to determine how much of the catheter should be inserted into the airway. Once done, turn on the suction unit and insert the suction catheter. Once fully inserted to the depth premeasured, apply suction and keep the catheter moving around the airway, gradually withdrawing from the airway. Suction should not be applied for more than 15 seconds at a time to allow for adequate ventilations. If suction is needed continuously, suction for 15 seconds alternating between 2 minutes of uninterrupted ventilations. It is a good idea to rinse the catheter with saline between suctioning to clear the tube.

ARTIFICIAL VENTILATION

When providing artificial ventilation for a patient, there should be equal rise and fall of both sides of the chest, the rate of ventilation should fall within the normal rate range for your patient, and you should see the patient's color and heart rate return to normal. Inadequate ventilations will not produce adequate rise and fall of the chest and the patient's color and heart rate will continue to be abnormal.

Studies have shown that the most effective means of providing ventilations of adequate volume are mouth-to-mask devices, two-person bag-valve masks, flow-restricted, oxygen-powered ventilation devices, and one-person bag-valve masks, in that order. After providing for body substance isolation, whatever the device, the most important and first point after opening the airway is to obtain and maintain a seal around the mouth. Using the thumb and forefinger to form a "C" around the base of the mask, holding it to the face and making a seal is the most effective one-handed method. If there are two EMTs, you can use both hands to ensure a seal. Having the device connected to an oxygen source increases the oxygen concentration of each ventilation. The mouth-to-mask device consists of a mask, a one-way valve that prevents the rescuer from coming in contact with the patient's expired air or airway secretions, and should also have a nipple to attach the oxygen supply. Bag-valve masks consist of a mask, a one-way valve, a self-inflating bag, and an oxygen reservoir. When attached to an oxygen supply of 15L per minute, ventilations of 95% to 100% oxygen can be obtained. It can be difficult for one EMT to maintain the seal and squeeze the bag. This is why mouth-to-mask and two-person bag-valve masks have better ventilation volumes. Bag-valve masks also come in child and infant sizes to limit the chance of overinflating the patient.

Flow-restricted oxygen-powered ventilators can provide 100% oxygen under pressure to ventilate the patient. The volume delivered still depends on an adequate seal. The device has a pressure relief valve designed to prevent over-inflation.

For patients who have stomas as airways you need to either seal around the stoma to ventilate (you will have to hold the mouth and nose closed also) or seal the stoma and have the patient breathe through the mouth and nose.

AIRWAY ADJUNCTS

You may find it necessary to use an airway adjunct to maintain an open airway. If the patient is unconscious and does not have an active gag reflex, you can use an oropharyngeal airway. Select the proper size by measuring from the corner of the mouth to the earlobe. Then insert it into the open mouth with the tip toward the roof of the mouth, rotating it as you insert. You may also insert the airway directly into position without needing to rotate if you hold the tongue down with a tongue blade.

For patients with a gag reflex, use a nasopharyngeal airway. Select a size that is small enough to fit the nostrils and measure the length it should be inserted from the nose to the earlobe. The insertion end is beveled and this bevel should face the center of the nose. Insert the airway allowing the curve of the device to approximate the curve of the airway and stop at the point determined by your measurement of the distance from the earlobe to the nose.

OXYGEN

D cylinders (350 liters) and E cylinders (625 liters) are most commonly used in portable oxygen delivery systems. The in-line oxygen in an ambulance is usually attached to an M cylinder (3,000 liters). G cylinders (5,300 liters) and H cylinders (6,900 liters) are also available. Safety includes handling this equipment carefully to avoid damaging the valve assembly and understanding that the contents are under pressure. While oxygen is not flammable, it will increase the intensity of flame if exposed to it.

When changing tanks, remove the assembly from the empty cylinder (2,000psi is full and anything less than 500psi is considered empty) and remove the protective seals from the full cylinder. Quickly open and shut the valve at the top of the tank. Attach the regulator to the tank and the oxygen delivery device to the regulator.

Equipment for Oxygen Delivery

Nonrebreathers allow for up to 90% oxygen delivery to the breathing patient. The oxygen flow rate to the device should be adjusted to keep the oxygen reservoir bag filled between breaths. This may require 15L/pm in the adult patient. This is the preferred device for patients showing signs of hypoxia.

Nasal cannulas can only accept 6L/pm of oxygen and will only assist in a slightly better than room air concentration of oxygen delivered. Its use should be limited to the patient who does not tolerate the nonrebreather mask.

Special Considerations

Special considerations are patients with stomas with or without tubes in place. You need to be prepared to suction, ventilate, and provide oxygen to these patients.

Infants and children may need padding behind their shoulders to keep the airway in-line and open because of the size of their head relative to their body. Gastric distension is also more common when ventilating infants and children. Bleeding can be significant with facial injuries, so keeping the airway clear may be a challenge. Airway obstructions may need to be cleared manually, using abdominal thrusts or back blows as appropriate for the age of the patient and whether they are conscious or unconscious. Also be aware of dental appliances. Generally, they will need to be left in place in order to get a seal with a mask around the mouth, but watch that they are secure and do not slip into the airway.

Scenario 1

You are on the scene with a nonbreathing patient. There is no history of injury. How should you proceed to aid this patient?

SOLUTION

As there is no history of head or neck injury, the airway should be opened using the head-tilt chin-lift method. Then the EMT should "look, listen, and feel" for respirations. If there are none, the EMT should clear the airway, using suction if necessary and provide artificial ventilation.

Scenario 2

You opened your patient's airway and are providing ventilations, but the chest does not appear to rise and your partner does not hear ventilations when he auscultates the chest. What should you do next?

SOLUTION

Reposition the airway and check the seal around the patient's mouth. An inadequate seal is the most common problem associated with inadequate ventilations.

Scenario 3

If your patient had a history of head and/or neck injury, what would you have done differently?

SOLUTION

In patients with possible neck injuries, the head and neck should be immobilized as you open the airway. The technique for opening the airway in a patient with possible head and neck injuries is the jaw-thrust method.

Review Questions

EXERCISES

The exercises in this review are designed to help reinforce your knowledge of the objectives for this chapter. If you find it difficult to meet any of the objectives stated, go back and review those materials again.

1. Name and label the major structures of the upper respiratory system on this diagram. (Objective 1)

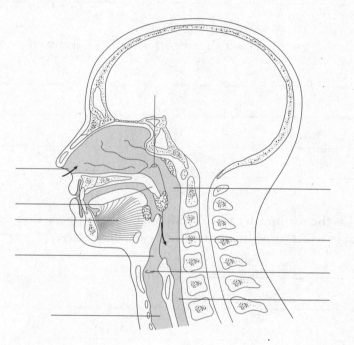

2. What are the indications that a patient is breathing adequately? (Objective 2)

_____

_____

_____

_____

3. What are the indications that a patient's breathing is inadequate? (Objective 3)

_____

_____

4. How is the head-tilt chin-lift maneuver performed? (Objective 4)

_____

_____

5. How does identification of mechanism of injury influence the selection of a manual airway maneuver to open the airway? (Objective 5)

_____

_____

6. How is the jaw-thrust maneuver performed? (Objective 6)

_____

_____

_____

_____

7. What is the reason why EMTs should always have a suction unit immediately available when providing emergency care? (Objective 7)

_____

_____

_____

_____

8. How is the skill of airway suctioning performed? (Objective 8)

_____

_____

_____

_____

9. How are ventilations delivered using a mouth to mask device? (Objective 9)

_____

_____

_____

_____

10. How is the bag-valve mask device used for ventilation while maintaining a jaw-thrust maneuver? (Objective 10)

_____

_____

_____

_____

11. List the parts of a bag-mask system. (Objective 11)

_____

_____

_____

_____

12. Differentiate the techniques of one-rescuer and two-rescuer bag-mask ventilations. (Objective 12)

_____

_____

_____

_____

13. What are the indications that bag-mask ventilations are adequate? (Objective 13)

_____

_____

14. How would you determine if bag-mask ventilations were not adequate? (Objective 14)

_____

_____

15. How is a flow-restricted, oxygen-powered ventilation device used to ventilate a patient? (Objective 15)

_____

_____

_____

_____

16. Differentiate the techniques of mouth-to-mouth and mouth-to-stoma ventilations. (Objective 16)

_____

_____

_____

_____

17. How is an oropharyngeal airway measured and inserted? (Objective 17)

_____

_____

_____

_____

18. How is a nasopharyngeal airway inserted and measured? (Objective 18)

_____

_____

_____

_____

19. Label the components of an oxygen delivery system on the drawing. (Objective 19)

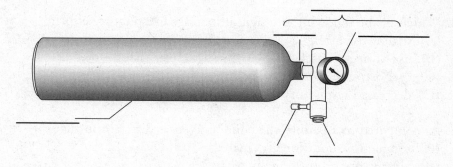

20. A non-rebreather mask requires an oxygen flow of _____ to _____ liters per minute. (Objective 20)

MULTIPLE-CHOICE QUESTIONS

1. The leaf-shaped structure that covers the trachea to protect the airway from liquids and food is the
   (A) alveoli.
   (B) epiglottis.
   (C) uvula.
   (D) thyroid cartilage.

2. During inspiration the intercostal muscles _____ and the diaphragm _____ .
   (A) contract; relaxes
   (B) relax; contracts
   (C) contract; contracts
   (D) relax; relaxes

3. The normal respiratory rate for adults is _____ breaths per minute.
   (A) 8 to 12
   (B) 12 to 20
   (C) 16 to 24
   (D) 18 to 30

4. The normal respiratory rate for a child is _____ breaths per minute.
   (A) 8 to 12
   (B) 12 to 20
   (C) 15 to 30
   (D) 20 to 40

5. Which of the following is a sign of increased respiratory effort?
   (A) shallow breathing
   (B) use of neck muscles
   (C) cyanosis
   (D) decreased respiratory rate

6. As compared to an adult, the child's airway is different in that the
   (A) tongue is proportionally smaller.
   (B) airways are proportionally narrower.
   (C) lungs are not as elastic.
   (D) ribs and cartilage are stiffer.

7. You arrive on the scene of a patient who has fallen 15 feet from a ladder onto solid ground. The patient is not responding to painful stimuli. The correct way to open this patient's airway is to use a _____ maneuver.
   (A) jaw-thrust
   (B) head-tilt chin-lift
   (C) head-tilt neck-lift
   (D) tongue–chin-lift

8. Each attempt to suction a patient's airway should be limited to _____ seconds.
   (A) 15
   (B) 30
   (C) 45
   (D) 60

9. Your patient is complaining of shortness of breath and is using accessory muscles to breathe, but is maintaining her own airway and moving an adequate amount of air. You should provide oxygen via a
    (A) nasal cannula.
    (B) bag-valve mask.
    (C) pocket mask.
    (D) nonrebreather mask.

10. Which of the following should be considered when managing the airway and ventilation of a small child?
    (A) Suction as long as necessary to clear the airway.
    (B) Hyperextend the head as far as possible.
    (C) Place padding under the shoulders to position the head.
    (D) Use a nasal cannula at a high flow rate to provide ventilations.

ANSWERS TO REVIEW QUESTIONS

Exercises

1.

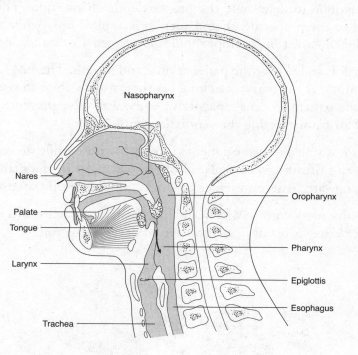

2. The adult respiratory rate should be between 12 and 20 per minute (15 to 30 for children and 25 to 50 for infants), the rhythm is regular, breath sounds are clear, breathing is effortless, and there is adequate expansion of the lungs.

3. Increased effort in breathing; an abnormally fast or slow rate; abnormal rhythm; unequal or inadequate inflation of the lungs; and pale, cool, or cyanotic skin.

4. Place one hand on the patient's forehead and the fingers of the other hand under the bony part of the chin. Simultaneously tilt the head back while lifting the chin upward.

5. Patients with a mechanism of injury that indicates the potential for spinal injury should have the airway opened with a jaw-thrust maneuver to avoid manipulation of the cervical spine.

6. From a position above the supine patient's head, rest your elbows on the ground on either side of the patient's head. Place your thumbs on the patient's cheek bones, with the fingers of each hand under the angles of the patient's mandible. Use the fingers to push the mandible upward.

7. In the event that a patient cannot protect his or her airway from vomit, blood, or secretions, the EMT must be able to immediately clear the airway to prevent the patient from aspirating fluids into the lungs.

8. The suction tip, either rigid or soft, is measured from the corner of the mouth to the earlobe to determine the proper depth of insertion. The catheter is inserted to the proper depth and suction is applied only while withdrawing the catheter. A suction attempt should not exceed 15 seconds in duration.

9. The mask is sealed over the patient's nose and mouth. The EMT exhales into the chimney of the mask, watching for the patient's chest to rise. The EMT allows the patient to exhale passively. A one-way valve prevents the patient's exhaled air from entering the ventilation port.

10. The mask is sealed over the patient's mouth and nose while the rescuer's third, fourth, and fifth fingers are placed under the angles of the mandible to displace it upward. A second rescuer provides ventilations by squeezing the bag.

11. A bag-valve mask consists of a flexible air chamber, attached to a face mask via a shutter valve. Most devices also have an oxygen reservoir.

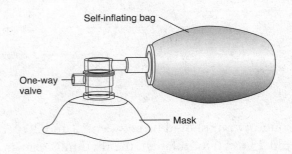

Self-inflating bag

One-way valve

Mask

12. With one rescuer, the rescuer forms a "C" with one hand to seal the mask over the nose and mouth, while using the other hand to squeeze the bag. With two rescuers, the first rescuer uses both hands to maintain a seal over the patient's mouth and nose, while the second rescuer squeezes the bag to ventilate the patient.

13. The rate should be in the normal range for the patient's age and there should be equal rise and fall of the chest. The patient's heart rate and skin color should be normal.

14. Chest rise and fall will not be adequate and the patient's skin color and heart rate will either become or remain abnormal.

15. Adequate ventilation depends on maintaining an adequate seal. The device is triggered to deliver the ventilation, but must have a relief valve to prevent over-inflation of the lungs.

16. The EMT should always use a barrier device when providing mouth-to-mouth or mouth-to-stoma ventilations. The device is placed either over the patient's mouth and nose or over the stoma. In the case of a partial laryngectomy, the EMT will need to close the patient's mouth and seal the nose to ensure that air enters the lungs instead of exiting through the upper airway.

17. The oropharyngeal airway is measured from the corner of the mouth to the earlobe. Preferably, the device is inserted with the distal tip curved upward, toward the roof of the mouth, and is rotated 180 degrees during insertion. A tongue depressor may be used to prevent the tongue from being pushed into the posterior pharynx, in which case it is not necessary to begin with the device rotated 180 degrees.

18. The nasopharyngeal airway is measured from the opening of the nare (nostril) to the earlobe. The diameter must be small enough to fit in the nare, but no smaller than necessary, so that an adequate airway passage is provided. The nasopharyngeal airway must be lubricated and is inserted with the bevel (slanted opening) toward the septum (center) of the nose. The device is inserted toward the posterior pharynx, not upward.

19.

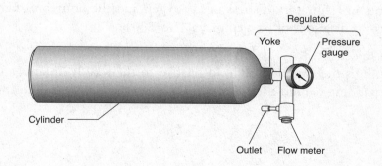

20. A nonrebreather mask requires an oxygen flow of **10 to 15** liters per minute.

Multiple-Choice Answers

1. **(B)** Objective 1
   The epiglottis is positioned over the trachea and esophagus. When one swallows, the epiglottis moves to close the trachea, keeping foreign bodies out of the lungs.

2. **(C)** Objective 2
   The primary muscles of breathing are the diaphragm and intercostal muscles. As these muscles contract, the lungs are pulled open to allow air to enter the lungs.

3. **(B)** Objective 2
   Normally, adults breathe 12 to 20 times per minute. More or less than that decreases the overall volume of breathing and the patient will become hypoxic.

4. **(C)** Objective 2
   Children breathe somewhat faster than adults, ranging from 15–30 times per minute normally.

5. **(B)** Objective 3
   Patients in respiratory distress will use their neck muscles and try to position themselves to make breathing easier.

6. **(B)** Objective 1
   Infant and child airways are proportionally narrower than an adult's.

7. **(A)** Objective 5
   A jaw thrust is used to open the airway of patients with possible spine injuries. The head-tilt method is inappropriate as it may make neck injuries worse.

8. **(A)** Objective 8
   Suctioning should be limited to 15 seconds or about as long as you can hold your breath. Your needing a breath is a good indication that the patient needs a breath too.

9. **(D)** Objective 20
   Patients in respiratory distress need oxygen and the nonrebreather mask can give concentrations of oxygen of 95% to 100%.

10. **(C)** Objective 13
    Because of the size of their head relative to their body, infants and children need padding behind their shoulders to keep the airway in-line and open.

Patient Assessment

 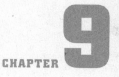

Section 1—Scene Size-Up

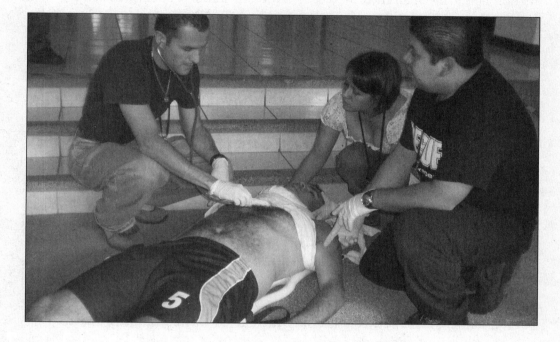

OBJECTIVES

This chapter and the review questions will help readers determine if they are able to

1. recognize hazards/potential hazards;

2. describe common hazards found at the scene of a trauma and to the medical patient;

3. determine if the scene is safe to enter;

4. discuss common mechanisms of injury/nature of illness;

5. discuss the reason for identifying the total number of patients at the scene;

6. explain the reason for identifying the need for additional help or assistance.

Scene size-up begins with BSI and scene safety. Before you enter the scene it is important to protect yourself from exposure by wearing gloves and eye protection and adding masks and gown as necessary. Then the scene needs to be evaluated to determine if there are threats to the rescuers or the patient. These threats will have to be stabilized before approaching the patient. This may involve fire or police personnel, depending on the nature of the scene. Fire or HAZMAT, unstable surfaces, and other unsafe conditions must be made safe for the EMT to enter. The EMT may also need turnout gear for working in hazardous environments.

As the EMT approaches the scene he or she should be observing for critical information about mechanism of injury or nature of illness. Patients, bystanders, and family can give you an idea about why you were called. You can observe the number of patients before you approach in order to call for additional help. Once you call for additional resources you can begin to triage multiple victims. Your observation of the scene and interviews with bystanders and family can help you to determine the mechanism of injury.

Section 2—Initial Assessment

OBJECTIVES

This chapter and the review questions will help readers determine if they are able to

1. summarize the reasons for forming a general impression of the patient;

2. discuss methods of assessing altered mental status;

3. differentiate between assessing the altered mental status in the adult, child, and infant patient;

4. discuss methods of assessing the airway in the adult, child, and infant patient;

5. state reasons for management of the cervical spine once the patient has been determined to be a trauma patient;

6. describe methods used for assessing if the patient is breathing;

7. state what care should be provided to the adult, child, and infant patient with adequate breathing;

8. state what care should be provided to the adult, child, and infant patient without adequate breathing;

9. differentiate between the patient with adequate or inadequate breathing;

10. distinguish between methods of assessing breathing in the adult, child, and infant patient;

11. compare the methods of providing airway care to the adult, child, and infant patient;

12. describe the methods used to obtain a pulse;

13. differentiate between obtaining a pulse in an adult, child, and infant patient;

14. discuss the need for assessing the patient for external bleeding;

15. describe normal and abnormal findings when assessing skin color;

16. describe normal and abnormal findings when assessing skin temperature;

17. describe normal and abnormal findings when assessing skin condition;

18. describe normal and abnormal findings when assessing skin capillary refill in the infant and child patient;

19. explain the reason for prioritizing patient care and transport.

The initial assessment is done to form a general impression. This is focused on the mechanism of injury or chief complaint. While noting the age, sex, and race of the patient you determine whether there are any obvious immediate life threats, treating them as you find them. We use the acronym ABCDE to make sure we evaluate the patient in order of the priorities of Airway, Breathing, Circulation, Disability, and Exposure.

A—Airway

The patient's mental status should be assessed next, keeping in mind that if the patient is unresponsive, airway and breathing need to be evaluated immediately. Alert and responsive patients imply open airway and a breathing patient. The acronym AVPU, Alert, Verbal, Painful, or Unresponsive is used to describe the levels of mental status.

In the unresponsive patient, in medical situations, you can examine the airway using the head-tilt, chin-lift maneuver and determine if the airway is clear or obstructed. Neck-injured patients should be evaluated using the trauma jaw thrust.

B—Breathing

Breathing is then evaluated. If the patient is breathing, supplemental oxygen may be used and if the patient is not breathing, ventilations should be provided by the EMT. Breathing patients with ineffective breathing (too many, too few, too weak) should also have ventilations provided by the EMT. You may need to use airway adjuncts (oro- or nasopharyngeal airways) to maintain an open airway.

C—Circulation

Circulation is checked by finding a pulse and evaluating its quality. In adult conscious patients the radial pulse is checked and in patients less than 1 year old the brachial pulse is used. If there is no pulse, CPR should begin immediately. If there is a pulse, it should be observed to determine strength, regularity, and general rate (fast or slow).

Next check for bleeding, controlling it as you find it. The patient's skin condition and color also give information about circulation. Check the nail beds and around the eyes if you can; you should normally see pink, dry, and warm skin. Pale or blue skin shows oxygen deficits; flushed or red can indicate hypertension, fever, or an allergic reaction; yellow skin or jaundice hints at liver problems. Cool or moist skin hints at inadequate circulation and hot dry skin may be fever associated with infection. In infants and children we also check capillary refill, which should be less than two seconds.

D—Disability

Determine the patient's ability to move extremities and whether they can feel you touching their feet and hands.

E—Exposure

Expose the patient fully to ensure injuries are not missed. This would also be the time to check the pupils to see if they are dilated or constricted, and equal and reactive to light (PERL).

The goal here is to determine priority patients. This would include patients with poor general impression, unresponsive patients or patients with inappropriate responses, patients with difficulty breathing or signs of inadequate perfusion (circulation to tissues), complicated childbirth, chest pain, uncontrolled bleeding, or severe pain. Transport should be expedited in priority patients and then focused history and physical exam can be done.

Section 3—The Focused History and Physical Exam: Trauma Patients

OBJECTIVES

This chapter and the review questions will help readers determine if they are able to

1. discuss the reasons for reconsideration concerning the mechanism of injury;

2. state the reasons for performing a rapid trauma assessment;

3. recite examples and explain why patients should receive a rapid trauma assessment;

4. describe the areas included in the rapid trauma assessment and discuss what should be evaluated;

5. differentiate when the rapid assessment may be altered in order to provide patient care;

6. discuss the reason for performing a focused history and physical exam.

The focused history and physical exam focuses on the mechanism of injury you isolated during your initial exam. Significant mechanisms like car crash rollovers, high speed, ejection, pedestrians struck by vehicles, motorcycle crashes, the death of another patient in the same vehicle, falls of over 20 feet, unresponsive trauma patients, or penetrations to head or trunk imply life-threatening potentials. Even restraint systems can cause injury that your patient should be evaluated for. Air bags can cause abrasions and other soft tissue injuries in average-size adults and can cause fatal injuries in pediatric patients who should be in car seats in the back seat of the car. Shoulder harnesses and seat belts can cause abrasions, contusions, and fractures in some situations.

In infants, consider falls of greater than 10 feet, and bicycle injuries and vehicle collisions of even moderate energy.

If you determine that there is a significant mechanism, perform a rapid trauma assessment while continuing support of the c-spine and the airway. If the patient is responsive and in minor to moderate distress, perform a more thorough survey to look for injuries. The acronym DCAPBTLS is meant to help you remember what to check for when assessing your patient. Working from the head to the toes, palpate, look, and feel for Deformities, Contusions, Abrasions, Punctures, Burns, Tenderness, Lacerations, or Swelling. The head, neck, and trunk are done first and then the extremities. As always, life threats should be treated as you find them. Remember to roll the patient to check the back.

Once the physical exam is done, vital signs should be obtained along with a SAMPLE history.

Section 4—The Focused History and Physical Exam: Medical Patients

OBJECTIVES

This chapter and the review questions will help readers determine if they are able to

1. describe the unique needs for assessing an individual with a specific chief complaint with no prior history;

2. differentiate between the history and physical exam that are performed for responsive patients with a known prior history;

3. describe the needs for assessing an individual who is unresponsive;

4. differentiate between the assessment that is performed for a patient who is unresponsive or has an altered mental status and other medical patients requiring assessment.

In the responsive medical patient, begin your focused assessment with the acronym OPQRST or Onset, Provocation, Quality, Radiation, Severity, and Time to describe pain, discomfort, or distress. Next is the SAMPLE history or Signs and Symptoms, Allergies, Medications, Pertinent past medical history, Last intake of food, and Events leading up to calling for help. Vital signs should then be obtained and care should be administered appropriate to your findings under the guidance of medical direction.

In unresponsive patients a rapid assessment is done. The airway should be opened and evaluated and breathing evaluated and/or supplemented as needed. A head to toe assessment is then done by palpating, looking, and feeling your way down the anterior and then the posterior of the body. Patient position should be such as to protect the airway as in the recovery position. SAMPLE history should be obtained from family or bystanders.

Section 5—Detailed Physical Exam

OBJECTIVES

This chapter and the review questions will help readers determine if they are able to

1. discuss the components of the detailed physical exam;

2. state the areas of the body that are evaluated during the detailed physical exam;

3. explain what additional care should be provided while performing the detailed physical exam;

4. distinguish between the detailed physical exam that is performed on a trauma patient and that of the medical patient.

The detailed physical exam is specific to your patient and his or her illness or injury. You will move from head to toe by palpating, looking, and feeling as with the focused exams but in the focused exams you were looking for life threats particular to the mechanism or complaint; here you will be doing a thorough evaluation in the absence of life threats requiring your attention. At the end of your detailed exam the vital signs should be reevaluated.

Section 6—Ongoing Assessment

OBJECTIVES

This chapter and the review questions will help readers determine if they are able to

1. discuss the reasons for repeating the initial assessment as part of the ongoing assessment;

2. describe the components of the ongoing assessment;

3. describe trending of assessment components.

The ongoing assessment is the continuous reassessment of your findings in the initial, focused, and detailed exams. Mental status, airway, breathing, and circulation should be reassessed along with the vital signs. Patient priorities may shift along with your findings in the ongoing assessments. Your treatments—oxygen, airways, and ventilation, for instance—should be reassessed as to their effectiveness at meeting the patient's needs.

Scenario 1

You are responding to a call involving a shooting victim. What precautions should you take in responding to this call?

SOLUTION

First, you should determine from dispatch whether police are on the scene and the scene is secure. If you arrive on the scene and the police are not there, you should park a block or so away from the scene and notify dispatch that you are "staging" until the scene is made safe for you to enter.

Scenario 2

Once the scene is made safe and you enter, what will you do as you make your scene size-up and initial assessment?

SOLUTION

As you move to the scene you continue to observe for the safety of the scene for you and your patient and start to get a sense of the patient's condition by how he or she is positioned and whether he or she is interacting with people or the environment. You are also making sure that there is just one patient. As you approach you are getting from either bystanders or the patient information that describes the mechanism of injury to enable you to continue your exam. You quickly determine that the patient is alert and the wound appears to be in and out of the right forearm. The patient is talking and breathing without effort but is understandably excited.

Scenario 3

How do you proceed with your assessment of this patient?

SOLUTION

You first do a rapid trauma assessment to look for immediate life threats.

Scenario 4

The injury appears to be isolated to the arm and the patient is not complaining of any other problems, nor are there any other obvious injuries. How do you proceed?

SOLUTION

You begin your focused trauma assessment. Given the mechanism, the focus is on the area of injury and quickly done.

Scenario 5

There are entrance and exit wounds in the arm with minimal bleeding but significant pain and swelling. As your partner dresses and splints the injured arm, what should you do next?

SOLUTION

Here is where you should get baseline vitals and start the patient on oxygen.

Scenario 6

The patient's vitals are HR = 96, RR = 20, and B/P 120/70. Skin condition is good, pupils are PERL and the patient is on high concentration oxygen with 15L to a nonrebreather mask. What is your next job with this patient?

SOLUTION

Next you should conduct a detailed physical exam, beginning with the patient's head and moving all the way to the feet.

Scenario 7

What are you checking for as you move through your detailed physical exam?

SOLUTION

DCAPBTLS. As you move from the head to the toes you are checking for Deformities, Contusions, Abrasions, Punctures/Penetrations, Burns, Tenderness, Lacerations, and/or Swelling. You should also reassess the baseline vital signs at the completion of the exam.

Scenario 8

You are now en route to the hospital. What should you do for the patient till you get to the hospital?

SOLUTION

The patient appears to be stable so vitals should be repeated at least every 15 minutes. Since the mechanism was a gunshot, however, you might want to treat him or her as a critical patient and repeat the vital signs every 5 minutes.

Review Questions

EXERCISES

The exercises in this review are designed to help reinforce your knowledge of the objectives for this chapter. If you find it difficult to meet any of the objectives stated, go back and review those materials again.

Section 1—Scene Size-Up

1. List at least five potential hazards that the EMT may encounter at the scene of an EMS call. (Objectives 1–3)

   _____

   _____

   _____

2. List the types of additional help an EMT may require at the scene of an EMS call. (Objectives 4–6)

   _____

   _____

   _____

Section 2—Initial Assessment

1. What is the purpose of forming a general impression of the patient's status? (Objective 1)

_____

_____

_____

2. Discuss how each component of the initial assessment contributes to forming an initial impression of a patient. (Objective 1)

_____

_____

_____

_____

3. What are some indications that a small child or infant has an altered mental status? (Objectives 2–4)

_____

_____

_____

_____

Section 3—The Focused History and Physical Exam: Trauma Patients

1. Explain the purpose of considering the mechanism of injury in trauma patients. (Objective 1)

_____

_____

2. What is the purpose of the rapid trauma assessment? (Objectives 2 and 3)

_____

_____

3. Explain the rapid trauma assessment process. (Objectives 4 and 5)

_____

_____

4. When would a trauma patient receive a focused history and physical exam? (Objective 6)

_____

_____

Section 4—The Focused History and Physical Exam: Medical Patients

1. Differentiate the applications of the focused history and physical exam for different types of medical patients. (Objectives 1–4)

_____

_____

_____

_____

Section 5—Detailed Physical Exam

1. Explain how you would conduct a detailed physical exam, including differences for medical and trauma patients. (Objectives 1–4)

_____

_____

_____

_____

Section 6—Ongoing Assessment

1. Discuss the purposes and process of ongoing assessment. (Objectives 1–3)

_____

_____

_____

_____

MULTIPLE-CHOICE QUESTIONS

1. You have been dispatched to respond for a sick person. Which of the following best describes the appropriate actions regarding the use of BSI?
   (A) Wear gloves before examining the patient regardless of the patient's condition.
   (B) Wear gloves only if there are visible body fluids present.
   (C) Wear gloves only if you have cuts or scrapes on your hands.
   (D) Gloves are not required as long as you practice good hand-washing after patient contact.

2. Whose safety is the highest priority on any EMS call?
   (A) the EMS crew
   (B) the patient
   (C) family and bystanders
   (D) the general public

3. You arrive on the scene of a motor vehicle collision. You are the first arriving unit and you can see immediately that you have at least four patients and that there are power lines involved. Which of the following should you do first?
   (A) Begin triage to determine how serious the injuries are.
   (B) Call for the power company.
   (C) Determine the exact number of patients.
   (D) Begin treating the most seriously injured patient.

4. You approach a patient who appears to be unconscious. The patient does not open his eyes when you speak to him, but tries to push your hand away when you pinch his shoulder. The patient's level of responsiveness is best described as
   (A) unresponsive.
   (B) responsive to verbal stimuli.
   (C) responsive to painful stimuli.
   (D) alert.

5. Which of the following patient situations should be considered a high priority for expedited transport?
   (A) 30-year-old female in active labor with her first child
   (B) 3-month-old infant with a fever and a rash
   (C) 50-year-old male who is alert but complaining of chest pain
   (D) 45-year-old female with nausea and vomiting

6. Which of the following is considered a significant mechanism of injury?
   (A) falling from a curb onto the street
   (B) 15 mph vehicle collision
   (C) stab wound to the hand
   (D) motorcycle collision

7. You performed an initial assessment and determined that your patient has a significant mechanism of injury. Which of the following should be performed next?
   (A) SAMPLE history
   (B) detailed physical exam
   (C) rapid trauma assessment
   (D) focused history and physical exam

8. You have been called to respond to a sick person in a residence. Your patient is a 65-year-old female who does not respond to verbal or painful stimuli. After the initial assessment, which of the following should be performed next?
   (A) SAMPLE history
   (B) detailed physical exam
   (C) rapid assessment
   (D) focused history and physical exam

9. Your patient is a 25-year-old male who was ejected from a vehicle during a high-speed collision. He is unresponsive to verbal and painful stimuli. Which of the following best describes what should be included in the detailed physical exam?
   (A) head, neck, chest, back, abdomen, pelvis
   (B) head, chest, abdomen, vital signs
   (C) chest, abdomen, pelvis, lower extremities
   (D) the entire body, from head to toe, anteriorly and posteriorly

10. Which of the following is assessed in the ongoing assessment?
    (A) mental status
    (B) vital signs
    (C) effectiveness of interventions
    (D) all of the above

ANSWERS TO REVIEW QUESTIONS

Exercises

SECTION 1—SCENE SIZE-UP

1. Potential hazards include fire, hazardous materials, explosion, communicable diseases, sharp objects, uncontrolled traffic, downed power lines, unstable vehicles and structures, and violence.

2. Additional resources needed may include special rescue crews (water, high angle, etc.), fire suppression, law enforcement, utility companies, and additional EMS personnel and transport vehicles.

SECTION 2—INITIAL ASSESSMENT

1. The general impression is formed from the scene size-up and initial assessment and is critical in determining the need for additional resources, such as an advanced life support response, and the patient's priority for treatment and transport.

2. Any abnormalities in the initial assessment, such as airway compromise, difficult or absent breathing, impaired or absent circulation, or neurological disability (such as altered mental status) should result in a general impression of an unstable patient in immediate need of intervention.

3. Small children and infants lack the verbal skills to communicate awareness of surroundings and will not be aware of day, time, place, or the role of strangers. However, after 2 to 3 months of age, the infant or child should be aware of the presence of strangers and react normally to their caregivers. Asking the caregiver for their impression of the infant's or child's level of orientation can provide valuable information.

SECTION 3—THE FOCUSED HISTORY AND PHYSICAL EXAM: TRAUMA PATIENTS

1. Knowing the mechanism of injury allows the EMT to develop an index of suspicion for injuries that are likely, but which may not be immediately obvious.

2. The rapid trauma assessment is performed after the initial assessment for unstable trauma patients in order to detect any potentially life-threatening conditions not found in the initial exam.

3. The areas checked include the head, neck, chest, abdomen, back, and extremities. The goal is not to find all injuries, but to detect potentially serious injuries.

4. A focused history and physical exam are indicated for conscious, stable patients with a minor and localized mechanism of injury.

SECTION 4—THE FOCUSED HISTORY AND PHYSICAL EXAM: MEDICAL PATIENTS

1. The focused history and physical exam are guided by the patient's chief complaint and past medical history. Therefore, the focused history and physical exam are tailored to the patient's needs.

SECTION 5—DETAILED PHYSICAL EXAM

1. The detailed physical exam is a head-to-toe assessment that is very thorough in unstable trauma patients and trauma patients with a significant mechanism of injury. The detailed physical exam for medical patients is guided by the history and chief complaint, and is most important in unresponsive patients in whom the problem has not been identified.

SECTION 6—ONGOING ASSESSMENT

1. The ongoing assessment includes repeating the initial assessment, vital signs, focused physical exam, and the effects of interventions to detect trends in the patient's condition and response to treatment.

Multiple-Choice Answers

1. **(A)** Section 1, Objective 1
   At a minimum, gloves should always be worn when approaching patients.

2. **(A)** Section 1, Objective 3
   The safety of the EMS crew must be assured before approaching a scene. When the scene is determined to be safe and precautions for continued safety of the team are taken, the scene can be entered and the safety of the patient determined.

3. **(C)** Section 1, Objective 5
   You should determine the exact number of patients before you approach in order to call for additional help.

4. **(C)** Section 2, Objective 1
   The patient is responsive to painful stimuli.

5. **(C)** Section 2, Objective 19
   The goal of the initial assessment is to determine priority patients, which would include patients with chest pain.

6. **(D)** Section 3, Objective 1
   A motorcycle collision is considered a significant mechanism of injury.

7. **(C)** Section 3, Objective 2
   If you've determined that there is a significant mechanism of injury, perform a rapid trauma assessment while continuing support of the c-spine and the airway.

8. **(C)** Section 4, Objective 3
   In unresponsive patients a rapid assessment is done.

9. **(D)** Section 5, Objective 1
   The entire body is thoroughly evaluated during a detailed physical exam.

10. **(D)** Section 6, Objective 2
    The ongoing assessment is the continuous reassessment of your initial exam findings. Your treatments are also reassessed as to their effectiveness in meeting the patient's needs.

Communications

 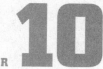

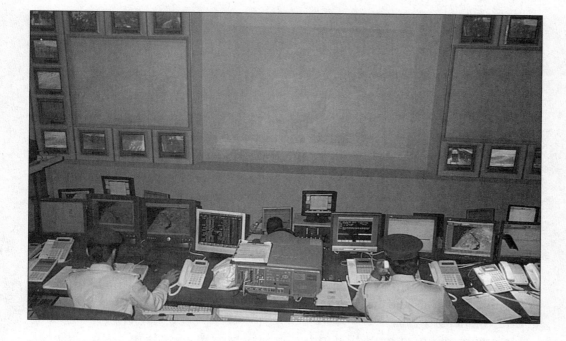

OBJECTIVES

This chapter and the review questions will help readers determine if they are able to

1. list the proper methods of initiating and terminating a radio call;

2. state the proper sequence for delivery of patient information;

3. explain the importance of effective communication of patient information in the verbal report;

4. identify the essential components of the verbal report;

5. describe the attributes for increasing effectiveness and efficiency of verbal communications;

6. state legal aspects to consider in verbal communication;

7. discuss the communication skills that should be used to interact with the patient;

8. discuss the communication skills that should be used to interact with the family, bystanders, and individuals from other agencies, while providing patient care, and the difference between skills used to interact with the patient and those used to interact with others;

9. list the correct radio procedures in the following phases of a typical call:

   - to the scene
   - at the scene
   - to the facility
   - at the facility
   - to the station
   - at the station

The components of a communication system include base stations, mobile radios in vehicles at lower watts (20–50) and portable hand-held units that are even lower power (1–5 watts). Repeater stations can boost the signals from mobiles and transmit to base stations. The Federal Communications Commission (FCC) assigns the frequencies used by emergency personnel. Digital radio equipment is also supplemented with cellular and satellite telephones.

The 911 centers or non-911 dispatch centers receive a call and then dispatch units to respond. Communication from the responding unit should include response, arrival on the scene, transport, and back-in-service information. Other communications should be directed to other services that are needed, like police and/or fire department.

Communication with medical direction may be over the MERCI radio network or cell phones. Medical direction is not necessarily at the receiving hospital, depending on system design and protocols. Any communication should be organized, concise, clear, and most importantly, accurate. Remember to pause 1 second before speaking after you press the push-to-talk button and speak with the microphone 2 to 3 inches from your mouth. Any order or transmission that is unclear should be repeated. Good communication makes certain that adequate resources are at the scene, appropriate orders are given for the patient's needs, and the hospital is prepared to receive the patient. Identify yourself and who you are talking to. Speak slowly and in a monotone voice. Use clear, plain English and avoid repetitive or useless phrases. Keep in mind that radio frequencies are monitored by private citizens, so refrain from using patient names or any unnecessary descriptions or generalizations. Profanity and slang are inappropriate. Avoid making a diagnosis; rather describe what you found and what you have done.

Verbal reports should include the identity of the care provider, time of arrival, patient's age and sex, patient complaint, brief pertinent history of present illness, major past illnesses, mental status, baseline vital signs, pertinent finding of exam, emergency medical care given, and the patient's response to your care.

After the report is given the EMT will continue monitoring the patient and adjusting care as needed based on those assessments. Changes in the patient's condition must be reported also.

The EMT must understand the responsibilities involved in maintenance of communications systems.

In giving the report directly to personnel at the hospital, summarize the chief complaint, history not transmitted previously, and any additional assessments or treatments en route.

In communicating with your patient, make and keep eye contact from a position lower than the patient if possible. Be aware of your body language while speaking slowly, clearly, and distinctly. Use the patient's proper name and do so while positioned in front of the patient with your lips visible in case your patient has trouble hearing. Be honest with your patient, move, speak, and act calmly and give your patient enough time to answer before repeating or moving on.

Special considerations the EMT must be prepared to deal with include visual or auditory disturbances and language barriers.

Scenario 1

Once you are dispatched, what events should you notify dispatch of?

SOLUTION

You should notify dispatch that you are en route, on the scene, leaving the scene for the hospital, arrived at the hospital, and back in service at the hospital returning to quarters.

Scenario 1

Once back in quarters, you are informed that it is difficult to understand what you are saying over the radio. What can you do to ensure that you are understood when using a radio?

SOLUTION

Make sure the radio is on and properly adjusted, listen to make sure the frequency is clear before you key the microphone, wait 1 second before speaking after keying the microphone, and speak with your lips 2 to 3 inches from the microphone.

Scenario 3

You are handing your patient over to the staff of the emergency department. What information should be a part of your verbal report?

SOLUTION

Chief complaint, any history not already given, any treatment provided en route, current vital signs, and any information you may have that was not already given over the radio or cell phone.

Review Questions

EXERCISES

The exercises in this review are designed to help reinforce your knowledge of the objectives for this chapter. If you find it difficult to meet any of the objectives stated, go back and review those materials again.

1. You are preparing to give a radio report to the receiving hospital. Describe how you will initiate and terminate the call. (Objective 1)

   _____

   _____

   _____

   _____

2. Describe how you will organize the patient information delivered in a radio report. (Objectives 2–5)

   _____

   _____

   _____

   _____

3. Describe at least one potential legal pitfall in radio communications. (Objective 6)

   _____

   _____

   _____

   _____

4. Discuss general principles of effective communication with patients and others at the scene. (Objectives 7 and 8)

_____

_____

_____

_____

5. What are the important events during an EMS call that should be marked by radio communication? (Objective 9)

_____

_____

_____

_____

MULTIPLE-CHOICE QUESTIONS

1. A hand-held radio communication device is referred to as a
   (A) base station.
   (B) mobile radio.
   (C) portable radio.
   (D) repeater.

2. A device that receives a signal from a low-power portable or mobile and transmits it at a higher power on another frequency is a
   (A) base station.
   (B) mobile two-way radio.
   (C) portable radio.
   (D) repeater.

3. Which of the following is **false** concerning radio communication?
   (A) Speak clearly and slowly in a monotone voice.
   (B) Keep transmission brief, less than 30 seconds.
   (C) Use plain English.
   (D) Use the patient's first and last name.

4. Online medical control should be accessed via
   (A) radio.
   (B) cell phone.
   (C) both radio and cell phones.
   (D) landlines only.

5. True or False: Giving a report over the radio makes the verbal report on arrival at the hospital unnecessary.
   (A) True
   (B) False

6. When communicating with your patient, you should
   (A) make and keep eye contact.
   (B) tell the patient what you think the diagnosis is.
   (C) always reassure the patient that everything will be alright.
   (D) both A and B

7. When communicating with patients, the EMT should
   (A) use the patient's name to show respect.
   (B) use nicknames or terms of endearment to put the patient at ease.
   (C) speak quickly to inspire the patient's confidence.
   (D) use medical terminology to gain the patient's trust.

8. When caring for special needs patients, the EMT should
   (A) avoid communicating with the patient to prevent misunderstanding.
   (B) speak slowly and clearly, positioned directly in front of the patient.
   (C) speak slowly and loudly.
   (D) communicate through a family member or caregiver.

9. When communicating with patients you should
   (A) be aware of your body language.
   (B) stand above the patient to convey authority.
   (C) show emotion to demonstrate that you recognize how serious the situation is.
   (D) avoid eye contact.

10. True or False: When you are communicating with a patient, body language can either set your patient at ease or make him or her uncomfortable or uncooperative.
    (A) True
    (B) False

ANSWERS TO REVIEW QUESTIONS

Exercises

1. Communication should be organized, concise, clear, and accurate. Pause 1 second before speaking after you press the push-to-talk button and speak with the microphone 2 to 3 inches from your mouth. Any order or transmission that is unclear should be repeated. Identify yourself and whom you are talking to. Speak slowly and in a monotone voice. Use clear, plain English avoiding repetitive or useless phrases.

2. Identify the care provider, time of arrival, patient's age and sex, patient complaint, brief pertinent history of present illness, major past illnesses, mental status, baseline vital signs, pertinent finding of exam, emergency medical care given, and the patient's response to your care.

3. Patient confidentiality, because patient names should never be used on the air.

4. Maintain eye contact from a position lower than the patient, if possible. Be aware of your body language and speak slowly, clearly, and distinctly. Use the patient's proper name and face the patient while speaking, be honest; move, speak, and act calmly, and give your patient enough time to answer.

5. Typically, EMTs notify dispatch when they are responding, when they arrive at the scene, when they are en route to the facility, when they arrive at the facility, and when they are back in service, and may also be required to notify dispatch of their location at other times. The codes or terms used to communicate these actions may vary from location to location.

Multiple-Choice Answers

1. **(C)** Objective 1
   Hand-held radios are carried on your person.

2. **(D)** Objective 1
   Hand-held and some portable radios transmit with a relatively weak signal. Repeaters pick up the weak signals and amplify them for improved reception within the communication system.

3. **(D)** Objective 1
   Patient confidentiality laws prohibit the use of patients' names over the air.

4. **(C)** Objective 1
   Online medical control involves actually speaking to the medical director or his or her agent via phone or radio.

5. **(B)** Objective 1
   While the radio report prepares the hospital to receive the patient, there should always be a report given during patient exchange. The person who received the radio report may not be the person who takes responsibility for the patient, and the patient's condition may have changed since the radio report.

6. **(A)** Objective 7

    In communicating with your patient, make and keep eye contact from a position lower than the patient.

7. **(A)** Objective 7

    The EMT should make eye contact and speak directly to the patient using the patient's proper name.

8. **(B)** Objective 7

    Speaking clearly and in clear sight of the patient is always important, but even more so with special needs patients.

9. **(A)** Objective 7

    In communicating with your patient, be aware of your body language.

10. **(A)** Objective 7

    Body language communicates to people whether we are passive or aggressive. Clenched fists and pacing communicate anger and agitation, while a relaxed posture and open palms imply a relaxed listener.

Documentation

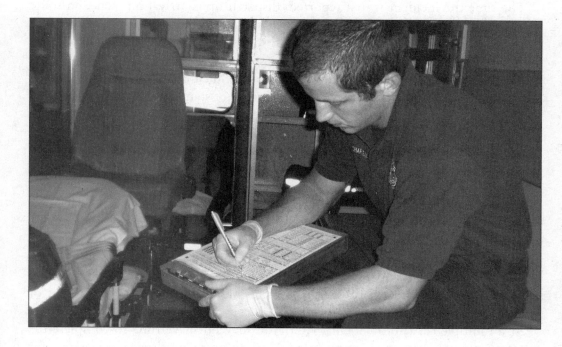

OBJECTIVES

This chapter and the review questions will help readers determine if they are able to

1. explain the components of the written report and list the information that should be included in the written report;

2. identify the various sections of the written report;

3. describe what information is required in each section of the prehospital care report and how it should be entered;

4. define the special considerations concerning patient refusal;

5. describe the legal implications associated with the written report;

6. discuss all state and/or local record and reporting requirements.

ocumentation is important, as it is the permanent record of the history of your patient and your actions with the patient. Continuing medical care and responses to allegations in the future depend on accurate, complete documentation. Also, the minimum data set is a national data set that will allow us to accumulate data for research to determine the future of prehospital care. Minimally this includes the chief complaint, level of consciousness (LOC), vital signs, including skin color, temperature, and condition, as well as quality of pulses and respiratory effort.

The time the incident is first reported, dispatch time, arrival on scene, en route to hospital, and the time care is turned over, all have to be documented. Clocks on the units must be synchronized with the dispatch center. The names of the crew members should be clearly listed.

All forms should be filled out completely, boxes filled in completely, and in narratives that avoid slang and abbreviations that are not standardized. Remember that these reports represent you and will be read by other health care professionals and possibly legal representatives. Make sure spelling and structure are accurate and professional. Any prehospital report is confidential patient information. Make sure you understand your state laws in regard to patient confidentiality.

If you make a mistake on a report, do not attempt to erase it, rather draw a line through the error, write the word "error," and initial it. Document any deviation from standard of care and the story behind it. Never falsify information on a report, as that is a criminal act. Also document patient refusals of care including that the patient was informed of possible complications if treatment or transport is withheld. Have the patient and a family member sign the documentation. Patients that have an altered mental state cannot refuse aid. When in doubt about consent or refusal, contact medical control.

At a multiple casualty incident (MCI) you may not have time to complete the report until after everyone is transported. Your disaster plan should have a plan for collecting important information temporarily like triage tags. Your system should also have addendum or special situation forms to document unusual events that call for additional explanation in case there are questions later. Documentation, when reviewed, should be a part of a continuous quality improvement program that allows us to improve our practice by monitoring our performance in the field and the documentation of that performance.

Scenario 1

At the end of your shift, you are at a local restaurant having breakfast with several coworkers, one of whom is showing a copy of the run report involving an embarrassing situation for the patient to the waitress and others at his table. Is this an acceptable activity?

SOLUTION

You should inform your coworker that he is violating patient confidentiality and breaking the law. It is not acceptable legally, morally, or ethically.

Scenario 2

While finishing your run report at the hospital, you notice that there are no vital signs. Is it acceptable to copy them from the patient's emergency room chart?

SOLUTION

That would be considered falsification of records. If you did not obtain the vital signs, they do not belong on your report.

Scenario 3

If you suspect abuse of a patient you have transported, what should you do?

SOLUTION

The EMT is required to report abuse to the facility he or she transports to. Check your state laws as some states may require that you report the suspected abuse directly to the state agency that investigates the class of abuse you suspect. In any case, you should tell the people that receive your patient and if you are concerned beyond that, you can report the event directly to the agency independently.

Review Questions

EXERCISES

The exercises in this review are designed to help reinforce your knowledge of the objectives for this chapter. If you find it difficult to meet any of the objectives stated, go back and review those materials again.

1. Describe the minimum data that should be included in a patient care report. (Objectives 1–3)

---

2. At the minimum, what information must be included when documenting a patient refusal? (Objective 4)

_____

_____

_____

_____

3. What are the legal considerations to be kept in mind when documenting patient care? (Objective 5)

_____

_____

_____

_____

MULTIPLE-CHOICE QUESTIONS

1. The minimum data set is established at the _____ level.
   (A) national
   (B) municipal
   (C) state
   (D) provider service

2. The EMS report form is
   (A) a legal document.
   (B) a part of the patient's medical record.
   (C) an educational tool.
   (D) all of the above

3. The section of the EMS form that includes date and times is the
   (A) run data.
   (B) patient data.
   (C) narrative.
   (D) check area.

4. When writing a narrative, it is important that the EMT do all of the following EXCEPT
   (A) describe the patient's condition.
   (B) include pertinent negatives.
   (C) include treatments provided.
   (D) provide a diagnosis of the patient's condition.

5. When an error is made on the report form, the EMT should
   (A) erase or use correction fluid to correct the error.
   (B) draw a line through the error, initial it, and write the correction.
   (C) black out the error with ink, initial it, and make the correction.
   (D) discard the report form and start over.

6. Which of the following is the best general course of action when a competent adult patient wants to refuse your care?
   (A) Once you are on the scene, you are obligated to transport the patient.
   (B) You should call for law enforcement assistance.
   (C) You should inform the patient of the potential risks of refusing treatment.
   (D) You should immediately leave the scene and mark in service.

7. Under which of the following circumstances may a written patient care report be released?
   (A) The patient provides written permission.
   (B) It is requested by an attorney.
   (C) The patient is deceased.
   (D) All of the above.

8. Which of the following requires mandatory reporting by health care personnel?
   (A) any patient with an infectious disease
   (B) elder, child, or dependent adult abuse
   (C) attempted suicide
   (D) use of illegal drugs

9. You have decided a patient is competent to refuse care. You should do all of the following EXCEPT
   (A) tell the patient he or she may call back if he or she changes his or her mind.
   (B) have the patient sign your report to acknowledge refusal of care.
   (C) have someone other than your partner sign the report as a witness.
   (D) make sure the patient understands that he or she may die and it will not be your fault.

10. The narrative portion of the report should include
    (A) a description of how the patient was found.
    (B) treatments given.
    (C) assessment findings.
    (D) all of the above

ANSWERS TO REVIEW QUESTIONS
Exercises

1. The chief complaint, LOC, vital signs, including skin color, temperature, and condition as well as quality of pulses and respiratory effort, the time the incident is first reported, dispatch time, arrival on scene, en route to hospital, and the time care is turned over.

2. The patient's mental status, that he or she was informed of possible complications if treatment or transport is not accepted, and that the patient may call back if he or she changes his or her mind. Have the patient and a family member sign the documentation.

3. All forms should be filled out completely, boxes filled in completely, and in narratives, avoid slang and nonstandard abbreviations, making sure spelling and grammar are accurate and professional. All prehospital reports are confidential. If you make a mistake on a report, draw a line through the error, write the word "error," and initial it. Document any deviation from the standard of care and the reason for it. Never falsify information on a report.

Multiple-Choice Answers

1. **(A)** Objective 1
   The federal government requires that EMS systems use the minimum data set on their report forms. It is further required that the information be collected by each state and reported to the federal government.

2. **(D)** Objective 1
   The EMS report form is a legal document, a part of the patient's permanent medical record, and a part of internal quality improvement and education for the healthcare providers involved in the patient's care.

3. **(A)** Objective 2
   Dates and times are in the section of the report that contains the run data.

4. **(D)** Objective 3
   The EMT should provide information that other health care providers can use to draw their own conclusions. This requires that the EMT describe rather than conclude, give positive and pertinent negative findings, and report all occurrences or findings required by the state.

5. **(B)** Objective 3

   When an error is made on a written report, a line should be drawn through the mistake with the word "error" written alongside and initialed by the person writing the report. Never erase or destroy a written report.

6. **(C)** Objective 4

   While competent adults can refuse care, we should always try to encourage them to be evaluated and treated and, at the very least, inform them of the possible ill effects of not seeking care.

7. **(A)** Objective 5

   The written report is a legal document, part of the patient's medical record, and protected by confidentiality rules. Release to anyone other than the patient requires the patient's (or the patient's documented agent) written permission, or a subpoena.

8. **(B)** Objective 6

   While each state has its own laws regarding mandatory reporting by public safety and healthcare workers, elder, child, and dependent adult abuse is always a required reporting situation.

9. **(D)** Objective 4

   Once you have determined that you will allow a person to refuse care, the patient refusing and a witness should sign your report.

10. **(D)** Objective 3

    The narrative portion of the report should be a brief accounting of the entire call. It should include what was found, assessments and treatments, results of that treatment, and any events that occur up to the time care is turned over to the hospital.

General Pharmacology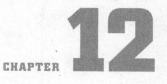

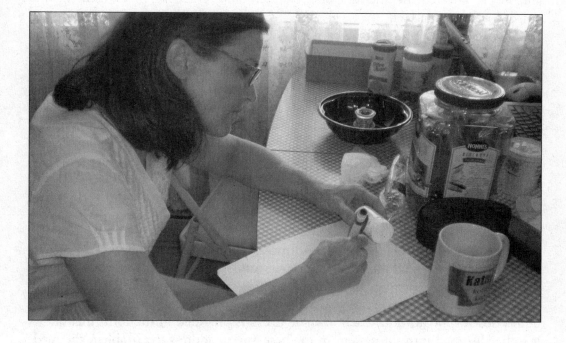

OBJECTIVES

This chapter and the review questions will help readers determine if they are able to

1. identify which medications will be carried on the unit;

2. state the medications carried on the unit by the generic name;

3. identify the medications that the EMT may assist the patient in administering;

4. state the medications the EMT can assist the patient with by the generic name;

5. discuss the forms in which the medications may be found.

The medications that the EMT must be familiar with include medications that are carried on the ambulance for the EMT to administer and medications prescribed by a physician to your patient that the EMT may be called upon to assist with.

The medications that are carried on the ambulance are activated charcoal, used in poisonings and overdose, oxygen, administered to assist patients with difficulty breathing or who may be hypoxic for other reasons such as trauma, and oral glucose for diabetic emergencies. Oxygen delivery is covered in the airway chapter, glucose is covered in the diabetic chapter, and charcoal is covered in the poison/overdose chapter.

The medications prescribed by a physician that the EMT may assist with include inhalers for chronic obstructive pulmonary disease (COPD) patients, nitroglycerin (for chest pain), and epinephrine (for allergic reactions). These are covered in depth in the respiratory, cardiac, and allergy chapters.

In general, medications are known by generic names, which identify all drugs of the same kind and trade names that are specific to the manufacturer. An example is ibuprofen, a widely used over-the-counter pain medication that is marketed as "Advil" by one manufacturer.

The reason a drug is given is called an "indication." For instance, difficulty breathing is an indication for oxygen. A contraindication for a medication is a reason not to give it. For instance, aspirin is contraindicated for patients with bleeding disorders or stomach problems.

Medications are provided in many forms. Nitroglycerin is supplied as a compressed powder (a small pill) or a sublingual (under the tongue) spray, epinephrine is a liquid for injection; we carry glucose as a gel, activated charcoal as a suspension; inhalers contain a fine powder, oxygen is a gas, and nebulizers provide a vaporized liquid dose of medication. Each of these drugs is provided in the form that allows it to be absorbed into the system in the best way to address the problem the medication is used for.

With each medication, the EMT should be familiar with the dose (how much to give) and the administration route (i.e., oral, injection, sublingual, etc.). The EMT should also know the actions of the medication or what the drug will do for the patient. An example is that nitroglycerin is for pain relief due to dilation of the coronary vessels. The EMT must know the contraindications of these medications or the reasons not to give them. For example, do not give nitroglycerin to a patient with a blood pressure less than 100 systolic.

Before you give any medication you should do a full set of baseline vital signs, and repeat as a part of ongoing assessment. Any changes in the patient condition after the medications are given must be documented and reported.

Scenario 1

A patient with chest pain possesses a prescription for nitroglycerin and his wife hands the pills to you. Are you allowed to give him the nitroglycerin?

SOLUTION

Nitroglycerin is considered a patient assist medication for the EMT. If the prescription is written for your patient, he is having chest pain, or the systolic pressure is over 100, you can assist the patient in taking his own medication.

Scenario 2

If your patient's blood pressure is 80/50 but he still has chest pain, could you give the nitroglycerin?

SOLUTION

Blood pressure less than 100 systolic is considered a contraindication or a reason not to give the medication.

Review Questions

EXERCISES

The exercises in this review are designed to help reinforce your knowledge of the objectives for this chapter. If you find it difficult to meet any of the objectives stated, go back and review those materials again.

1. What medications may be carried on a BLS ambulance for use by EMTs? (Objective 1)

    _____

    _____

    _____

    _____

2. Match the generic medication name on the left with the indication for use on the right. (Objective 2)

    _____ Oral glucose   (A) Hypoxia

    _____ Activated charcoal   (B) Hypoglycemia

    _____ Oxygen   (C) Ingested poisons

3. List the medications that EMTs may assist patients in using. (Objective 3)

_____

_____

_____

_____

4. Match the generic medication name on the left with the indications for use on the right. (Objective 4)

_____ Metered dose inhaler   (A) Chest pain

_____ Epinephrine   (B) Difficulty breathing in COPD

_____ Nitroglycerin   (C) Severe allergic reaction

5. Match each medication on the left with the form in which it used by the EMT on the right. Choices on the right may be used more than once. Some items have more than one correct answer. (Objective 5)

_____ Nitroglycerin   (A) Gel

_____ Epinephrine   (B) Powder

_____ Oxygen   (C) Liquid

_____ Activated charcoal   (D) Suspension

_____ Metered dose inhaler   (E) Gas

_____ Oral glucose   (F) Tablet

MULTIPLE-CHOICE QUESTIONS

1. Which of the following medications may be carried on a BLS ambulance for administration by an EMT?
   (A) aspirin
   (B) epinephrine
   (C) albuterol
   (D) glucose

2. Which of the following medications may be carried on a BLS ambulance for administration by an EMT?
   (A) activated charcoal
   (B) nitroglycerin
   (C) acetaminophen
   (D) sodium bicarbonate

3. Your 65-year-old male patient is complaining of chest pain. His heart rate is 60 and blood pressure is 94/68. He states he has taken two of his nitroglycerin tablets. Which of the following medications should you administer?
   (A) another nitroglycerin tablet
   (B) oxygen
   (C) both nitroglycerin and oxygen
   (D) none of the above

4. Which of the following best describes the trade name of a medication?
   (A) the common name that is used by all manufacturers of a medication
   (B) the name under which a specific company markets its brand
   (C) the chemical make-up of the drug
   (D) the official name of the drug as it is listed in Food and Drug Administration (FDA) publications

5. A reason that a medication normally used to treat a patient's condition would be withheld is a
   (A) mechanism of action.
   (B) therapeutic effect.
   (C) contraindication.
   (D) side effect.

6. Nitroglycerin works by
   (A) relaxing the small airways.
   (B) dilating coronary arteries.
   (C) increasing oxygen levels in the blood.
   (D) raising blood sugar levels.

7. Before giving any medication you should
   (A) ask about allergies.
   (B) get a complete set of vital signs.
   (C) ask about other medications the patient is taking.
   (D) all of the above

8. Which of the following is **not** a route by which the EMT administers drugs?
   (A) intravenously
   (B) orally
   (C) sublingually
   (D) inhalation

9. Which of the following should be done after administering a medication to a patient?
   (A) document the name of the medication, the dose, and the route
   (B) recheck vital signs
   (C) ask the patient about effects and side effects of the medication
   (D) all of the above

10. A young man with difficulty breathing has emptied one of his inhalers and is attempting to use a second inhaler. He is still wheezing. He is also shaking and cannot guide the inhaler to his mouth on his own. His blood pressure is 130/90, heart rate is 112, and respirations are 28. You should
    (A) assist the patient with the second inhaler.
    (B) administer oxygen by nonrebreather mask.
    (C) both A and B
    (D) none of the above

ANSWERS TO REVIEW QUESTIONS
Exercises

1. Although some states may expand or restrict the EMT's scope of practice, the usual medications allowed on a BLS ambulance are oral glucose, oxygen, and activated charcoal.

2. **Oral glucose:** (B) hypoglycemia
   Activated charcoal: (C) ingested poisons
   Oxygen: (A) hypoxia

3. Although some states may restrict or expand the EMT's scope of practice, the drugs most EMTs are allowed to assist patients in using include metered dose inhalers for respiratory difficulty, epinephrine auto-injectors, and nitroglycerin.

4. **Metered dose inhaler:** (B) difficulty breathing in COPD
   Epinephrine: (C) severe allergic reaction
   Nitroglycerin: (A) chest pain

5. **Nitroglycerin:** (F), (C), Liquid, Tablet
   Epinephrine: (C) Liquid
   Oxygen: (E) Gas
   Activated charcoal: (D) Suspension
   Metered dose inhaler: (B) Powder
   Oral glucose: (A) Gel

Multiple-Choice Answers

1. **(D)** Objective 1
   The EMT will carry glucose on the ambulance for hypoglycemic patients.

2. **(A)** Objective 1
   The EMT will carry activated charcoal on the ambulance to treat poison ingestions.

3. **(B)** Objective 3
   It is contraindicated to give a patient nitroglycerin tablets when he or she has already taken several of them.

4. **(B)** Objective 2
   Trade names are specific to the manufacturer.

5. **(C)** Objective 5
   A contraindication for a medication is a reason not to give it.

6. **(B)** Objective 3
   Nitroglycerin is a powerful medication that causes a coronary vasodilator response.

7. **(D)** Objective 4
   Before giving any medication the EMT should have a full set of baseline vital signs and be aware of any contraindications.

8. **(A)** Objective 4
   An EMT must be a paramedic in order to be qualified to administer drugs intravenously.

9. **(D)** Objective 4
   Any changes in the patient's condition after the medications are given must be documented and reported.

10. **(B)** Objective 4
    Oxygen is administered to assist patients who have difficulty breathing.

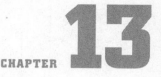

Respiratory Emergencies

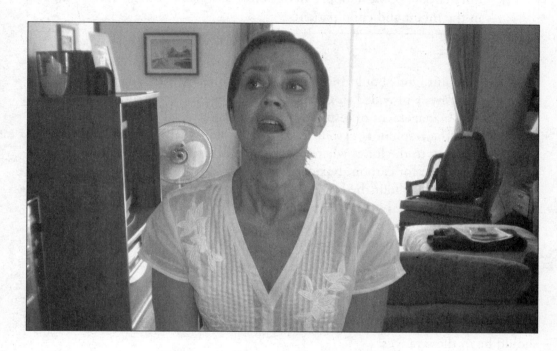

OBJECTIVES

This chapter and the review questions will help readers determine if they are able to

1. list the structure and function of the respiratory system;

2. state the signs and symptoms of the patient with breathing difficulty;

3. describe the emergency medical care of the patient with breathing difficulty;

4. recognize the need for medical direction to assist in the emergency medical care of the patient with breathing difficulty;

5. describe the emergency medical care of the patient with breathing distress;

6. establish the relationship between airway management and the patient with breathing difficulty;

7. list signs of adequate air exchange;

8. state the generic name, medication forms, dose, administration, action, indications, and contraindications for a prescribed inhaler;

9. distinguish between the emergency medical care of the infant, child, and adult patient with breathing difficulty;

10. differentiate between upper airway obstruction and lower airway disease in the infant and child patient.

By this point, you should be comfortable with respiratory anatomy. A review of anatomy is provided in Chapter 5 . Here we focus on function, dysfunction, and our management of respiratory emergencies.

The job of the respiratory system is to take in air, which is conducted through the upper airways to the lungs where oxygen is taken from the alveoli into the capillaries in exchange for carbon dioxide. The reverse takes place in the capillaries at the tissue level throughout the body.

The active part of breathing is **inhalation**. The diaphragm and intercostal muscles contract, pulling the lungs into expansion. The passive part of breathing is **exhalation** as the diaphragm and intercostals muscles relax, the lungs contract, and air leaves the chest.

INADEQUATE BREATHING

Breathing efficiency is measured by rate, rhythm, and quality. Respiratory rates should be in these ranges:

- Adult: 12–20 breaths per minute
- Child: 15–30 breaths per minute
- Infant: 25–50 breaths per minute

Any rates less or more may indicate inadequate breathing. The breathing must also have a steady regular rhythm. Irregular breathing is indicative of inadequate breathing. The quality of respirations should also be assessed. Breath sounds should be present and equal, and chest expansion and the depth of each breath should be adequate. Respiratory effort is a key assessment. Breathing should be effortless. Generally, if you think about it, you do not notice people are breathing unless they are in distress. Noisy breathing, use of accessory muscles (usually in children), or a patient who appears to be working hard to breathe indicate inadequate breathing. The harder it looks for them, the more severe their distress. Inability to speak or speaking in short bursts is another indication of serious respiratory distress. A patient in respiratory distress will also use positioning to assist breathing, including the tripod position (leaning forward on arms), sitting upright with legs dangling, and standing. An inability to lie down on the back is common. Patients with long histories of chronic obstructive pulmonary disease (COPD) may develop a barrel chest appearance.

Noisy breathing is a sign of distress and it can give you an idea of where the problem is in the respiratory anatomy. Stridor, crowing, gurgling, and snoring are caused by obstruction of the upper airway (above the larynx). Wheezing or crackles are lower airway obstructions heard when auscultating the lungs with your stethoscope.

Inadequate respirations are unable to provide adequate oxygenation of the body's tissues and carbon dioxide levels will build. As this worsens, there will be observable changes in the patient's condition.

The earliest sign may be a change in the level of consciousness (LOC) or mental status of your patient. The patient becomes increasingly hypoxic the longer he or she is in respiratory distress. Early changes in LOC may be nervousness, agitation, or confusion. This will worsen along with increasing hypoxia, eventually causing a loss of consciousness if uncorrected.

Skin condition changes as hypoxia worsens. The skin may be pale, blue, and or clammy. The circulatory system responds to the lack of oxygen in the blood by speeding up the heart rate.

The respiratory rate may speed up in early phases of distress. If the respiratory rate becomes gasping and sporadic, it is an indication that respiratory arrest is imminent.

Special considerations for the pediatric patient include anatomical differences. The airways are smaller and more easily obstructed and the head is larger causing hyperflexion when the patient is supine. Infant's and children's tongues are proportionately larger than those of adults and take up more space in the airway. Their tracheas are narrower and softer, more flexible and more easily obstructed, and their cartilage is less developed and less rigid. Their chest walls are softer and they depend more on their diaphragm for breathing. Infants and children are subject to respiratory fatigue if they are in respiratory difficulty for too long. They can actually become "too tired to breathe."

ARTIFICIAL VENTILATION

If the EMT is providing adequate artificial ventilation, the chest should rise and fall with each ventilation at a sufficient rate of about 12 times per minute in the adult and 20 breaths per minute in infants and children. Improving mental status, skin color, and a heart rate that returns to normal are indications of adequate ventilation.

If the chest does not rise and fall at an adequate rate or if the rate is too fast, the artificial ventilations will be inadequate. Poor skin color and condition and a heart rate that continues to be fast are indications of inadequate ventilation.

Inhalers

Patients suffering from COPD such as asthma may have prescribed inhalers. Patients will know how to use their inhaler but in some cases may require assistance. Before using the inhaler the EMT must ensure that the patient is in respiratory distress, that the inhaler is prescribed for this patient, and that medical direction has instructed you to assist. In requesting permission to assist from medical control, the EMT should note the expiration date on the inhaler and report to medical control how many times it was used prior to EMS arrival at the scene. Once the order is confirmed the inhaler should be shaken. The EMT should ask the patient to exhale, place the inhaler in the patient's mouth, and spray the inhaler as the patient takes a deep breath. Encourage the patient to hold his or her breath if possible to ensure absorption of the medication.

Scenario 1

You are presented with a 70-year-old unresponsive male. Your partner tells you that his respirations are shallow at about 30 breaths per minute. How will you manage this patient?

SOLUTION

These respirations are inadequate, so maintain his airway in an open position; you should ventilate him with a bag-valve mask connected to an oxygen source at a rate of 12–20 breaths per minute.

Scenario 2

You were called for a patient with difficulty breathing and on arrival you find a 16-year-old male who tells you that he is fine. You can hear audible wheezing and he is posturing but says he is fine. Is the young man "fine" like he says?

SOLUTION

Breathing is supposed to be effortless. Any time breathing is remarkable because it is noisy or the patient is working hard to breathe, it is evidence of distress.

Scenario 3

Are there any clues as to the origin of respiratory distress a patient may be experiencing?

SOLUTION

Noise or distress on inspiration indicates upper airway obstruction or obstruction above the larynx, as with laryngeal edema or choking. Noise on expiration indicates lower airway obstructions, as with asthma or emphysema.

Review Questions

EXERCISES

The exercises in this review are designed to help reinforce your knowledge of the objectives for this chapter. If you find it difficult to meet any of the objectives stated, go back and review those materials again.

1. Match the name of the respiratory structure on the left with its description on the right. (Objective 1)

_____ Nose	(A)	Large airways that enter each lung
_____ Nasopharynx	(B)	Warms, filters, and humidifies air
_____ Pharynx	(C)	Contracts, increasing the size of the thorax
_____ Oropharynx	(D)	Site of gas exchange with the capillaries
_____ Epiglottis	(E)	Conducting portion of the airway immediately below the larynx
_____ Trachea	(F)	Small airways leading to the terminal air sacs
_____ Diaphragm	(G)	Protects the airway during swallowing
_____ Bronchi	(H)	Also known as the throat
_____ Bronchioles	(I)	Immediately posterior to the nasal passages
_____ Alveoli	(J)	Posterior to the oral cavity

2. Describe the signs and symptoms that would allow you to recognize difficulty breathing. (Objective 2)

_____

_____

_____

_____

3. List the primary concerns in the care of patients with difficulty breathing. (Objective 3)

_____

_____

_____

_____

4. Describe the circumstances under which you should consult medical control when caring for a patient with difficulty breathing. (Objective 4)

_____

_____

_____

_____

5. Describe the importance of airway management in the patient with difficulty breathing. (Objective 5)

_____

_____

_____

_____

6. What are the indications of adequate air exchange? (Objective 7)

_____

_____

_____

_____

7. List the drug profile of a prescribed inhaler for relief of difficulty breathing. (Objective 8)

Generic name: _____

Medication form: _____

Dose: _____

Administration: _____

_____

Action: _____

Indications: _____

_____

Contraindications: _____

_____

MULTIPLE-CHOICE QUESTIONS

1. The voice box is also known as the
   (A) trachea.
   (B) larynx.
   (C) pharynx.
   (D) epiglottis.

2. The windpipe is also known as the
   (A) trachea.
   (B) larynx.
   (C) pharynx.
   (D) epiglottis.

3. The dome-shaped muscle that participates in breathing is the
   (A) intercostal.
   (B) sternocleidomastoid.
   (C) latisimus.
   (D) diaphragm.

4. True or False: The muscles of respiration contract during inspiration.
   (A) True
   (B) False

5. The normal respiratory rate for an adult is _____ breaths per minute.
   (A) 12–20
   (B) 15–30
   (C) 25–50
   (D) 30–60

6. True or False: Respiratory problems should be suspected in patients with behavioral changes.
   (A) True
   (B) False

7. Special considerations in infant and child airways include
   (A) smaller structures more easily obstructed.
   (B) tongue and head proportionately larger.
   (C) softer cartilage easily kinked if hyperflexed or extended.
   (D) all of the above.

8. In which of the following positions would it be least likely that you would find an adult patient with difficulty breathing?
   (A) standing
   (B) sitting straight up
   (C) sitting up, leaning forward on the arms
   (D) lying down

9. The medication with which the EMT can assist the patient in respiratory distress is
   (A) albuterol.
   (B) nitroglycerin.
   (C) advair.
   (D) flovent.

10. A barrel chest appearance is associated with
    (A) asthma in infants.
    (B) congestive heart failure.
    (C) COPD.
    (D) pneumonia.

ANSWERS TO REVIEW QUESTIONS

Exercises

1. **Nose:** (B) Warms, filters, and humidifies air
   Nasopharynx: (I) Immediately posterior to the nasal passages
   Pharynx: (H) Also known as the throat
   Oropharynx: (J) Posterior to the oral cavity
   Epiglottis: (G) Protects the airway during swallowing

Trachea: (E) Conducting portion of the airway immediately below the larynx
Diaphragm: (C) Contracts, increasing the size of the thorax
Bronchi: (A) Large airways that enter each lung
Bronchioles: (F) Small airways leading to the terminal air
Alveoli: (D) Site of gas exchange with the capillaries

2. Signs and symptoms include cyanosis, changes in mental status, a respiratory rate that is faster or slower than normal, inadequate depth of breaths, irregular breathing pattern, inability to speak in full sentences, increased effort or use of accessory muscles, and noisy breathing.

3. The primary concerns are ensuring an open airway, ensuring adequate rate and depth of ventilations, assisting with a bag mask as necessary, and providing supplemental oxygen. In some cases, such as COPD or asthma, assisting with a prescribed inhaler may help increase the size of the smaller airways by relaxing bronchial smooth muscles.

4. In most cases it is necessary to consult with medical control prior to assisting a patient with a prescribed inhaler.

5. Having a patent airway is critical to maximize ventilation and oxygenation.

6. Breathing is normally regular, effortless and quiet, with a normal rate and volume of respirations.

7. **Generic name:** albuterol
Medication form: aerosolized powder
Dose: provided by metered-dose inhaler, usually 1 to 2 inhalations
Administration: shake the inhaler, have the patient put the inhaler to the lips, exhale maximally, begin inhalation, depress the canister of the inhaler, continue inhaling, have the patient briefly hold his or her breath if possible
Action: relaxes the smooth muscle of the small airways, increasing airflow
Indications: EMTs may assist patients who have an inhaler prescribed to them when they are in respiratory distress, and when authorized by medical direction
Contraindications: Patient has exceeded maximum dose

Multiple-Choice Answers

1. **(B)** Objective 1
   The voice box is the larynx, the trachea is the windpipe, the pharynx is that part of the digestive tract that connects the mouth cavity to the esophagus, and the epiglottis is the leaf-shaped muscle flap that moves to cover the trachea when one swallows and the esophagus when one breathes.

2. **(A)** Objective 1
   The trachea is the windpipe, the larynx is the voice box, the pharynx connects the mouth cavity to the esophagus, and the epiglottis is a leaf-shaped muscle flap that covers the trachea when one swallows and the esophagus when one breathes.

3. **(D)** Objective 1

The diaphragm is the dome-shaped muscle that forms the base of the chest cavity and the upper limits of the abdomen. The intercostal muscles between the ribs also assist in breathing. The gluteus is the muscle that forms the buttock and the latisimus is a muscle on the superior aspect of the anterior chest.

4. **(A)** Objective 1

The muscles of respiration contract to pull the lungs open, causing air to enter the lungs during inspiration. When these muscles relax, the chest cavity shrinks and air leaves the lungs during expiration.

5. **(A)** Objective 1

12–20 breaths per minute are normal for adults. Respiratory rates that are much slower or faster than these limits decrease the overall volume of air being exchanged, causing hypoxia, meaning that oxygen levels in the blood drop and the carbon dioxide levels rise.

6. **(A)** Objective 2

The earliest sign of inadequate respirations may be a change in the mental status of your patient. Early changes in behavior may be nervousness, agitation, or confusion.

7. **(D)** Objective 2

Infants and children have anatomical differences that affect management of airway and respiratory problems. The head is larger and when they are supine, its size causes flexion and compression of the airway. The shoulders should be padded to maintain a neutral line with an open airway. The tongue is also proportionately larger compared to that of adults and can easily obstruct the airway, particularly if the neck is flexed. The airways are also shorter and narrower, hence more easily obstructed.

8. **(D)** Objective 2

A patient in respiratory distress will use positioning to assist breathing, including leaning forward on his or her arms, sitting upright with legs dangling, or standing. An inability to lie down on the back is common.

9. **(A)** Objective 2

Albuterol is an example of a prescribed inhaler that patients with asthma may use.

10. **(C)** Objective 2

Typically a sign of COPD, barrel chest results from augmented lung volumes due to chronic airflow obstruction.

Cardiac Emergencies

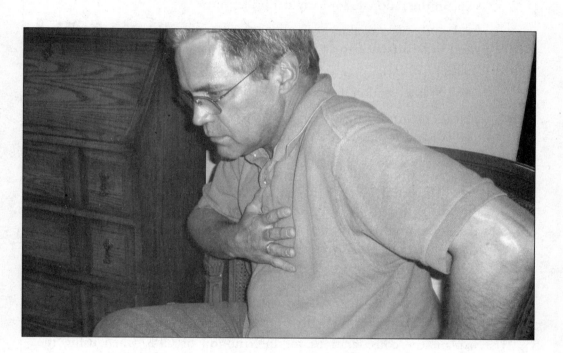

OBJECTIVES

This chapter and the review questions will help readers determine if they are able to

1. describe the structure and function of the cardiovascular system;

2. describe the emergency medical care of the patient experiencing chest pain/discomfort;

3. list the indications for automated external defibrillation;

4. list the contraindications for automated external defibrillation;

5. define the role of the EMT in the emergency cardiac care system;

6. explain the impact of age and weight on defibrillation;

7. discuss the position of comfort for patients with various cardiac emergencies;

8. establish the relationship between airway management and the patient with cardiovascular compromise;

9. predict the relationship between the patient experiencing cardiovascular compromise and BLS;

10. discuss the fundamentals of early defibrillation;

11. explain the rationale for early defibrillation;

12. explain that not all chest pain patients result in cardiac arrest and do not need to be attached to an automated external defibrillator;

13. explain the importance of prehospital advanced cardiac life support (ACLS) intervention if it is available;

14. explain the importance of urgent transportation to a facility with ACLS if it is not available in the prehospital setting;

15. discuss the various types of automated external defibrillators;

16. differentiate between the fully automated and the semiautomated defibrillator;

17. discuss the procedures that must be taken into consideration for standard operations of the various types of automated external defibrillators;

18. state the reasons for assuring that the patient is pulseless and apneic when using the automated external defibrillator;

19. discuss the circumstances that may result in inappropriate shocks;

20. explain the considerations for interruption of CPR when using the automated external defibrillator;

21. discuss the advantages and disadvantages of automatic external defibrillators;

22. summarize the speed of operation of automatic external defibrillation;

23. discuss the use of remote defibrillation through adhesive pads;

24. discuss the special considerations for rhythm monitoring;

25. list the steps in the operation of the automated external defibrillator;

26. discuss the standard of care that should be used to provide care to a patient with persistent ventricular fibrillation and no available ACLS;

27. discuss the standard of care that should be used to provide care to a patient with recurrent ventricular fibrillation and no available ACLS;

28. differentiate between single rescuer and multirescuer care with an automated external defibrillator;

29. explain the reason for pulses not being checked between shocks with an automated external defibrillator;

30. discuss the importance of coordinating ACLS-trained providers with personnel using automated external defibrillators;

31. discuss the importance of postresuscitation care;

32. list the components of postresuscitation care;

33. explain the importance of frequent practice with an automated external defibrillator;

34. discuss the need to complete the automated defibrillator: Operator's Shift Checklist;

35. discuss the role of the American Heart Association (AHA) in the use of automated external defibrillation;

36. explain the role medical direction plays in the use of automated external defibrillation;

37. state the reasons why a case review should be completed following the use of an automated external defibrillator;

38. discuss the components that should be included in a case review;

39. discuss the goal of quality improvement in automated defibrillation;

40. recognize the need for medical direction protocols to assist in the emergency medical care of a patient with chest pain;

41. list the indications for the use of nitroglycerin;

42. state the contraindications and side effects for the use of nitroglycerin;

43. define the function of all controls on an automated external defibrillator, and describe event documentation and battery defibrillator maintenance.

ANATOMY AND PHYSIOLOGY REVIEW

The heart is a four-chambered muscle that pumps blood to the lungs and out to the body. The right atria receives blood from the vena cava and pumps it to the right ventricle. The right ventricle pumps the blood to the lungs through the pulmonary artery (the only artery that carries unoxygenated blood). The lungs exchange oxygen for carbon dioxide between the alveoli and capillary beds and return the oxygenated blood to the left atria through the pulmonary vein (the only vein that carries oxygenated blood). The left atria pumps the blood to the left ventricle and the left ventricle pumps the oxygenated blood out to the body through the aorta.

The heart's muscle is highly specialized in that it conducts its own electrical impulses, which travel across the muscle causing the contractions that pump the blood out to the lungs and the body.

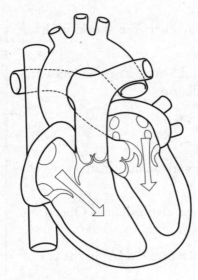

The right atrium receives blood
from the vena cava and pumps it to
the right ventricle, which pumps
blood to the lungs from the
pulmonary artery.

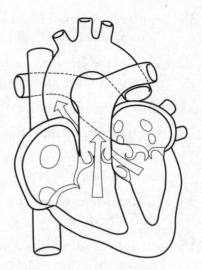

The left atrium pumps the blood
to the left ventricle, which pumps
the oxygenated blood to the body
through the aorta.

The arteries carry oxygenated blood throughout the body, and the veins return the blood to the heart for return to the lungs to exchange carbon dioxide for oxygen. Capillaries exchange oxygen and nutrients for carbon dioxide and waste from tissue cells. Blood flows into the capillaries from arterioles and out through venules.

Plasma carries the other parts of circulating blood. Red blood cells carry oxygen or carbon dioxide, white blood cells help to fight infection, and platelets help to form clots.

Obtainable pulses are created when an artery runs over muscle and/or bone and is close to the skin's surface. Important central pulses are carotid (neck) and femoral (groin). Important peripheral pulses are brachial (anticubital fossa), radial (wrists), posterior tibial (ankle), and dorsalis pedis (top of foot).

Blood pressure consists of systolic pressure and diastolic pressure. Systolic is the first pulse felt or auscultated, brought about by the pressure exerted against the walls of the artery when the ventricle contracts. Diastolic is the last pulse auscultated and represents the pressure in the arteries during the relaxation of the ventricles.

Inadequate circulation brings about shock or hypoperfusion and depresses the vital functions of the body. This inadequate circulation can be recognized as pale, cyanotic, cool, and clammy skin, rapid weak pulses, rapid shallow breathing, restlessness and anxiety, and nausea and/or vomiting.

EMERGENCY CARE FOR CARDIAC PATIENTS

Cardiac problems may be evidenced by patients experiencing chest pain, difficulty breathing, or changes in their mental status. Signs and symptoms of shock may also be present; irregular pulses and complaints of a feeling of impending doom are also common.

Emergency care for cardiac patients includes position of comfort, oxygen, a full assessment, and baseline vital signs. Any complaint of pain or breathing difficulty can be assessed using OPQRST.

O	=	Onset
P	=	Provocation
Q	=	Quality
R	=	Radiation
S	=	Severity
T	=	Time

Nitroglycerin is a medication the cardiac patient may have and require an EMT's assistance with. Nitroglycerin is a medication that relaxes blood vessels and in a patient with chest pain it may open the blood vessels to better circulate the heart muscle. The EMT may give one dose to a patient with chest pain if it is prescribed to the patient and if the systolic pressure is over 100. It can be given every 3 to 5 minutes, up to three doses, and vitals should be assessed before and after each dose. Side effects include headaches, hypotension, and pulse rate changes.

Cardiac patients who go into full cardiopulmonary arrest will be supported by the EMT performing CPR. The EMT should be familiar with both one- and two-rescuer CPR. The EMT should also be familiar with the use of automatic external defibrillators (AEDs). EMTs should know when ALS back-up might be beneficial. The use of airway adjuncts, bag-valve masks, suction, and other airway devices can be used to keep the airway open and ventilate the patient.

Scenario 1

You arrive at the scene where a 49-year-old male is complaining of chest pain. After you determine the scene to be safe and have donned PPE, what will you do for this patient?

SOLUTION

After performing your assessments, you should place the patient in a position of comfort and provide oxygen. Further history should be done to determine the OPQRST or the Onset, Provocation, Quality, Radiation, Severity, and Time of the patient's complaints.

Scenario 2

The patient has nitroglycerin tablets that were prescribed to him. He just took one but is still having a lot of pain. Can you give him another one?

SOLUTION

First, contact medical control. If his pressure remains above 100 systolic and he is still in pain, you will probably be ordered to give another tablet 3 to 5 minutes after the first.

Scenario 3

You come upon an unresponsive woman lying in the street. Should you apply the AED immediately?

SOLUTION

Before applying the AED, you must first determine that the patient has no pulses and/or respirations.

Review Questions

EXERCISES

The exercises in this review are designed to help reinforce your knowledge of the objectives for this chapter. If you find it difficult to meet any of the objectives stated, go back and review those materials again.

1. Label the great vessels in the diagram. (Objective 1)

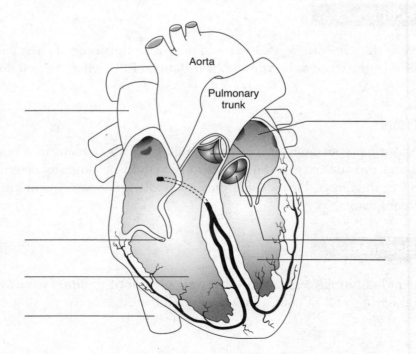

Aorta

Pulmonary
trunk

2. Complete each sentence below to describe the function of the cardiovascular system. (Objective 1)

The blood vessels that transport blood away from the heart are collectively called _____.

The microscopic blood vessels that exchange oxygen, nutrients, and wastes with the cells of the body are called _____.

The largest, thickest artery in the body is the _____.

Deoxygenated blood from the body returns to the _____ (left/right) _____ (atrium/ventricle) of the heart.

The right ventricle pumps blood through the _____ (name of vessel) to the _____ .

The phase in which the heart muscle contracts is called _____ , while the phase in which the heart muscle relaxes is called _____ .

3. List at least two reasons why nitroglycerin should not be administered to a patient complaining of chest pain. (Objectives 2–43)

_____

_____

4. List the signs and symptoms that are commonly associated with cardiac problems. (Objectives 2–43)

_____

_____

5. List the indications for use of an automated defibrillator. (Objectives 2–43)

_____

_____

6. The two cardiac dysrhythmias that an automated defibrillator is designed to treat are _____ and _____ . (Objectives 2–43)

7. The preferred position of transport for most patients experiencing chest pain

   or discomfort is _____ .
   (Objectives 2–43)

MULTIPLE-CHOICE QUESTIONS

1. Which of the following is the intended effect when administering sublingual nitroglycerin to a patient with a possible heart attack?
   (A) lowered blood pressure
   (B) increased oxygenation of the heart muscle
   (C) decreased patient anxiety
   (D) increased strength of heart contraction

2. Which of the following best explains the reason for giving oxygen to a patient complaining of chest pain?
   (A) relief of pain
   (B) decrease the patient's anxiety
   (C) maximize oxygenation of the heart muscle
   (D) relieve nausea and prevent vomiting

3. Which of the following best explains how defibrillation works?
   (A) restarts the heart when it has stopped, restoring electrical activity to the heart
   (B) causes the heart muscle to contract more effectively, restoring a pulse
   (C) increases the heart rate, resulting in better circulation
   (D) stops chaotic electrical activity, allowing the heart's own pacemaker to take over again

4. Which of the following best explains the role of defibrillation in the treatment of children?
   (A) Children require smaller defibrillation pads and less energy than adults.
   (B) Defibrillation is rarely indicated in children.
   (C) Automated defibrillators are typically not designed for use in children.
   (D) All of the above.

5. Which of the following vessels supply blood to the head and brain?
   (A) jugular veins
   (B) subclavian veins
   (C) carotid arteries
   (D) subclavian arteries

6. Which of the following best describes the primary function of red blood cells?
   (A) help fight infection
   (B) help in forming blood clots
   (C) carry oxygen
   (D) carry glucose

7. Which of the following components of the blood is responsible for initially stopping bleeding?
   (A) platelets
   (B) plasma
   (C) white blood cells
   (D) red blood cells

8. Which of the following best explains the cause of a heart attack?
   (A) The electrical system of the heart dysfunctions.
   (B) The blood supply to the heart muscle is disrupted.
   (C) One or more chambers of the heart rupture.
   (D) A blood clot forms in one of the chambers of the heart.

9. Which of the following best describes how a fully automatic defibrillator is used?
   (A) The EMT applies it to the patient and turns it on.
   (B) The EMT manually triggers defibrillation by depressing a button on the machine in response to a command from the machine.
   (C) The machine responds to the EMT's voice commands.
   (D) The EMT must interpret the patient's cardiac rhythm and determine whether defibrillation is necessary.

10. Which of the following is a contraindication to the use of an AED?
    (A) The patient responds to painful stimuli.
    (B) The patient has a pulse.
    (C) The patient is breathing.
    (D) All of the above.

ANSWERS TO REVIEW QUESTIONS
Exercises

1.

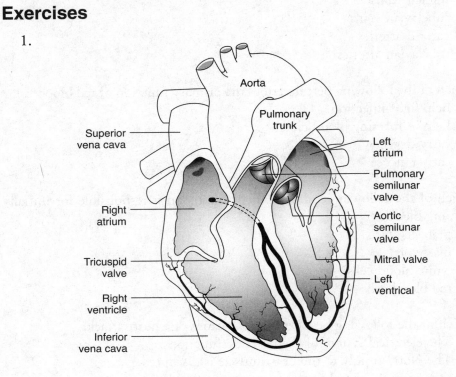

Aorta

Pulmonary trunk

Superior vena cava

Left atrium

Pulmonary semilunar valve

Right atrium

Aortic semilunar valve

Tricuspid valve

Mitral valve

Left ventrical

Right ventricle

Inferior vena cava

2. The blood vessels that transport blood away from the heart are collectively called **arteries**.

The microscopic blood vessels that exchange oxygen, nutrients, and wastes with the cells of the body are called **capillaries**.

The largest, thickest artery in the body is the **aorta**.

Deoxygenated blood from the body returns to the **right atrium** of the heart.

The right ventricle pumps blood through the **pulmonary artery** to the **lungs**.

The phase in which the heart muscle contracts is called **systole**, while the phase in which the heart muscle relaxes is called **diastole**.

3. A systolic blood pressure of less than 100 mm Hg; the patient has exceeded the total dose; the patient takes a medication for erectile dysfunction, such as Viagra, Levitra, or Cialis.

4. Signs and symptoms include chest pain, pain in the neck, arms, or jaw; difficulty breathing, nausea, vomiting, profuse sweating, pale skin, irregular pulse, and anxiety or a feeling of impending doom.

5. The patient must be unresponsive, pulseless, apneic, and meet the age and weight requirements established by your medical director.

6. The two cardiac dysrhythmias that an automated defibrillator is designed to treat are **Ventricular fibrillation** and **Ventricular tachycardia (pulseless)**.

7. The preferred position of transport for most patients experiencing chest pain or discomfort is **sitting up**.

Multiple-Choice Answers

1. **(B)** (Objective 41)
   Although nitroglycerin may lower the blood pressure and result in relief of chest pain, the reason why it is given is to dilate the coronary arteries, increasing the supply of oxygenated blood to the heart muscle.

2. **(C)** (Objective 2)
   Oxygen is given to increase the concentration of oxygen in the blood so that more oxygen reaches the tissues, including the heart muscle.

3. **(D)** (Objective 11)
   The purpose of defibrillation is to momentarily interrupt chaotic, ineffective electrical activity in the heart in hopes that the normal pacemaker of the heart's own electrical system will resume functioning and re-establish a regular heart rhythm.

4. **(D)** (Objective 3)
   When children are in cardiac arrest, the primary cause is usually not ventricular fibrillation. If ventricular fibrillation does occur in children, their small bodies require (and can only tolerate) lesser amounts of energy distributed over a smaller surface area of the body. Automated defibrillators are not designed for this purpose.

5. **(C)** (Objective 21)
   The carotid arteries, along with the vertebral arteries, supply oxygenated blood to the head and brain.

6. **(C)** (Objective 1)
   Although red blood cells are found trapped in blood clots, their role is to carry oxygen, and to a lesser degree, carbon dioxide, in the blood stream.

7. **(A)** (Objective 1)
   The first step in blood clotting is that platelets are attracted to damaged areas of blood vessels to form a plug.

8. **(B)** (Objective 1)
   A heart attack, or myocardial infarction, is caused when an area of the heart muscle is deprived of oxygenated blood, usually by a blood clot in one of the coronary arteries. As a result of the damage to the heart muscle, the electrical system can dysfunction, and the weakened area of the heart can rupture, but these two events are not the cause of a heart attack. A blood clot in a chamber of the heart can be ejected and cause problems elsewhere in the body, but is not the cause of a heart attack.

9. **(A)** (Objective 16)

A defibrillator that requires any other action by the EMT than placing the pads on the patient and turning it on is not fully automated.

10. **(D)** (Objective 35)

Because some heart rhythms that are recognized by AEDs, e.g., ventricular tachycardia, may occur with a pulse, the AED must not be applied unless the patient is in cardiac arrest.

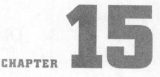
Diabetes/Altered Mental Status

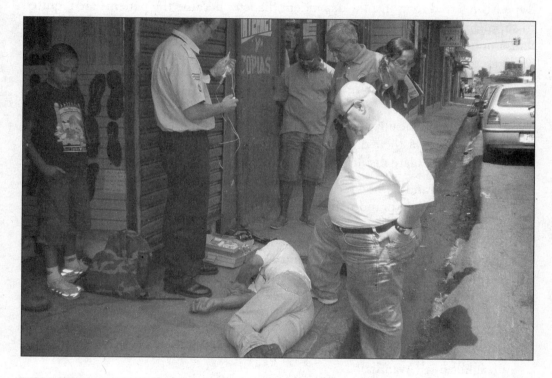

OBJECTIVES

This chapter and the review questions will help readers determine if they are able to

1. identify the patient taking diabetic medications with altered mental status and the implications of a diabetes history;

2. state the steps in the emergency medical care of the patient taking diabetic medicine with an altered mental status and a history of diabetes;

3. establish the relationship between airway management and the patient with altered mental status;

4. state the generic and trade names, medication forms, dose, administration, action, and concentrations for oral glucose;

5. evaluate the need for medical direction in the emergency medical care of the diabetic patient.

DIABETES

Other than head injuries, diabetes is the most common cause of unconsciousness. Patients with histories of diabetes who experience rapid onset altered mental status should be evaluated to determine if meals were missed or insulin was given and patient is vomiting, or if there is a history of unusual work, exercise, or stress. Hypoglycemic patients can appear intoxicated with elevated heart rate, cold, clammy skin, hunger, or seizures.

Type I Diabetes

Type I is referred to as insulin-dependent diabetes because the patients are required to supplement with insulin, as their pancreas no longer produces adequate consistent amounts of insulin. Type I is often called "juvenile diabetes" because it is typically identified in childhood. It can, however, come on later in life.

Type II Diabetes

Type II diabetes typically comes on later in life and is noninsulin dependent. These patients can control their disease through diet, exercise, or oral pancreatic stimulants that help regulate insulin production. Examples of these medications are:

- acarbose (brand name Precose)
- chlorpropamide (brand name Diabinese)
- glimepiride (Amaryl)
- glipizide (brand names Glucotrol and Glucotrol XL)
- glyburide (Micronase, Glynase, and Diabeta)
- meglitol (Glyset)
- metformin (brand name Glucophage)
- nateglinide (Starlix)
- pioglitazone (ACTOS)
- repaglinide (brand name Prandin)
- rosiglitazone (Avandia)
- sitagliptin (Januvia)

You may find Diabinese, Orinase, or Micronase in the patient's house (often in the refrigerator). Uncharacteristic, anxious, or combative behavior is possible.

When confronted with a known insulin-dependent diabetic patient with sudden onset altered mental status, the EMT may administer glucose gel between the cheek and gum.

SEIZURES

Another frequent cause of altered mental status is seizures. While chronic seizure disorders are rarely fatal, all seizures, including febrile seizures in children, should be considered life threatening. The key thing to remember in treating seizure disorders is to protect and not restrain the patient. In general the seizure activity will stop and then the EMT can clear and maintain the airway, deliver oxygen, and transport.

The preferred position to place patients with altered mental status is in the recovery position. This allows saliva and other material to drain from the airway and allows for free and easy breathing.

Scenario 1

A patient has slurred speech, a staggering gate, and a fruity acetone odor to her breath. Your partner thinks she is intoxicated but what else might it be?

SOLUTION

This is a classic presentation of an acute diabetic patient. Specifically, this patient is hyperglycemic.

Scenario 2

A patient complains of a sudden onset of weakness and nausea. During your history, the patient tells you that he is an insulin-dependent diabetic and although he took his insulin today, he has not eaten since last night. What should you do for this patient?

SOLUTION

Your protocols call for you to administer glucose gel to any medication-dependent diabetic patient with an altered mental status as long as he is able to swallow and you keep an eye on the airway. This patient shows classic history and symptoms of hypoglycemia and should respond quickly to the glucose.

Scenario 3

You arrive on the scene where a group of friends are holding down a patient who appears to be having a seizure and trying to insert a spoon into his mouth. Are they treating him appropriately?

SOLUTION

Many people are under the mistaken impression that they must restrain the patient and jam something/anything between his teeth. This is not true. Your priority is to protect, not restrain. The seizure will end after a few moments; just get everything out of the patient's way so he does not get hurt during the seizure by striking something.

Review Questions

EXERCISES

The exercises in this review are designed to help reinforce your knowledge of the objectives for this chapter. If you find it difficult to meet any of the objectives stated, go back and review those materials again.

1. List at least three medications, other than insulin, that indicate a history of diabetes. (Objective 1)

_____

_____

_____

2. Describe the steps in the management of a diabetic patient with an altered mental status. (Objective 5)

_____

_____

_____

_____

MULTIPLE-CHOICE QUESTIONS

1. You are on the scene of an unconscious adult without any indication of trauma. The most common cause of this situation is
   (A) diabetes.
   (B) heart attack.
   (C) seizures.
   (D) stroke.

2. Your patient is a known diabetic who took his insulin but has not eaten as scheduled. He is confused and uncooperative. You should suspect:
   (A) diabetic coma
   (B) seizure
   (C) hyperglycemia
   (D) hypoglycemia

3. Which of the following is indicated in the treatment of a patient having a seizure?
   (A) restrain the arms and legs
   (B) move things out of the patient's way
   (C) insert an oral airway
   (D) place a tongue blade between the teeth

4. Which of the following is true of oral medications taken for diabetes?
   (A) they are oral forms of insulin
   (B) they are taken to increase the blood sugar level
   (C) they stimulate the pancreas to secrete insulin
   (D) they reduce the body's need for glucose

5. You are caring for a patient who is having a seizure. His family states he has never had a seizure before. Which of the following questions can provide important information?
   (A) Has the patient recently suffered an injury to the head?
   (B) Has the patient ever suffered an injury to the head?
   (C) Has the patient been ill?
   (D) All of the above.

6. Your patient is a 50-year-old male who takes Orinase. His family reports a two-day history of progressive lethargy. The patient's skin is warm, flushed, and dry. Which of the following is most likely?
   (A) hypoglycemia
   (B) hyperglycemia
   (C) a problem not related to diabetes
   (D) allergic reaction to Orinase

7. Which of the following signs and symptoms are NOT consistent with hypo-glycemia?
   (A) rapid onset
   (B) frequent urination
   (C) cool, clammy skin
   (D) seizures

8. Which of the following best describes the action of insulin?
   (A) increases the level of sugar in the blood
   (B) stimulates the pancreas
   (C) allows sugar to enter the cells for energy
   (D) breaks down fats for use as energy

9. The source of insulin in the human body is the
   (A) spleen.
   (B) pancreas.
   (C) liver.
   (D) thyroid.

10. Which of the following best characterizes Type 1 diabetes?
    (A) insulin dependent
    (B) noninsulin dependent
    (C) overweight
    (D) onset in adulthood

ANSWERS TO REVIEW QUESTIONS

Exercises

1. Orinase, Diabeta, Micronase, Avandia, Glucophage, and Glucotrol

2. As with all patients with altered mental status, scene safety is critical. Hypo-glycemic patients can become violent. The patient's airway must be protected. If the patient's level of consciousness is decreased, the patient should be placed in the recovery position and suctioned as necessary. If the patient is able to protect his or her airway, oral glucose gel can be placed between the cheek and gum.

Multiple-Choice Answers

1. **(A)** Objective 1
   Aside from head injury, diabetes is the most common cause of unconscious-ness. However, there are other causes and if allowed in your scope of practice, always check the blood glucose level to determine if hyperglycemia or hypo-glycemia is the cause of the patient's unresponsiveness.

2. **(D)** Objective 2
   Insulin lowers the blood sugar level by facilitating the entry of glucose into the cells. If the patient has not eaten, he will have an inadequate amount of glucose remaining. Sudden onset of confusion and uncooperative behavior frequently accompany hypoglycemia.

3. **(B)** Objective 3
   Restraining the arms and legs can result in injury to the patient, as can attempting to insert anything into the mouth during an active seizure. The best way to protect the patient during a seizure is to move objects away from him or her.

4. **(C)** Objective 4

   Many oral antihyperglycemics work by stimulating the pancreas to increase the production of insulin. However, there are a few medications that work by increasing the cell's receptivity to insulin.

5. **(D)** Objective 1

   New-onset seizures can be caused by a variety of problems, including new or old injury to the brain either from trauma or stroke, medications, illness, or metabolic disorders.

6. **(B)** Objective 1

   The onset of hypoglycemia is rapid. The typical progression of hyperglycemia occurs over several hours to days. Warm, flushed, dry skin is an indication of the dehydration that accompanies hyperglycemia.

7. **(B)** Objective 1

   Hypoglycemia typically has a rapid onset, resulting in cool, clammy skin and, sometimes, seizures. Frequent urination is associated with untreated diabetes and hyperglycemia.

8. **(C)** Objective 4

   Insulin is a naturally occurring hormone secreted by the pancreas. One of its actions is to bind to cells and make it easier for sugar molecules to enter the cell as a source of energy.

9. **(B)** Objective 4

   The islets of Langerhans of the pancreas have specialized cells that produce insulin.

10. **(A)** Objective 1

    The best way of characterizing Type I diabetes is as insulin dependent. Although Type II diabetics are commonly overweight, noninsulin dependent, and middle-aged or older adults, this is not always the case. The primary way of differentiating types of diabetes is by dependence on insulin.

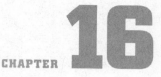

CHAPTER 16

Allergies and Poisoning/Overdose

Section 1—Allergies

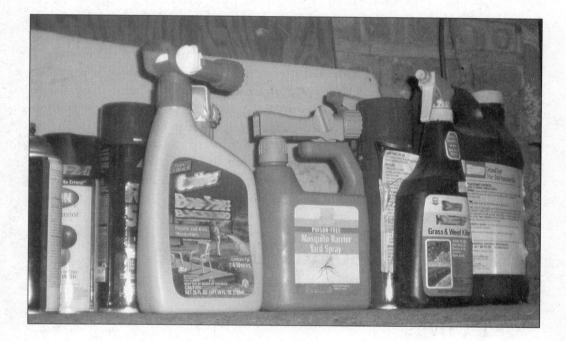

OBJECTIVES

This chapter and the review questions will help readers determine if they are able to

1. recognize the patient experiencing an allergic reaction;

2. describe the emergency medical care of the patient with an allergic reaction;

3. establish a relationship between the patient with an allergic reaction and airway management;

4. describe the mechanisms of allergic response and the implications for airway management;

5. state the generic and trade names, medication forms, dose, administration, action, and contraindications for the epinephrine auto-injector;

6. evaluate the need for medical direction in the emergency medical care of the patient with an allergic reaction;

7. differentiate between the general category of those patients having an allergic reaction and those patients having an allergic reaction and requiring immediate medical care, including immediate use of the epinephrine auto-injector.

Allergic reactions are a frequent cause of medical emergencies. People can have reactions to almost anything. Insect bites, food, plants, and medications can cause even fatal reactions. The typical allergic response ranges from itching, hives, flushed red skin, and swelling in the face and hands. A serious allergic response can result in difficulty breathing due to swelling and inflammation of the airways. A coughing, wheezing patient with noisy respirations or a hoarse voice has possibly been exposed to an allergen. Other symptoms can include an increase in heart rate, itchy, watery eyes, headache, and a runny nose. As the reaction advances without intervention, mental status can decrease and hypoperfusion (shock) can result.

The treatment of allergic reactions consists of early recognition, airway and oxygen therapy, and if the patient has a history and an Epipen auto-injector, administration of epinephrine. Side effects of epinephrine include increased heart rate, pallor, dizziness, chest pain, and headaches.

Section 2—Poisoning/Overdose

OBJECTIVES

This chapter and the review questions will help readers determine if they are able to

1. list various ways that poisons enter the body;

2. list signs/symptoms associated with poisoning;

3. discuss the emergency medical care for the patient with possible overdose;

4. describe the steps in the emergency medical care for the patient with suspected poisoning;

5. establish the relationship between the patient suffering from poisoning or overdose and airway management;

6. state the generic and trade names, indications, contraindications, medication forms, dose, administration, actions, side effects, and reassessment strategies for activated charcoal;

7. recognize the need for medical direction in caring for the patient with poisoning or overdose.

Poisonings and overdose are common causes of medical emergencies. The EMT needs to determine what substance the patient took or was exposed to, when it was taken or exposed, over what time it was taken or exposed, what if any interventions were taken, and what the patient's weight is.

Poison can enter the body via ingestion, injection, inhalation, or absorption. Emergency medical care includes maintaining airway and breathing and identifying the substance.

Activated charcoal can be administered to patients who have ingested poison. Adults and children can be given 1 gram/kg; the usual adult dose is 25 to 50 grams and the usual infant or child dose is 12.5 to 25 grams. Activated charcoal prevents poison from being absorbed into the body. Side effects include black stools and possibly nausea and vomiting. The dose should be repeated if the patient vomits after administration.

Scenario 1

You are called to evaluate a 25-year-old female complaining of "feeling funny." On arrival, you find the patient to have flushed skin and complaints of itching and tingling sensations all over her body. She says that it started not long after a wasp stung her. What do you suspect is the nature of her problem?

SOLUTION

It looks very much like the patient is having an allergic reaction. The fact that her complaints came on not long after the sting makes it likely.

Scenario 2

Hives, itching, and swelling may not be life threatening but if the reaction progresses it can become a life threat. What should the EMT watch for?

SOLUTION

One of the most common allergic responses is difficulty breathing in the form of asthma-like presentation. The patient wheezes and possibly presents with stridor if the edema settles into the upper airways. The EMT should monitor the patient's airway and breathing closely.

Scenario 3

You are caring for a patient who claims to have taken numerous pills and the hospital has ordered activated charcoal. How much should you give to this 150-pound male?

SOLUTION

Activated charcoal is dosed at 1gm/kg body weight. The typical adult dose is 25 to 50 grams. This patient weighs 150 pounds so the full 50 grams should be given.

Review Questions

EXERCISES

The exercises in this review are designed to help reinforce your knowledge of the objectives for this chapter. If you find it difficult to meet any of the objectives stated, go back and review those materials again.

Section 1—Allergic Reactions

1. Describe the indications that someone is experiencing an allergic reaction. (Objective 1)

   _____

   _____

   _____

2. Describe the indications that the airway is compromised in a patient having an allergic reaction. (Objectives 3 and 4)

   _____

   _____

   _____

   _____

3. Describe the benefits of giving epinephrine to a patient having a severe allergic reaction. (Objective 5)

_____

_____

_____

4. Under what circumstances should epinephrine be withheld in the treatment of a patient having an allergic reaction? (Objective 5)

_____

_____

MULTIPLE-CHOICE QUESTIONS

1. All of the following indicate a severe allergic reaction requiring prehospital treatment by the EMT EXCEPT
   (A) labored breathing.
   (B) itching.
   (C) stridor.
   (D) hypotension.

2. Which of the following statements regarding epinephrine auto-injectors is true?
   (A) They are available over the counter.
   (B) They are carried on the ambulance for use in patients with or without prior allergic reactions.
   (C) They are available in adult and pediatric dosages.
   (D) They can be used to prevent an allergic reaction if exposure to an allergen is anticipated.

3. In administering the auto-injector it should be positioned midway between the hip and knee on the _____ aspect of the thigh.
   (A) lateral
   (B) medial
   (C) anterior
   (D) posterior

4. True or False: Once a severe allergic reaction is treated with epinephrine the patient does not require further treatment.
   (A) True
   (B) False

5. True or False: All patients with an epinephrine auto-injector who are experiencing an allergic reaction should be assisted in administering their auto-injector.
   (A) True
   (B) False

6. Which of the following are the intended actions of epinephrine when administered for a severe allergic reaction?
   (A) dilating the bronchioles and blood vessels
   (B) constricting the bronchioles and blood vessels
   (C) dilating the bronchioles and constricting the blood vessels
   (D) constricting the bronchioles and dilating the blood vessels

7. A patient has had skin exposure to a toxin. The route of entry for the toxin is
   (A) absorption.
   (B) inhalation.
   (C) ingestion.
   (D) injection.

8. In the case of ingested poisons the EMT should consider
   (A) administering syrup of ipecac.
   (B) manually inducing vomiting.
   (C) administering activated charcoal.
   (D) having the patient drink large quantities of milk or water

9. The pediatric dose of activated charcoal is typically _____ grams.
   (A) 5 to 12.5
   (B) 12.5 to 25
   (C) 25 to 50
   (D) 50 to 100

10. Activated charcoal works by
    (A) preventing absorption of some poisons.
    (B) inducing vomiting.
    (C) serving as an antidote to some poisons.
    (D) coating the lining of the stomach to reduce irritation.

ANSWERS TO REVIEW QUESTIONS

Exercises

SECTION 1—ALLERGIES

1. Allergic reactions can range from mild to severe. Signs and symptoms can include itching, hives, swelling, nausea, vomiting, diarrhea, hoarseness, wheezing, and hypotension.

2. Airway compromise should be anticipated or suspected with a complaint of itching of the throat, swelling of the tongue, hoarseness, coughing, stridor, wheezing, complaint of difficulty breathing, obvious signs of respiratory distress, decreased oxygen saturation reading, or cyanosis.

3. Epinephrine can reduce swelling and improve blood pressure through vasoconstriction and can relax bronchial smooth muscle to improve gas exchange in the lungs.

4. Epinephrine is not given for mild allergic reactions without respiratory distress, airway compromise, or hypotension.

Multiple-Choice Answers

1. **(B)** Section 1, Objective 1
Although itching and hives can accompany severe allergic reactions, by themselves, they are not indicative of a severe allergic reaction.

2. **(C)** Section 1, Objective 5
Epinephrine auto-injectors are only available by prescription to patients with a history of severe allergic reaction. The EMT may assist a patient with the patient's auto-injector, but does not carry auto-injectors on the ambulance. Epinephrine is not used to prevent an allergic reaction. Both adult and pediatric dosages are available.

3. **(A)** Section 1, Objective 5
The auto-injector is administered at the outer (lateral) aspect of the thigh.

4. **(B)** Section 1, Objective 7
Epinephrine has only a short-term effect and does not treat all of the mechanisms of severe allergic reactions.

5. **(B)** Section 1, Objective 7
Epinephrine is only administered if the allergic reaction is severe. Epinephrine is a potent drug that can have side effects, such as increasing the oxygen demands of the heart. Therefore, it is only given when clearly needed.

6. **(C)** Section 1, Objective 6
Epinephrine relaxes the smooth muscle of the bronchioles, but causes constriction of the smooth muscle in blood vessels. While this seems paradoxical, epinephrine has different properties that allow it to have different effects on different types of tissue in the body.

7. **(A)** Section 2, Objective 4
Some toxins can be absorbed directly through the skin or mucus membranes. Inhalation refers to breathing in the toxin, ingestion means swallowing the toxin, and injection refers to introducing the toxin into the tissues below the surface of the skin, such as by a needle or insect bite or sting.

8. **(C)** Section 2, Objective 6
The treatment of ingested toxins varies depending on the toxin, the amount ingested, the age of the patient, and the length of time since ingestion. The EMT should always consult medical direction or Poison Control with as much information about the poisoning as possible. The EMT may be advised to give activated charcoal for some poisons, but it is not indicated in all situations. Inducing vomiting by any means is no longer a recommended treatment for ingested poisons. Only rarely would the EMT be advised to dilute the poison by having the patient drink fluids.

9. **(B)** Section 2, Objective 6
The dosage of activated charcoal is weight-based. It is preferred that the patient's weight is known. Most pediatric patients will receive dosages in the rage of 12.5 to 25 grams of activated charcoal.

10. **(A)** Section 2, Objective 6
Activated charcoal can bind some poisons, preventing them from being absorbed through the gastrointestinal tract.

Environmental Emergencies

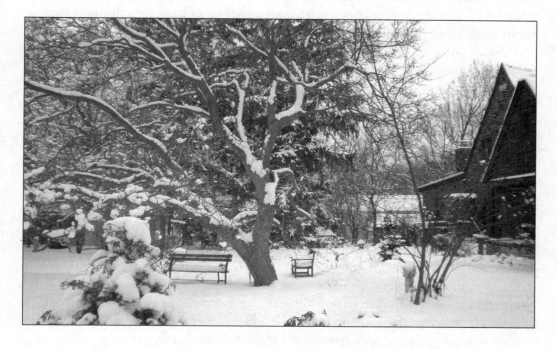

OBJECTIVES

This chapter and the review questions will help readers determine if they are able to

1. describe the various ways that the body loses heat;

2. list the signs and symptoms of exposure to cold;

3. explain the steps in providing emergency medical care to the patient exposed to cold;

4. list the signs and symptoms of exposure to heat;

5. explain the steps in providing emergency care to the patient exposed to heat;

6. recognize the signs and symptoms of water-related emergencies;

7. describe the complications of near drowning;

8. discuss the emergency medical care of bites and stings.

TYPES OF ENVIRONMENTAL EMERGENCIES

Environmental emergencies include exposure to heat and cold. The body can lose heat via radiation, convection, conduction, evaporation, and breathing or respiration creating hypothermia. If the heat gained by the body exceeds the heat lost by the body, hyperthermia can occur.

Any environmental exposure calls for the EMT to determine the source, the environment, if there was or is a loss of consciousness, and whether the effects are general or local.

Generalized hypothermia can be caused by immersion (soaked as in a rain) or submersion (as in being underwater). Infants and children might actually be at greater risk as they have a larger surface area relative to their overall mass, making them more susceptible. Less body fat also places them at risk.

Patients who are compromised by other problems such as shock, injury, burns, infection, diabetes, or other disease or injury are also more susceptible.

Treatment of Generalized Hypothermia

Generalized hypothermia is treated first with removal from the environment. Get rid of wet or restrictive clothing. Do not let the patient walk or exert himself or herself and if hypothermia is profound, administer warm humidified oxygen if available.

Cold Injuries

Superficial injury exposure can be recognized by blanching of the skin with palpation and normal color does not return. There is loss of feeling and sensation, skin remains soft, and tingles with rewarming. Signs of late or deep injury include white waxy skin, firm to frozen feeling, blisters, and mottling with rewarming. Care includes removing the patient from the environment, protecting from further injury, removing wet or restrictive clothing, and administering oxygen.

Remove clothing and jewelry and keep the patient warm and dry. If transport is exceedingly long, immerse the body part in warm water until color returns and then dress patient with dry sterile dressings.

Heat Exposure

Climate, exercise, activity, and the age and general physical condition of the patient can contribute to the potential for problems associated with heat exposure. Muscle cramps, weakness, exhaustion, dizziness, faintness, moist pale skin with normal to cool temperature, and rapid heart rate are examples of heat cramps and heat exhaustion, while hot dry skin and altered mental status are signs of heat stroke or severe heat exposure.

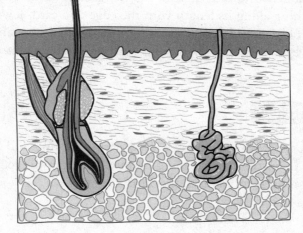

A cross-section of a subcutaneous view of the skin showing a hair follicle and sweat gland.

Patients with heat exposure should be removed from the environment, given oxygen, have clothing loosened or removed, and cooled by fanning. If the patient is alert and not nauseated, cool liquids can be administered. If the patient is vomiting, transport the patient to the hospital.

Cool packs to the neck and groin are appropriate for the patient with hot dry skin and altered mental status.

Drowning

Drowning or near-drowning victims should be removed from the water with attention to the potential for spinal injuries once safety of the rescuers is assured. Contrary to what is generally supposed, drowning victims don't take a large amount of water into the lungs. What actually happens is that the water entering the airway stimulates the gag reflex, closing the airway and causing the patient to suffocate. The water temperature also causes the patient to become hypothermic. Treatment of the drowning victim centers on creating and protecting an airway and considering that the patient will need to be warmed and ventilated for a time before resuscitation can be successful. CPR should be performed if the patient is without a pulse and is not breathing. The EMT should also consider head and neck injuries. Often, such injuries cause the patient to sink under the water. This further explains why many drowning victims succumb in less than five feet of water.

Bites and Stings

Bites and stings are included in environmental injuries. Pain, redness, swelling, and associated weakness, dizziness, chills, fever, nausea, or vomiting can indicate a possible serious reaction to the bite or sting. If the stinger is visible, it can/should be removed by brushing along its length with the edge of a card. Jewelry and restrictive clothing should be removed before swelling makes this impossible. These patients should be observed for respiratory difficulty or signs of shock associated with allergic response.

Scenario 1

You are called for a "man down" on a cold damp evening and find a man in his underwear lying in an alley. Once you determine whether the man is breathing and has pulses, what is your immediate concern?

SOLUTION

Hypothermia. The patient should be removed as soon as possible from the environment that brought about the hypothermia.

Scenario 2

Once moved to the warm ambulance, how else can you treat the hypothermia?

SOLUTION

Remove any wet clothing and cover the patient with warm, dry blankets.

Scenario 3

You are working with an unresponsive heat exposure patient. She is breathing and has a rapid, shallow respiratory rate. Her skin is hot and dry to the touch. What treatments are you considering for this patient?

SOLUTION

Remove restrictive clothing, administer oxygen, apply cool packs to the neck, groin, and armpits and keep the skin moist with a sponge or wet towel.

Review Questions

EXERCISES

The exercises in this review are designed to help reinforce your knowledge of the objectives for this chapter. If you find it difficult to meet any of the objectives stated, go back and review those materials again.

1. Describe each of the ways by which the body loses heat. (Objective 1)

   _____

   _____

   _____

   _____

2. You are caring for a patient who was found unresponsive in an alley. It is very chilly outside and it is unclear how long the patient has been there. How would you recognize if the patient is suffering from exposure to the cold? (Objective 2)

   _____

   _____

   _____

   _____

3. What are they key considerations in providing care for the patient who is suffering from cold exposure? (Objective 3)

   _____

   _____

   _____

   _____

4. You have been called to respond to a person who became ill while mowing the lawn. It is very hot and humid outside. What are the indications that the patient's problem is related to the heat? (Objective 4)

_____

_____

_____

_____

5. What are the key considerations in caring for patients with heat-related emergencies? (Objective 5)

_____

_____

_____

_____

6. What types of problems should you anticipate in caring for the patient who has been rescued from submersion in water? (Objectives 6 and 7)

_____

_____

_____

_____

7. What is the general prehospital care for bites and stings? (Objective 8)

_____

_____

_____

_____

MULTIPLE-CHOICE QUESTIONS

1. Losing heat from an uncovered head in cool weather with a light breeze is an example of
   (A) conduction.
   (B) convection.
   (C) radiation.
   (D) evaporation.

2. Heat loss through wet clothing is
   (A) conduction.
   (B) convection.
   (C) radiation.
   (D) evaporation.

3. Your patient is found outdoors in cold weather with rain-soaked clothing. The specific terminology for this is _____ hypothermia.
   (A) waterborne
   (B) wet
   (C) submersion
   (D) immersion

4. To assess the general body temperature of the patient the EMT should
   (A) place the back of the hand on the patient's forehead.
   (B) place the back of the hand between the patient's clothing and abdomen.
   (C) place the back of the hand in the patient's palm.
   (D) place the back of the hand in the small of the patient's back.

5. Which of the following is true of treating cold injuries to the extremities?
   (A) Fingers and toes should be rubbed vigorously.
   (B) Cold water should be run over the extremity.
   (C) Encourage the patient to walk on cold injured feet.
   (D) The patient should be handled gently.

6. Early or superficial cold injury is evidenced by
   (A) tingling sensation when rewarmed.
   (B) blisters.
   (C) flushed skin.
   (D) white waxy skin.

7. Rewarming affected parts by immersing in warm water should only be done in the prehospital setting if
   (A) it is a late or deep cold injury.
   (B) the injury is superficial.
   (C) transport is long or delayed.
   (D) a physician is on the scene.

8. Exercise and heat can work together to cause the loss of _____ of perspiration per hour.
   (A) 50 mL
   (B) 500 mL
   (C) 1 liter
   (D) 2 liters

9. The progression of heat-related illness, from mildest to most severe is
   (A) heat cramps, heat exhaustion, heat stroke.
   (B) heat exhaustion, heat stroke, heat cramps.
   (C) heat stroke, heat cramps, heat exhaustion.
   (D) heat cramps, heat stroke, heat exhaustion.

10. Your patient was riding his bicycle in hot, humid weather. He is now complaining of weakness and nausea. His skin is pale, cool, and clammy and he has a rapid heart rate. This is most consistent with
    (A) heat cramps.
    (B) heat exhaustion.
    (C) heat stroke.
    (D) heat rash.

ANSWERS TO REVIEW QUESTIONS

Exercises

1. Radiation: Loss of heat into still air; convection: loss of heat as warmed from radiation is replaced with cooler air; evaporation: loss of heat associated with loss of body water into the air; respiration: loss of heat via air that has been warmed by the body in the respiratory system, then exhaled; conduction: loss of heat from contact with an object or substance below body temperature.

2. Suspicion will increase if the patient has any risk factors for hypothermia, such as being wet, having little body fat, or having a preexisting illness. Local cold injuries are noted by blanching of the skin or a firm waxy sensation of the skin, and possibly in the deeper tissues. Generalized cold exposure might be suspected with cold skin, shivering, lack of responsiveness, nonreactive pupils, or weak or absent peripheral pulses.

3. Because this is an environmental emergency, the first consideration is removing the patient from the environment that caused the problem. The patient's airway, breathing, and circulation must all be maintained. Remove any damp clothing, and prevent further heat loss by increasing the temperature in the ambulance, and cover the patient with blankets. Active rewarming is typically delayed until arrival at the hospital. Local cold injuries are treated by gentle handling, using bulking bandages to protect the area, not allowing the patient to use the affected part, and not attempting to actively rewarm the part unless transport is long or delayed.

4. The presentation of heat-related problems depends on the severity of heat exposure. The patient may complain of weakness, nausea, or muscle cramps. The patient's skin may be pale, cool, and clammy, or may be hot, dry, and flushed. Altered mental status is a sign of a serious heat-related problem.

5. The patient must be removed from the hot environment and heavy clothing should be removed. If the patient is alert and not complaining of nausea, sips of cool water can be provided. If the patient has an altered mental status and hot, dry, skin, cold packs can be applied to the neck, groin, and armpits.

6. Depending on the way in which the patient entered the water, spinal injury may be present. Even submersion in relatively warm water can lead to hypothermia.

7. Reactions to bites and stings can be localized or generalized. Treatment of local reactions includes scraping away the stinger, if present, and removing jewelry and restrictive clothing from the affected area. Generalized reactions may include allergic reactions, which should be treated accordingly. Treatment of marine animal and snake envenomations should be guided by local protocol, as recommendations can change.

Multiple-Choice Answers

1. **(B)** (Objective 1)
   Heat is lost due to convection when air warmed by heat from the body is replaced with cooler air, causing the body to lose more heat to warm the air around it.

2. **(A)** (Objective 1)
   Losing body heat to cold, wet clothing is an example of conduction because of the body's direct contact with the clothing. If the skin was wet and heat was being lost as the water dried, this would be an example of evaporation.

3. **(D)** (Objective 2)
   Submersion hypothermia occurs in near-drowning incidents when the entire body, including the head, is under water. Immersion hypothermia occurs when the body is wet, but not under water.

4. **(B)** (Objective 3)
   The skin on the back of the hand is sensitive to changes in temperature and the abdomen is close to the core of the body.

5. **(D)** (Objective 3)
   Ice crystals can form in frozen tissues and damage adjacent tissues with rubbing or use of the extremity. No attempt at rewarming affected extremities is made in the prehospital setting except in extenuating circumstances.

6. **(A)** (Objective 3)
Superficial frostbite recovers quickly and is evidenced by tingling, maybe even a painful stinging sensation as the tissue warms and the nerve ends respond to the superficial soft tissue damage.

7. **(C)** (Objective 3)
Rewarming must be carried out under circumstances where the temperature of the water can be carefully controlled. Rewarming is extremely painful and should be delayed until the patient can receive pain medication, unless the transport time is so long that the risk of further damage is greater than the consideration for the patient's discomfort.

8. **(C)** (Objective 4)
Depending on the environment and degree of exertion, up to a liter of perspiration can be lost in an hour.

9. **(A)** (Objective 4)
First, heat cramps occur as dehydration and loss of salt cause muscle spasms. Second, with heat exhaustion, the patient becomes diaphoretic, pale, clammy, dizzy, and nauseated. Finally, in heat stroke, the body's heat-regulating mechanisms are overwhelmed and the body temperature rises. The patient loses consciousness and may have seizures. The skin will be red, hot, and dry at this point.

10. **(B)** (Objective 4)
These signs and symptoms are consistent with heat exhaustion. With heat stroke, the mental status is altered and the skin may be cool and clammy.

CHAPTER 18

Behavioral Emergencies

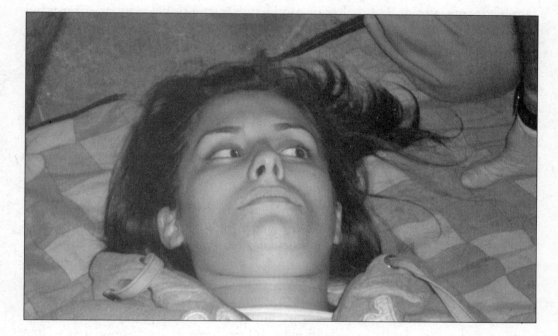

OBJECTIVES

This chapter and the review questions will help readers determine if they are able to

1. define behavioral emergencies;

2. discuss the general factors that may cause an alteration in the patient's behavior;

3. state the various reasons for psychological crises;

4. discuss the characteristics of an individual's behavior, which suggests that the patient is at risk for suicide;

5. discuss special medical/legal considerations for managing behavioral emergencies;

6. discuss the special considerations for assessing the patient with behavioral problems;

7. discuss the general principles of an individual's behavior that suggests that he or she is at risk for violence;

8. discuss methods to calm behavioral emergency patients.

BEHAVIOR

The manner in which a person acts or performs is behavior. A behavioral emergency is a situation where a person's behavior is unacceptable to the patient, family, or community. This behavior can be due to emotional extremes or psychological or physical conditions.

Factors that can cause changes in behavior include stresses, illness, psychiatric problems, or drugs. Low blood sugar, hypoxia, poor cerebral blood flow, head injuries, or environmental extremes of heat or cold can cause changes in behavior also.

Psychological crises include panic, agitation, bizarre thinking and behavior, danger to self and self-destructive behavior, suicide, danger to others, threatening behavior, and violence.

Assessing for suicide risk includes recognizing depression, such as sad, tearful people with thoughts of death or taking one's own life. Risk factors for suicidal gestures include individuals over 40, single, widowed, or divorced, and alcoholic or depressed. A defined lethal plan of action may have been verbalized. There may be signs of an unusual gathering of articles that can cause death like guns, pills, and so on. Look for a previous history of suicidal attempts, recent diagnosis of serious illness, loss of a loved one, arrest, or job loss. Look for patients in unsafe surroundings, exhibiting self-destructive behavior.

The EMT should size up the scene, determine safety, and perform a patient assessment. Calm the patient and do not leave him or her alone. These patients must be restrained if necessary. Police should help and can provide legal support as well as physical support. If drugs or poisons are used, bring them along to the hospital.

Remember that if you are treating and transporting against a disturbed patient's will, you must be able to describe the risk to the patient or others. When in doubt seek advice from medical control. It is also important to document accurately your assessments and justifications for your treatment.

Communication is important when dealing with disturbed patients. Identify yourself and show a willingness to listen and help. Use a calm reassuring voice. Do not judge but accept what the patient tells you without scolding. You can show that you are listening by rephrasing what the patient says. Acknowledge the patient's feelings and assess his or her mental status by assessing appearance, speech, activity, and orientation to time, person, and place.

Scenario 1

You are called to attend to a suicidal patient. What is your first concern?

SOLUTION

Determining scene safety. If police are not yet on the scene, you should stage at a safe distance until the scene has been made safe.

Scenario 2

In addressing the patient, what can you do in your approach to help set the patient at ease and gain his or her trust?

SOLUTION

Maintain a passive stance, palms open, and face forward at a safe distance out of the patient's personal space. Speak slowly and in a calm, reassuring voice, listen carefully to the patient, and rephrase what he or she says occasionally to show that you are listening.

Scenario 3

If the patient is unwilling to go to the hospital, can you allow a suicidal patient to refuse care?

SOLUTION

This is one of the few situations where restraining the patient is advisable. With the advice and consent of medical control and the assistance of police, the patient should be restrained and transported even if against his or her will.

Review Questions

EXERCISES

The exercises in this review are designed to help reinforce your knowledge of the objectives for this chapter. If you find it difficult to meet any of the objectives stated, go back and review those materials again.

1. Define behavior. (Objective 1)

   _____

   _____

2. Define a behavioral emergency. (Objective 1)

   _____

   _____

3. What are three general factors that may predispose a patient to a behavioral emergency? (Objective 2)

   _____

   _____

4. Within the three general factors you listed in Question 3, what are some specific reasons for behavioral emergencies? (Objective 3)

   _____

   _____

5. You are on the scene of a patient whose spouse called because she fears her husband may be suicidal. During your history and assessment, what would increase your index of suspicion that the spouse is correct? (Objective 4)

   _____

   _____

   _____

   _____

6. In order to transport a patient with a behavioral emergency against his or her will, you must be able to document that he or she is a risk to _____ or _____ . (Objective 5)

7. Describe how you can assess the mental status of an individual with a behavioral emergency. (Objective 6)

_____

_____

8. You and your partner, an experienced EMT, are responding to a call for a behavioral emergency. Your partner asks you to explain how you would assess the risk of violent behavior. How do you respond? (Objective 7)

_____

_____

9. Your patient is a 32-year-old female who is very distraught and threatening to jump from a bridge. How should you attempt to calm the patient? (Objective 8)

_____

_____

MULTIPLE-CHOICE QUESTIONS

1. You are on the scene of a motor vehicle collision. Your patient, a 50-year-old male, is out of the vehicle and sitting on the ground. When you approach him he throws a rock at you and screams that you better not get near him. Which of the following should you assume to be cause of the patient's behavior?
   (A) psychiatric illness
   (B) hypoxia
   (C) hypoglycemia
   (D) all of the above

2. Which of the following is a risk factor for suicide?
   (A) being divorced
   (B) being female
   (C) having a large family
   (D) age 30 or younger

3. Which of the following principles should be used when managing a disturbed patient?
    (A) Let the patient know you want to help.
    (B) Ensure that law enforcement has restrained the patient before speaking to him or her.
    (C) Only say what is necessary to conduct your physical exam.
    (D) Tell the patient you know how he or she feels.

4. Which of the following is the correct response to a disturbed patient's hallucinatory thoughts?
    (A) "You are experiencing hallucinations because you are mentally ill."
    (B) Go along with the hallucination to comfort the patient.
    (C) Rephrase what the patient has said in your own words to show you are listening.
    (D) Point out that it is not possible to see or hear what the patient says he or she is seeing or hearing.

5. Which of the following applies when seeking consent for treatment of a disturbed patient?
    (A) Consent is not necessary for patients with a behavioral emergency.
    (B) Consent is only necessary if you must restrain the patient.
    (C) Consent is preferred, but implied consent may be used if the patient is a threat to himself, herself, or others.
    (D) There is nothing you can do if the patient refuses treatment and transport.

6. Which of the following situations is most clearly a behavioral emergency?
    (A) A woman calls for an ambulance to take her son to a drug rehabilitation program because he smokes marijuana.
    (B) A man calls 911 because his mother, who has Alzheimer's disease, is wandering through the house late at night disturbing other family members and is uncooperative.
    (C) A patient with a history of depression calls for an ambulance because she has a severe headache.
    (D) Any call for a patient with a history of a mental illness is considered a behavioral emergency.

7. Which of the following is an indication that violent behavior may occur?
    (A) yelling or screaming
    (B) use of profanity
    (C) clenched fists
    (D) all of the above

8. You have been called to an office building for a person "acting strangely." According to coworkers the 40-year-old woman seemed confused and "shaky," looked pale, and then began sweating profusely. On your arrival the patient is swearing and uncooperative with a coworker who is trying to get her to sit down. The coworkers state that this is very uncharacteristic of the woman, with whom they have worked for 12 years. Which of the following should be determined first?
   (A) Ask whether the patient has a history of diabetes.
   (B) Ask if the patient has a history of depression.
   (C) See if something has happened to upset the patient.
   (D) Ask if the patient has threatened to hurt herself or anyone else.

9. Your patient's family feels he may be at risk for suicide. Which of the following would increase this risk?
   (A) The patient has been charged with burglary and is awaiting trial.
   (B) The patient's girlfriend broke up with him.
   (C) The patient has previously attempted suicide.
   (D) All of the above.

10. Distrust, jealousy, seclusiveness, and hostile, uncooperative behavior are all indications that your patient suffers from
   (A) anxiety.
   (B) depression.
   (C) phobias.
   (D) paranoia.

ANSWERS TO REVIEW QUESTIONS

Exercises

1. The manner in which a person acts or performs is behavior.

2. A situation where a person's behavior is unacceptable to the patient, family, or community.

3. Emotional extremes or psychological or physical conditions.

4. Stresses, illness, psychiatric problems, drugs, low blood sugar (hypoglycemia), hypoxia, poor cerebral blood flow, head injuries, or environmental extremes of heat or cold.

5. Depression, sadness, tearfulness, thoughts of death or suicide; the patient is over 40, single, widowed, or divorced, alcoholic or has a history of depression; a lethal plan of action, gathering of articles that can cause death like guns, pills, and so on; history of suicide attempts, recent diagnosis of serious illness, loss of a loved one, arrest or job loss.

6. In order to transport a patient with a behavioral emergency against his or her will, you must be able to document that he or she is a risk to **himself/herself** or **others**.

7. Mental status can be assessed by noting the patient's appearance, speech, activity, and orientation to time, person, and place.

8. Indications of impending violence include agitated behavior, pacing, clenched fists, self-destructive behavior, destruction of property, yelling, threats, profanity, and possession of a weapon.

9. Identify yourself, be willing to listen, and state you would like to help. Use a calm, reassuring voice, accept what the patient tells you without being judgmental, and acknowledge the patient's feelings.

Multiple-Choice Answers

1. **(D)** Objective 2
   Any of the responses listed could be a cause of the patient's behavior. He could have a preexisting psychiatric condition that either caused the collision (e.g., attempted suicide) or was aggravated by the situation. The patient may have a medical condition that led to hypoxia and perhaps caused the collision, or he could be a diabetic and hypoglycemia could have caused the collision. Additionally, he could have suffered an injury in the collision that is causing hypoxia. Whatever the cause, after ensuring your own safety, first assess for and treat potentially life-threatening causes, such as hypoxia and hypoglycemia.

2. **(A)** Objective 4
   Of the choices given, only being divorced is a factor that increases the risk of suicide. However, given the right circumstances, anyone can be at risk for suicide. It should not be assumed that the patient without known risk factors will not commit suicide.

3. **(A)** Objective 5
   It is critical to identify yourself, be willing to listen to and communicate with the patient, and let him or her know you would like to help. However, it is not advisable to tell the patient you know how he or she feels. As far as the patient is concerned, he or she may feel that no one understands how he feels and to say so will damage your credibility with the patient.

4. **(C)** Objective 6
   While you should not go along with the patient's hallucination, you should demonstrate that you are listening to what he or she says is going on. Telling the patient he or she is mentally ill will not help. Do not tell the patient he or she cannot be experiencing the hallucination. The hallucination is actually occurring. Finally, the patient with a history of mental illness may be quite aware that what he or she is experiencing does not exist outside his or her own mind, and attempting to go along with the hallucination will damage your credibility with the patient, who needs to be able to trust you.

5. **(C)** Objective 6

Remember, consent laws and medical direction regarding the treatment of disturbed patients can vary according to your location and employer. However, in general, consent always applies, even if it is implied consent for persons incompetent to give expressed consent. Whenever possible, it is preferable to have the patient's expressed consent. If the patient refuses care and is not obviously incompetent to do so, involve medical control, the patient's family, and if necessary, law enforcement.

6. **(B)** Objective 1

Just because someone disagrees with the behavior of another (e.g., using drugs) does not mean there is a behavioral emergency. If the patient is not a threat to himself, herself, or others, or otherwise interfering with the rights of others or experiencing psychological distress, it is not a behavioral emergency. The patient with Alzheimer's disease is causing a disruption of the household and is not cooperative. Finally, the term "mental illness" technically applies to a wide variety of disorders from anxiety to depression to personality disorders and schizophrenia. Many of these disorders are well controlled with medication and therapy. Merely having a history of mental illness does not constitute a behavioral emergency.

7. **(D)** Objective 7

The more agitated the patient's behavior, the more you should anticipate violent behavior. Being loud, pacing, clenching the fists, making threats, using profanity, destroying property, and engaging in self-destructive behavior are all indications of impending violence.

8. **(A)** Objective 2

Although all are valid questions, you must first determine if there are any immediately life-threatening causes of the patient's sudden change in behavior, such as hypoglycemia—which you can treat.

9. **(D)** Objective 4

The history of recent arrest, loss of a relationship, and previous attempts at suicide would all increase the patient's risk for suicide.

10. **(D)** Objective 3

Distrust, jealousy, and seclusive, hostile, uncooperative behavior all characterize paranoia, but are not characteristic of the other conditions listed.

Obstetrics/Gynecology

 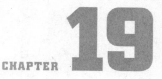

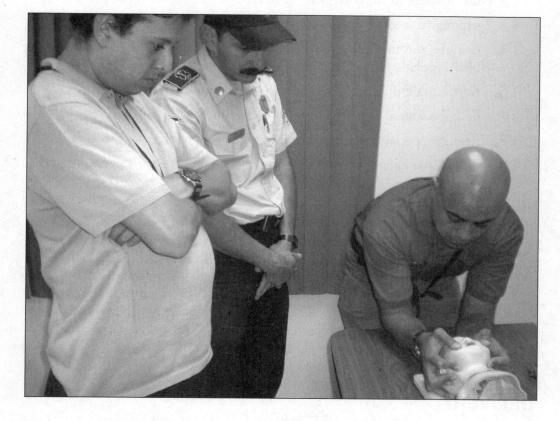

OBJECTIVES

This chapter and the review questions will help readers determine if they are able to

1. identify the following structures: uterus, vagina, fetus, placenta, umbilical cord, amniotic sac, and perineum;

2. identify and explain the use of the contents of an obstetric kit;

3. identify predelivery emergencies;

4. state indications of an imminent delivery;

5. differentiate the emergency medical care provided to the patient with predelivery emergencies from a normal delivery;

6. state the steps in the predelivery preparation of the mother;

7. establish the relationship between BSI and childbirth;

8. state the steps to assist in the delivery;

9. describe care of the baby as the head appears;

10. describe how and when to cut the umbilical cord;

11. discuss the steps in the delivery of the placenta;

12. list the steps in the emergency medical care of the mother post-delivery;

13. summarize neonatal resuscitation procedures;

14. describe the procedures for the following abnormal deliveries: breach birth, prolapsed cord, and limb presentation;

15. differentiate the special considerations for multiple births;

16. describe special considerations of meconium;

17. describe special considerations of a premature baby;

18. discuss the emergency medical care of the patient with a gynecological emergency.

ANATOMY

The fetus grows in the **uterus**, getting its life-giving nutrients through the umbilical cord from the **placenta**. To be born, it must move down the birth canal. When the child is born, emerging from the vagina, it may be covered by the **amniotic sac** that protected it while in the uterus. Deliveries can expose the EMT to lots of blood and body fluids, so gloves, eye protection, a mask, and even a gown should be worn to protect from the fluids.

DELIVERY

As the baby's head emerges, the face should be cleaned and the airway suctioned before the baby breathes and inhales fluids and debris that came out with it. When the rest of the baby is delivered, hold the baby below the vaginal opening to prevent blood from the baby from flowing back into the placenta, which has probably detached from the uterine wall. After drying and warming the baby, and the cord stops pulsating, the cord should be clamped four finger widths from the infant and again a couple of inches beyond that. The cord can be cut between the clamps. Wrap the baby in dry towels and allow the mother to hold the baby to her chest. The baby may be able to hear her heartbeat, which can soothe the baby. If the baby suckles to the mother's breast, it may assist in creating contractions that will control bleeding in the mother and deliver the placenta. If the placenta delivers, wrap it in a towel and bring it to the hospital. If it does not deliver within a few minutes, transport.

Complications

✔ If the baby is breech and the head is undelivered, insert a gloved hand into the vaginal opening and create an airway in case the baby tries to breathe before the head is delivered. Be prepared as inserting your hand may stimulate a contraction to expel the baby the rest of the way out.

✔ If an arm or a leg presents first, the baby cannot be delivered in the field and you should elevate the mother's hips and expedite transport.

✔ The APGAR score is a method of determining the baby's condition. It should be done at 1 minute and 5 minutes in the field and it will be repeated at the hospital to determine the infant's development after birth. A number is assigned for each of five assessments.

Sign	0	1	2
Appearance Skin color	Blue, Pale	Normal body,* Blue Extremities	Normal*
Pulse (Heart) Rate	Absent	<100 per minute	>100 per minute
Grimace Irritability	No Response	Grimace	Cough, Sneeze, Cry
Activity Muscle tone	Limp	Some Flexion	Active Motion
Respirations Respiratory Effort	Absent	Slow, Irregular	Good, Crying

*Based on race.

If the baby does not breathe spontaneously, open and clear the airway and begin artificial ventilations. After 30 seconds, reassess. If the baby's heart rate is less than 100, continue ventilations; if it is less than 60, begin compressions. Reassess and adjust resuscitation every 30 seconds.

Some bleeding is normal after delivery. Up to 500 mL is common without creating a danger to the mother. Fundal massage (massaging the abdomen over the uterus) and allowing the baby to suckle at the mother's breast can encourage uterine contraction to control bleeding from the mother. Loose dressing can be applied to the vaginal opening but the EMT should never attempt to pack dressing into the vagina.

A prolapsed cord is another situation that you cannot deliver in the field. Insert a gloved hand to keep the baby's head from pressing on the cord, elevate the mother's hips, and transport.

Gynecological emergencies with bleeding from trauma or internal problems can present with significant bleeding. The EMT should never pack the vagina but place dressings over the vagina and transport. Consider the need for psychological care in assault patients and use female technicians when possible and be reassuring and considerate when it is not possible.

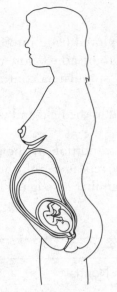

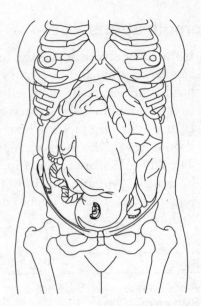

In the normal position, the fetus will lie head down in the uterus.

Even with normal presentations, complication can result from the position of the umbilical cord during the birth process.

Scenario 1

You are called to assist a 22-year-old female with abdominal pain in the pelvis area. On exam you notice that she is crowning. What should the EMT do at this point?

SOLUTION

Address BSI and prepare for the birth of the baby.

Scenario 2

After preparing for the birth of the baby you notice that the cord is prolapsed. What should the EMT do at this point?

SOLUTION

Elevate the mother's hips and transport. You cannot deliver a prolapsed cord birth in the field.

Scenario 3

You cleared the baby's airway, dried and rewarmed the baby, and the heart rate is less than 100. What should you do next?

SOLUTION

Begin artificial respirations and recheck the heart rate in 30 seconds.

Review Questions

EXERCISES

The exercises in this review are designed to help reinforce your knowledge of the objectives for this chapter. If you find it difficult to meet any of the objectives stated, go back and review those materials again.

1. Identify predelivery emergencies and complete the table below. (Objective 3)

	Placenta Previa	Abruptio Placentae	Eclampsia
Description of the Problem			
Signs and Symptoms			
Treatment			

2. What signs and symptoms indicate that you should immediately prepare to assist with delivery? (Objective 4)

_____

_____

_____

_____

3. You have examined your patient, a 25-year-old pregnant female, and you believe that delivery is imminent. Describe how you will prepare the patient for delivery, how you will manage each step of the delivery, and how you will care for the mother after delivery. (Objectives 5–12)

Preparing the patient for delivery:

_____

_____

_____

_____

Managing the delivery:

_____

_____

_____

_____

Post-delivery care of the mother:

_____

_____

_____

_____

4. You just delivered an infant who is not crying, has cyanosis of the body, and is limp. He has a brachial pulse of 92. Explain what you will do to manage this situation. (Objective 13)

_____

_____

_____

_____

5. How would you manage each of the following situations? (Objective 14)

During a delivery you notice that the buttocks are the presenting part:

_____

_____

_____

_____

While checking for crowning, you notice that the umbilical cord is the presenting part:

_____

_____

_____

_____

During a delivery you notice that an arm is the presenting part:

_____

_____

_____

_____

6. Explain how the care of infants from a multiple birth differs from that of a single infant. (Objective 15)

_____

_____

7. Upon delivery of an infant, the amniotic sac ruptures and the escaping fluid is stained with dark green material. How should you prepare to handle the situation? (Objective 16)

_____

_____

8. What are the primary concerns in caring for a preterm newborn? (Objective 17)

_____

_____

9. What are the primary concerns in the general care of a patient with a gyne-cological emergency? (Objective 18)

_____

_____

MULTIPLE-CHOICE QUESTIONS

1. Which of the following structures is the site of development of the fetus throughout pregnancy?
   (A) placenta
   (B) uterus
   (C) ovary
   (D) fallopian tube

2. The skin between the vagina and the anus that may tear during delivery is the
   (A) urethra.
   (B) perineum.
   (C) vulva.
   (D) cervix.

3. If an infant is crowning but undelivered after 10 minutes
   (A) gently stretch the vaginal opening to facilitate delivery.
   (B) insert your gloved hands on either side of the infant's head and apply gentle traction to facilitate delivery.
   (C) transport the mother to the hospital without further delay, but do not attempt to manually facilitate delivery.
   (D) wait up to an additional 10 minutes before taking any action.

4. Which of the following best describes the proper way to clamp and cut the umbilical cord?
   (A) Place a clamp as close to the baby's abdomen as possible and cut the cord on the side of the clamp closest to the mother.
   (B) Place a clamp as close to the placenta as possible and cut the cord on the side of the clamp closest to the baby.
   (C) Place a clamp about four finger widths from the baby; place a second clamp about 2 inches closer to the mother and cut the cord between the clamps.
   (D) Place a clamp as close to the baby's abdomen as possible, place a second clamp 6 to 8 inches closer to the mother, and cut the cord between the clamps.

5. Bleeding of up to_____is normal following delivery.
   (A) 100 mL
   (B) 500 mL
   (C) 1,000 mL
   (D) 1,500 mL

6. You just delivered an infant in the field. You notice the mother has brisk vaginal bleeding. All of the following are recommended ways of managing this problem EXCEPT
   (A) packing the vagina with gauze.
   (B) massaging the uterus.
   (C) placing a sanitary napkin over the perineal (vaginal) area.
   (D) encouraging the mother to nurse the infant.

7. One minute after the complete delivery of an infant, his fingers and toes are bluish in color, the heart rate is 140, his arms and legs are flexed, and he is crying. The APGAR score is
   (A) 7.
   (B) 8.
   (C) 9.
   (D) 10.

8. Resuscitative measures should be implemented if a newborn's heart rate is less than
   (A) 60.
   (B) 70.
   (C) 80.
   (D) 100.

9. When resuscitating a newborn, heart rate should be reassessed every
   (A) 5 minutes.
   (B) 2 minutes.
   (C) minute.
   (D) 30 seconds.

10. Which of the following best explains the significance of greenish colored amniotic fluid?
    (A) It is atypical, but nothing to worry about.
    (B) The infant requires aggressive suctioning as soon as the head is delivered.
    (C) The fetus died during the last trimester and the mother must be advised of this.
    (D) It is an indication of abruption placentae.

ANSWERS TO REVIEW QUESTIONS
Exercises

1.

	Placenta Previa	Abruptio Placentae	Eclampsia
Description of the Problem	The placenta is implanted partially or completely over the cervix and begins to separate prematurely from the uterine wall as the cervix dilates during labor.	The placenta may be implanted in a normal location, but completely or partially detaches from the uterine wall during the last trimester of pregnancy.	A disorder of pregnancy diagnosed with the onset of seizures in a pregnant woman with a history of a hypertensive disorder of pregnancy.
Signs and Symptoms	Typically painless, bright red bleeding. Shock may occur.	May be induced by trauma or physiological stress, often painful; bleeding may be internal. Shock may occur.	Signaled by the onset of seizures. Prior history of vision disturbances, hypertension, edema (swelling) of the hands, face, and feet, and protein in the urine.
Treatment	Ensure an adequate airway, ventilations, and oxygenation. Place the mother on her left side for transport. Transport without delay. Call for ALS intercept if transport time is long.	Ensure an adequate airway, ventilations, and oxygenation. Place the mother on her left side for transport. Transport without delay. Call for ALS intercept if transport time is long.	Manage the patient for seizure. Protect the airway, ensure adequate ventilation, apply high-flow oxygen by nonrebreather mask, dim the lights, prevent agitation, and place the mother on her left side for transport. Transport without delay. Call for ALS intercept if transport time is long.

2. Typically, the contractions are very strong and close together; upon questioning, the mother may state that she feels the need to move her bowels; the amniotic sac may or may not have broken; upon inspection, the perineum may be bulging; or the infant's scalp may be visible at the vaginal opening during contractions.

3. **Preparing the patient for delivery:** The patient should be placed supine with support under the shoulders, garments covering the lower half of the body should be removed, a folded towel is placed under the buttocks to elevate them slightly, the thighs and knees are flexed, and the feet are apart. If time permits, the lower abdomen and thighs are draped.

   Managing the delivery: The EMT must wear gloves, gown, face mask, and eye protection. A gloved hand is used to place gentle pressure over the vaginal opening to control the head as it is delivered. The mouth and then nose are suctioned with a bulb syringe. The head is supported and gently guided downward to facilitate delivery of the upper shoulder, then gently guided upward to facilitate delivery of the lower shoulder. The body is supported as the delivery is completed. The baby is kept at the level of the vagina until the cord stops pulsating. It is then clamped and cut. The infant is dried and wrapped in a blanket. The APGAR score is assessed at 1 and 5 minutes after the complete delivery. If resuscitation of the mother or infant is not required, the baby, wrapped in a blanket, is given to the mother. Perform ongoing assessment.

   Post-delivery care of the mother: Typically, the placenta will deliver on its own within 30 minutes of the delivery. It is not necessary to wait on the scene for the placenta to deliver. Never apply traction to the umbilical cord to hasten delivery of the placenta. If there is more than 500 mL (16 oz or 2 cups) of bleeding following delivery, the uterus is massaged, applying firm pressure with the side of one hand just above the pubic bone to support the uterus. Use the fingertips of the other hand to locate and massage the top (fundus) of the uterus, which is located at about the level of the umbilicus. Cover the vaginal area with a sanitary napkin, lower the mother's legs, and prepare for transport. Perform ongoing assessment.

4. Most infants will respond to tactile stimulation, such as rubbing the back, drying, and warming. If the infant's condition does not improve, oxygen is administered by "blow-by." If this is not effective, ventilations are assisted by bag-valve mask. Finally, if these measures have failed to improve the infant's condition and the heart rate drops below 60, chest compressions are started.

5. **During a delivery you notice that the buttocks are the presenting part:** Some breech presentations will deliver spontaneously in the field, but in some cases the head cannot deliver spontaneously. This situation is not corrected by the EMT in the field. The mother is placed in knee-chest position, or with pillows elevating the hips in a supine position, oxygen is applied to the mother, and transport is begun without delay. If the body has delivered, but the head has not, the EMT should place two fingers in a "V" shape around

the infant's nose to push the vaginal wall away from the face and create an airway in case the infant begins breathing before delivery is complete. If possible, ALS intercept should be requested.

While checking for crowning, you notice that the umbilical cord is the presenting part: This is the only instance in which the EMT attempts to restrict delivery by placing the mother in knee-chest position or elevating the hips in supine position, and placing a gloved hand in the vagina to keep the infant's head from compressing the umbilical cord. The protruding cord should be covered with a sterile saline dressing, oxygen is applied to the mother, and transport is begun without delay. If possible, ALS intercept should be requested.

During a delivery you notice that an arm is the presenting part: This situation cannot be managed in the field. The mother is placed in knee-chest position, or with pillows elevating the hips in a supine position, oxygen is applied to the mother, and transport is begun without delay. If possible, ALS intercept should be requested.

6. The primary difference is that infants from multiple gestation are smaller, and less able to preserve body heat. They may also be premature and have difficulty breathing.

7. The EMT must be prepared to aggressively suction the mouth and nose as the head emerges, before the infant takes a breath.

8. Preterm infants are less able to conserve body heat and must be kept warm. The are also prone to respiratory problems and may need ventilatory support.

9. The primary concerns are anticipating and treating for shock, protecting the patient's privacy, and transporting to the hospital for care.

Multiple-Choice Answers

1. **(B)** Objective 1
The uterus, or womb, is where the fetus develops throughout pregnancy. The placenta is a temporary organ of pregnancy that is attached to the uterine wall and to the infant, via the umbilical cord. The ovary releases eggs, which are transported to the uterus by the fallopian tube.

2. **(B)** Objective 1
The perineum is the region between the genitals and anus. The urethra is the passageway for urine to be emptied from the bladder; the vulva is the external female genitalia; and the cervix is the lower end of the uterus.

3. **(C)** Objective 4
This situation cannot be managed in the field.

4. **(C)** Objective 10

The cord must be clamped far enough away from the baby to allow for reclamping if bleeding should occur from the cut end. The cord must be clamped in two places to prevent bleeding from both ends.

5. **(B)** Objective 11

Bleeding over 500 mL in the period immediately following delivery is considered excessive.

6. **(A)** Objective 11

Both massaging the uterus and allowing the infant to nurse will cause the uterus to contract and minimize bleeding. A sanitary napkin over the perineum is sufficient for most bleeding. Gentle pressure can be applied over the sanitary napkin to control external bleeding from perineal tears. The EMT never places dressing material into the vaginal opening.

7. **(C)** Objective 13

Each item on the APGAR scale is worth 0, 1, or 2 points, for a total of up to 10 points. In this case, the infant only loses 1 point for appearance, due to the cyanosis of the fingers and toes, which is typical immediately following birth.

8. **(A)** Objective 13

In most cases, drying and warming the infant are effective resuscitation measures. However, if the infant's respirations are inadequate, the central part of the body is cyanotic, or the heart rate is less than 100, then oxygen is administered and ventilations are begun, if tactile stimulation and oxygen are not immediately effective. If the heart rate is below 60, chest compressions are begun.

9. **(D)** Objective 13

Infants may improve rapidly and should be assessed every 15 to 30 seconds.

10. **(B)** Objective 16

Greenish-black or greenish-brown discoloration of the amniotic fluid indicates the presence of meconium, the infant's first bowel movement, which may occur before birth in response to physiological stress. If the infant breathes in the meconium, it can lead to respiratory distress and pneumonia.

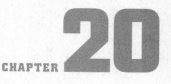
Bleeding and Shock

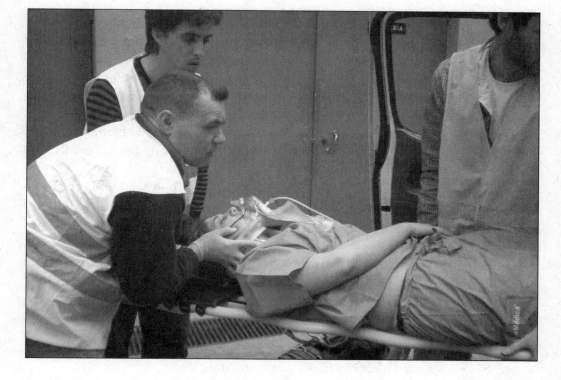

OBJECTIVES

This chapter and the review questions will help readers determine if they are able to

1. list the structures and functions of the circulatory system;

2. differentiate between arterial, venous, and capillary bleeding;

3. state methods of emergency medical care of external bleeding;

4. establish the relationship between BSI and bleeding;

5. establish the relationship between airway management and the trauma patient;

6. establish the relationship between mechanism of injury and internal bleeding;

7. list the signs of internal bleeding;

8. list the steps in the emergency medical care of the patient with signs and symptoms of internal bleeding;

9. list signs and symptoms of shock (hyperperfusion);

10. state the steps in the emergency medical care of the patient with signs and symptoms of shock (hypoperfusion).

THE CIRCULATORY SYSTEM

The circulatory system consists of the heart, which pumps blood into the arteries and out to the capillaries where oxygen and nutrients are exchanged for carbon dioxide and waste. The blood then returns through the veins to the heart where it is pumped to the lungs. In the lungs the carbon dioxide is exchanged for oxygen between the capillaries and alveoli in the lungs.

The EMT must protect himself or herself from exposure to blood and body fluids by practicing BSI. This includes gloves, eye protection, gowns, masks, and hand washing between patient contacts.

The sudden loss of a liter of blood in the adult, 500 cc in the child, or 100 to 200 cc in an infant constitutes serious bleeding. The patient's signs and symptoms will illustrate the severity of the blood loss.

BLEEDING

While clotting is the body's natural response to minimize bleeding, serious injury may prevent clotting from being effective. Uncontrolled bleeding leads to hypoperfusion or shock and death.

✔ *Arterial bleeding* is bright red in color (oxygen) and spurts or pulses.
✔ *Venous bleeding* is darker red (low in oxygen) and flows.
✔ *Capillary bleeding* is dark red and oozing.

EMTs must take full precautions for exposure to blood when approaching patients with external bleeding. Bleeding is primarily controlled by the application of direct pressure and the application of a pressure dressing. In the past, training included the use of elevation and pressure points to assist in slowing the bleeding, but there is no evidence that this is helpful and it is no longer recommended.

Bleeding in the face and head is a special problem. The EMT should not attempt to stop the flow of blood from the ears or nose if it is the result of trauma. Loose dressings should collect the blood. To treat nosebleeds place the patient in a sitting position leaning slightly forward. Apply pressure by pinching the fleshy portion of the nostrils together.

Internal bleeding can result in hidden, severe, and deadly blood loss from large blood vessels or internal organs. Knowledge of the mechanism of injury or illness along with the patient's signs and symptoms are the clues to internal bleeding. Pain, tenderness, swelling, discoloration, bleeding from the mouth, rectum, or vagina, vomiting bright red or coffee-ground-colored blood, dark, tarry, or bright flecked stools, and tender or rigid abdomen are all signs of possible internal bleeding. Early on in the bleeding patient, nervousness or agitation may reflect developing hypoxia. As the condition worsens the mental status worsens. As the bleeding continues or worsens, the patient's condition deteriorates and the vital signs begin to reflect that. Pale, cool, and clammy skin, rapid breathing and heart rate, and ultimately a falling blood pressure and shock will result. In infants and children capillary refill of greater than 2 seconds is also a sign of developing shock.

In some cases of internal bleeding, as in bleeds below the diaphragm in the abdomen and pelvis, the pneumatic antishock garment (PASG) may be indicated to limit the bleeding.

Tourniquets

While in the past tourniquets have been used as a last resort, recent studies have shown them to be effective and not the risk they were previously thought to be. They are recommended in situations in which direct pressure is impossible or ineffective. There are tourniquets available for purchase from medical suppliers, but they can be made up with common materials as well. Tourniquets should be at least 4 inches wide and wrapped around the extremity twice proximal to the bleeding site, but as close to the wound as possible. Tie a knot in the bandage being used as a tourniquet, place a stick over the knot and tie a knot over the stick. Turn the stick until the bleeding stops and secure the stick in place. Leaving a blood pressure cuff inflated in place may also work as a tourniquet until bleeding stops. Once in place a tourniquet should not be removed and the EMT must be certain to alert medical staff as to its location.

Note

As this book is going to print, the standards on bleeding control are changing slightly. New trauma guidelines have suggested eliminating elevation and pressure point from bleeding control as there is no evidence that they are effective. The new standard is direct pressure, pressure dressing, and if necessary, tourniquet. As we are writing this, the National Registry exams and many state exams still call for elevation and pressure points, so before you test, find out from your instructor or the testing agency as to whether the exam has been updated to the new guidelines.

Scenario 1

You are called to the scene of a stabbing. After staging until the scene is made safe, you ensure BSI and approach the patient and find that bright red blood is spurting from a wound in his right upper arm. How will you manage this patient?

SOLUTION

After ensuring that there are no other serious life threats, the EMT should apply direct pressure to the wound followed by a pressure dressing. Before and after placing the dressing, pulses and sensations below the dressing should be checked. Before transport, splinting the arm will limit the possibility of the dressing coming loose and increased bleeding.

Scenario 2

You are called to the scene to evaluate a patient who was struck in the abdomen by a 55-gallon drum. After determining that the scene is safe and donning PPE you find a drowsy man with cold, clammy skin, rapid pulse and respirations, clutching his abdomen. What do you think is going on here and what will you do for this patient?

SOLUTION

Your initial evaluation should tell you that this patient is in critical condition and expedited transport is a goal of your treatment. The skin condition, altered mental status, and rapid heart and respiratory rate all indicate hypoperfusion and developing shock. You need to do a quick trauma assessment and get this patient to the hospital as quickly as possible.

Scenario 3

Your focused rapid trauma assessment shows a rigid tender abdomen with abrasions from the 55-gallon drum. The patient is only responding to pain now. What will you do in preparing this patient for transport?

SOLUTION

Provide 15 liters of oxygen via a nonrebreather and monitor airway and ventilations as your first priority. Place the patient on a trauma board and secure him to prevent further injury and worsening the bleed. You may also use the PASG to manage the internal bleeding.

Review Questions

EXERCISES

The exercises in this review are designed to help reinforce your knowledge of the objectives for this chapter. If you find it difficult to meet any of the objectives stated, go back and review those materials again.

1. Your patient is a 14-year-old boy whose arm went through the glass of a storm door. He has a large laceration on the inside (medial aspect) of his right upper arm. Describe the bleeding you would expect to find if each of the following types of vessels were injured. (Objective 2)

   Arterial: _____

   Venous: _____

   Capillary: _____

2. Your patient is a 10-year-old boy who was mauled by a large dog. He has a wound on the inside of his right thigh with profuse bleeding. Explain, in order, the steps that are taken to control this type of bleeding. (Objective 3)

_____

_____

_____

_____

3. Explain the importance of good airway management in the patient with significant trauma. (Objective 5)

_____

_____

_____

_____

4. List at least four mechanisms of injury that place the patient at risk for internal injury and bleeding. (Objective 6)

_____

_____

_____

5. Your patient is a 25-year-old female who was thrown from, and then stepped on, by a horse. She has minor abrasions, but no significant external bleeding. First, describe what you will specifically look for in your assessment to determine if there is internal bleeding. Then, describe how you will treat the patient if you suspected internal bleeding and shock. (Objectives 7–10)

_____

_____

_____

_____

_____

MULTIPLE-CHOICE QUESTIONS

1. In an adult patient, the loss of _____ of blood is considered serious.
   (A) 500 mL
   (B) 1,000 mL
   (C) 1,500 mL
   (D) 2,000 mL

2. True or False: Your patient has fallen about 15 feet from a ladder to the ground. He is awake and alert, complaining of pain in his left thigh. His pulse is 88, respirations are 18, and blood pressure is 128/88. Therefore, you can rule out the possibility of internal bleeding and shock.
   (A) True
   (B) False

3. True or False: Your patient is an 8-year-old female who was accidentally stabbed in the thigh by her brother. You estimate she has lost 2 cups of blood. This amount of bleeding is of no concern in a child this age.
   (A) True
   (B) False

4. The primary method of bleeding control is
   (A) tourniquet.
   (B) pressure point.
   (C) direct pressure.
   (D) application of ice.

5. Which of the following statements concerning tourniquets is true?
   (A) EMTs are never permitted to use tourniquets.
   (B) Tourniquets are generally contraindicated for bleeding below (distal to) the knee or elbow.
   (C) Tourniquets are now favored as the first method of bleeding control for all arterial bleeding.
   (D) Tourniquets must never be used with penetrating trauma.

6. Your patient is a 19-year-old male who was beaten with a metal pipe. He is unresponsive, but you are managing his airway. He has bleeding from his right ear canal. Which of the following is an acceptable method of managing bleeding from this patient's ear?
   (A) Lightly cover the ear with an absorbent dressing.
   (B) Pack gauze into the ear.
   (C) Allow the ear to drain freely without covering it.
   (D) Cover the ear with an occlusive dressing, such as petroleum gauze.

7. Which of the following is typically the earliest indication of shock (hypoperfusion) due to blood loss?
   (A) nervousness and agitation
   (B) loss of consciousness
   (C) drop in blood pressure
   (D) slow pulse rate

8. Which of the following signs would you expect to see in a patient with ongoing blood loss?
   (A) increased heart rate
   (B) increased respiratory rate
   (C) cool, pale skin
   (D) all of the above

9. True or False: A falling blood pressure is one of the earliest signs of shock (hypoperfusion).
   (A) True
   (B) False

10. In which of the following age groups is capillary refill time most useful as an indicator of impaired perfusion, or shock?
   (A) young adults and the elderly
   (B) children and young adults
   (C) infants and children
   (D) all of the above

ANSWERS TO REVIEW QUESTIONS

Exercises

1. **Arterial:** bright red in color, spurts from the wound with each pulse wave through the artery.

   Venous: darker red in color, bleeding may be profuse, but does not spurt from the wound.

   Capillary: Between arterial and venous blood in color, oozes from the wound.

2. The first step, after ensuring scene safety, an open airway, and adequate breathing, is to immediately apply direct pressure to the wound. If this is not effective, the right lower extremity should be elevated. If necessary, pressure should be applied to the femoral artery in the groin. Finally, if earlier steps fail to control bleeding, a tourniquet should be applied above the wound.

3. Many mechanisms of injury may result in a compromised airway due to facial injury, bleeding, vomiting, or decreased level of consciousness. Without an open airway, it is not possible to achieve adequate breathing or ventilation, in order to supply the lungs with adequate oxygen and allow for elimination of carbon dioxide.

4. Falls from a height of more than 15 feet, or three times the patient's height, pedestrian being struck by a vehicle, being struck by an object, such as a pipe, bat, or fists, during an assault, gunshot wounds, stab wounds, or high-impact motor vehicle collisions.

5. One of the earliest indications of shock is a change in mental status. The patient may be restless or agitated. Later, the level of responsive may diminish. The skin may become cool, mottled, pale, or clammy due to vasoconstriction and stimulation of the "fight or flight" functions of the nervous system. Early on, the pulse is increased, the blood pressure is normal to slightly increased, and respirations are increased. However, as bleeding continues, the blood pressure will eventually drop. Other indications of internal bleeding would be bruises or abrasions over the torso, fractures of the pelvis or femurs, or multiple long bone fractures. The patient should be treated by stabilizing the cervical spine, ensuring an open airway, assisting ventilations if necessary, providing high flow oxygen, immobilizing the spine along with any other suspected fractures, and keeping the patient warm. If the transport time is prolonged, ALS intercept or aeromedical transport should be considered. The patient should be transported to the nearest hospital capable of providing trauma care.

Multiple-Choice Answers

1. **(B)** Objective 8
   The average adult has 5,000 to 6,000 mL (5 to 6 L) of blood. 1,000 mL is about 20% of the blood volume of an adult, representing significant hemorrhage.

2. **(B)** Objective 7
   The patient has significant mechanism of injury and is complaining of pain in his left thigh, which may indicate a femur fracture. The patient is at risk of ongoing blood loss that may result in shock.

3. **(B)** Objective 7
   Two cups is equivalent to 500 mL, a significant loss of blood for a child.

4. **(C)** Objective 3
   Most external bleeding can be controlled by direct pressure. Pressure points and application of ice are sometimes used as adjuncts in the control of bleeding, but are not effective by themselves. Tourniquets are used when all other methods are ineffective in controlling bleeding.

5. **(B)** Objective 3
   Tourniquets may be used by EMTs for bleeding proximal to the elbow or knee that cannot be controlled by other means.

6. **(A)** Objective 3
   This type of bleeding indicates a skull fracture. The amount of blood that will escape from the ear is not likely to be life threatening. However, the bleeding indicates an opening through the skull that may put the patient at risk for infection. Additionally, stopping the escape of blood, which is likely mixed with cerebral spinal fluid, from the ear can theoretically result in an increase in intracranial pressure.

7. **(A)** Objective 9

The nervous system responds quickly to injury and blood loss. The release of adrenalin from the adrenal glands results in nervousness and agitation. The choices listed are all late signs of shock.

8. **(D)** Objective 9

All of these findings are related to the body's attempts to compensate for blood loss.

9. **(B)** Objective 9

The body first compensates by constricting the blood vessels and increasing the heart rate. This results in a normal to slightly increased blood pressure. Only as blood loss continues and vasoconstriction and increased heart rate are no longer adequate to compensate, does the blood pressure drop.

10. **(C)** Objective 7

Factors other than systemic hypoperfusion can affect capillary refill in adults, including the elderly, making it a less reliable indicator of shock than it is in children and infants.

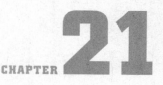

Dealing with Injuries

Section 1—Soft Tissue Injuries

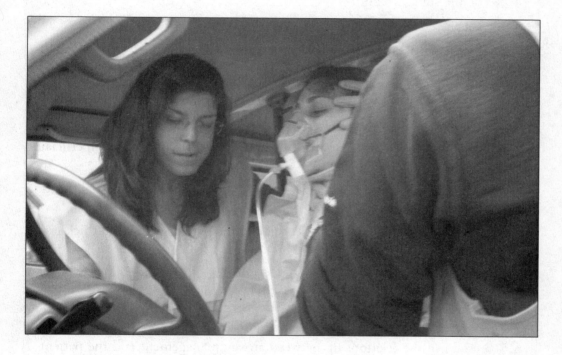

OBJECTIVES

This chapter and the review questions will help readers determine if they are able to

1. state the major functions of the skin;

2. list the layers of the skin;

3. establish the relationship between BSI and soft tissue injuries;

4. list the types of closed soft tissue injuries;

5. describe the emergency medical care of the patient with an open soft tissue injury;

6. state the types of open soft tissue injuries;

7. describe the emergency medical care of the patient with an open soft tissue injury;

8. discuss the emergency medical care considerations for the patient with a penetrating chest injury;

9. state the emergency medical care considerations for the patient with an open wound to the abdomen;

10. differentiate the care of an open wound to the chest from an open wound to the abdomen;

11. list the classifications of burns;

12. define superficial burn;

13. list the characteristics of a superficial burn;

14. define partial thickness burn;

15. list the characteristics of a partial thickness burn;

16. define full thickness burn;

17. list the characteristics of a full thickness burn;

18. describe the emergency medical care of the patient with a superficial burn;

19. describe the emergency medical care of the patient with a partial thickness burn;

20. describe the emergency medical care of the patient with a full thickness burn;

21. list the functions of dressing and bandaging;

22. describe the purpose of a bandage;

23. describe the steps in applying a pressure dressing;

24. establish the relationship between airway management and the patient with chest injury, burns, and blunt and penetrating injuries;

25. describe the effects of improperly applied dressings, splints, and tourniquets;

26. describe the emergency medical care of the patient with an impaled object;

27. describe the emergency medical care of the patient with an amputation;

28. describe the emergency care for a chemical burn;

29. describe the emergency care for an electrical burn.

THE SKIN

The skin serves us by keeping fluids in, regulating body temperature, and keeping bacteria out. Any significant disruption in the skin will cause possible loss of temperature regulation, infection, and loss of fluids. The skin's layers are the **epidermis** (outer) and the **dermis** (inner).

Soft Tissue Injuries

Soft tissue injuries can be open or closed. Closed soft tissue injuries include contusions, hematoma, and crushing injuries. Open soft tissue injuries include abrasions, lacerations, avulsions, puncture/penetrations, amputations, and some crush injuries. Treatment centers on bleeding control and immobilization.

Burns are classified as superficial, partial, or full thickness. The severity of a burn is determined by evaluating the depth, total body surface area, the location of the burn, along with the age and general physical condition of the patient. The rule of nines is used to determine the total body surface area. In treating chemical burns, after the safety of the rescuer is assured, the chemical needs to be removed from the body to stop the burning. Dry chemicals should first be brushed off, then rinsed off. The patient will also need to be treated for the chemical's toxic effects. Electrical burns cause deep tissue death and there is generally more damage than is apparent on the surface. The biggest concern with electrical burns is cardiac arrest. In general, after some initial cooling, burns should be dressed in clean dry dressings.

Section 2—Musculoskeletal Injuries

OBJECTIVES

This chapter and the review questions will help readers determine if they are able to

1. describe the function of the muscular system;

2. describe the function of the skeletal system;

3. list the major bones or bone groupings of the spinal column, the thorax, the upper extremities, the lower extremities;

4. differentiate between an open and a closed painful, swollen, deformed extremity;

5. state the reasons for splinting;

6. list the general rules of splinting;

7. list the complications of splinting;

8. list the emergency medical care for the patient with a painful, swollen, deformed extremity.

Mechanisms that can cause musculoskeletal injuries include direct, indirect, or twisting forces. Bone or joint injuries can be open or closed. Signs and symptoms of bone injuries include pain, swelling, deformity, tenderness, discoloration, and limited movement. Treatment includes BSI, ice, splinting, and elevation.

Proper splinting should prevent movement of bone fragments to limit further injury to nerves, blood vessels, and soft tissues and should be done before the patient is moved, if hazards permit. Before and after splints are applied, pulses and sensation should be checked distal to the injury. Splints include rigid, traction, pneumatic, improvised (pillows and blankets), and PASG (for pelvic injuries). When splinting joints, the bone above and below should be immobilized, and when splinting bones, the joint above and below the injury should be immobilized. Traction splints are only indicated for mid-shaft femur fractures (Thomas, Hare, or Sager). Recently, sheets tied around the pelvis or commercially available "pelvic slings" have been suggested for use with pelvic fractures and are in use in some protocols.

Scenario 1

You arrive on the scene of a motorcycle collision and the man you are looking at has extensive abrasions over much of his body. How will you tend to these wounds?

SOLUTION

After rinsing the debris of the wounds with saline, dress the wounds in dry sterile dressings. Keep in mind that hypothermia due to the loss of skin and exposure to the elements is a possibility.

Scenario 2

Your patient has burns to his face and hands. He is able to speak and walk but is in a great deal of pain. How serious are these burns and how will you treat them?

SOLUTION

These burns should be considered critical because of the possible airway involvement and the burns to the hands and feet. After light initial cooling, dry sterile dressings, and oxygen at 15 liters into a nonrebreather mask, you would transport to the appropriate facility as directed by medical control.

Scenario 3

You arrive on the scene where a young man has severed the index finger of his right hand. How will you care for this patient?

SOLUTION

Apply a pressure dressing to the hand, locate the severed finger, wrap it in a sterile dressing, wrap or bag it in plastic, and keep it cool. Transport the finger along with the patient to the appropriate facility as directed by medical control.

Scenario 4

You are on the scene with a young woman complaining of a painful, swollen right forearm. How will you treat her?

SOLUTION

After BSI and checking distal pulses and sensation, you should splint the injury to include the wrist and elbow. The addition of a sling will further protect and relieve some of the discomfort of this injury.

Scenario 5

While examining the pelvis of a trauma patient, you compress the pelvic wings together and notice a sensation of crepitus and an increase in pain for the patient. What do you suspect and how will you treat it?

SOLUTION

Your patient may have a pelvic fracture. The patient should be immobilized to a spine board. Using the PASG will help to immobilize the broken pelvis and could help to control the bleeding that accompanies this type of life-threatening fracture.

Scenario 6

You are preparing to splint a deformed right forearm injury. While checking the arm distal to the injury you notice that it appears cyanotic and swollen. The patient has decreased sensation and you do not feel pulses distal to the injury. How should the EMT address this?

SOLUTION

While splinting this extremity, the EMT should apply gentle traction while trying to realign the deformity in an attempt to return circulation distal to the injury.

Review Questions

EXERCISES

The exercises in this review are designed to help reinforce your knowledge of the objectives for this chapter. If you find it difficult to meet any of the objectives stated, go back and review those materials again.

Section 1—Soft Tissue Injuries

1. What are the consequences of losing or damaging large areas of the skin? (Objectives 1 and 2)

   _____

   _____

   _____

2. Match the description on the left with the terms below by writing the letter of the term in the blank next to the description. (Objectives 3–7)
   (A) Laceration
   (B) Abrasion
   (C) Avulsion
   (D) Burn
   (E) Hematoma
   (F) Contusion

   _____ Damaged tissue as a result of heat or chemical exposure

   _____ Linear tear in the skin caused by blunt or sharp trauma

   _____ Closed injury consisting of discoloration and tenderness without significant swelling

   _____ Superficial areas of skin are removed from friction against an object

   _____ Closed injury with swelling due to a collection of blood beneath the skin

   _____ A piece of skin is torn away, but may be attached by a small bit of skin

3. Your patient is a 35-year-old female with stab wounds to the anterior chest and abdomen. Assuming the patient's airway and breathing are being managed, how will you care for these wounds? (Objectives 8–10)

_____

_____

_____

_____

_____

_____

_____

4. Your patient is a 40-year-old female who poured charcoal lighter fluid onto a burning pile of yard debris. Her face is red, but without blisters, although her eyebrows are singed. She has redness and blisters on her right hand and forearm. First, classify the burns according to severity, then specify how you will treat the burns. (Objectives 11–20)

	Severity	Treatment
Face		
Right Hand and Forearm		

5. Describe the special considerations in caring for patients with chemical and electrical burns. (Objectives 21–29)

Chemical: _____

_____

Electrical: _____

_____

Section 2—Musculoskeletal Injuries

1. Your patient is a 12-year-old female who injured her arm while doing a cartwheel in her yard. Her arm is swollen, deformed, and painful just above the elbow. Respond to the following. (Objectives 1–8)

Why should this injury be splinted?

_____

_____

How should this injury be splinted?

_____

_____

What complications may occur as a result of splinting the injury?

_____

_____

MULTIPLE-CHOICE QUESTIONS

1. Your patient has a jagged piece of glass embedded in a wound on the palm of his left hand. Which of the following best describes the proper management of this wound?
   (A) Apply a pressure dressing over the object to stabilize it and control bleeding.
   (B) Place bulking dressing material around the object and bandage it in place to stabilize the object.
   (C) Remove the object before applying a pressure dressing to the wound.
   (D) Use an occlusive dressing, such as petroleum gauze, to seal the edges of the wound around the object.

2. For which of the following fracture locations is a traction splint indicated?
   (A) pelvis
   (B) femur
   (C) knee
   (D) tibia

3. You are preparing to transport a patient whose arm has been amputated just above the wrist. You have retrieved the amputated part. Which of the following best describes the proper care of it during transport?
   (A) Wrap it in a dry, sterile dressing and place it next to the patient to keep it warm.
   (B) Place it in a container of ice.
   (C) Cover it with a sterile dressing, place in a plastic bag, and place the bag in a container of cooled water.
   (D) Wrap it in a sterile dressing moistened with saline, then place it in a container of ice.

4. Your patient is complaining of pain in the right ankle after tripping on a step. The ankle is swollen, deformed, and tender. Which of the following best describes the assessment of circulation in relationship to splinting?
   (A) Check the pedal pulse, splint the ankle, recheck the pedal pulse.
   (B) Check the popliteal pulse, splint the ankle, recheck the pedal pulse.
   (C) Check both the pedal and popliteal pulses, splint the ankle, recheck both the pedal and popliteal pulses.
   (D) It is not necessary to check pulses when treating a joint injury.

5. In open fractures with bone protruding from the wound, the EMT should
   (A) push the bone back in.
   (B) pull on the extremity until the bone drops back into place.
   (C) splint the injury in a way that protects the bone end.
   (D) cover the bone end but do not splint.

6. Your patient is a 42-year-old male who received a knife wound to the abdomen in a bar fight. As you approach you see that he has a loop of intestine protruding from the wound. Which of the following is the highest priority in the treatment of this patient?
   (A) Cover the exposed intestine with a sterile, moist dressing.
   (B) Ensure adequate breathing.
   (C) Control bleeding from the wound.
   (D) Arrange spinal immobilization.

7. A hip injury caused when a knee strikes the dashboard is an example of
   (A) direct force.
   (B) indirect force.
   (C) twisting force.
   (D) traction force.

8. Which of the following best describes the depth of a burn that only involves the epidermis?
   (A) full thickness
   (B) partial thickness
   (C) superficial
   (D) moderate

9. Using the rule of nines, what is the percentage of body surface area involved if there are burns of the chest and the anterior surface of one arm?
   (A) 9%
   (B) 13.5%
   (C) 18%
   (D) 27%

10. Your patient is a 14-year-old boy who crashed his bicycle while riding downhill at approximately 20 miles per hour. He has abrasions to his hands, posterior forearms, chest, and knees. These injuries should be treated as if they are
    (A) contusions.
    (B) hematomas.
    (C) fractures.
    (D) burns.

ANSWERS TO REVIEW QUESTIONS

Exercises

SECTION 1—SOFT TISSUE INJURIES

1. The skin plays important roles in protecting the body against changes in environmental temperature, loss of water, and invasion by microorganisms. Intact skin is critical to our survival.

2. **(D) Burn:** Damaged tissue as a result of heat or chemical exposure

   (A) Laceration: Linear tear in the skin caused by blunt or sharp trauma

   (F) Contusion: Closed injury consisting of discoloration and tenderness without significant swelling

   (B) Abrasion: Superficial areas of skin are removed from friction against an object

   (E) Hematoma: Closed injury with swelling due to a collection of blood beneath the skin.

   (C) Avulsion: A piece of skin is torn away, but may be attached by a small bit of skin

3. The chest wounds should be managed first if there is evidence of air movement at the site of injury since an open pneumothorax or "sucking chest wound" interferes with breathing. These wounds are managed by placing an occlusive dressing sealed on three sides only over each wound. If there is significant bleeding from any of the wounds, they should be treated with direct pressure. If any of the abdominal wounds have abdominal contents protruding from them, they should be covered with a moist, nonadherent, sterile dressing, then covered by an occlusive dressing secured in place.

4.

	Severity	Treatment
Face	Superficial	No immediate treatment required due to the superficial nature and the implications of bandaging the face, but the airway should be monitored.
Right Hand and Forearm	Partial thickness	The area burned is small enough that a moist, sterile dressing can be used. However, whenever in doubt, use a dry sterile dressing.

5. **Chemical:** Ensure that it is safe for you to approach the patient; involve the hazardous material team if necessary. Most chemical exposures are treated by first removing the clothing that either contains the chemical or can absorb the chemical during decontamination, irrigating the affected area with copious amounts of water, then treating the burns as any other burn would be treated. Dry chemicals should always be brushed away before irrigating with copious amounts of water.

Electrical: Ensure that the source of electricity is off. In addition to treating the burns that can be seen, realize that internal injury may be massive. Anticipate respiratory and cardiac problems.

SECTION 2—MUSCULOSKELETAL INJURIES

1. **Why should this injury be splinted?** Splinting can prevent further damage from broken bone ends and reduce pain and bleeding.

   How should this injury be splinted? A sling and swathe would work well for this injury.

   What complications may occur as a result of splinting the injury? Manipulation of the extremity may result in further injury, including injury to blood vessels and nerves, and pain. If applied incorrectly, the splint may restrict circulation.

Multiple-Choice Answers

1. **(B)** Section 1, Objective 5
   Impaled objects are only removed if they interfere with the airway. Otherwise, they are carefully stabilized in place without applying pressure to the object, which will result in further injury.

2. **(B)** Section 2, Objective 5
   A traction splint is used only for femur fractures in order to overcome the strong contraction of the thigh muscles and allow gross alignment of the bone ends.

3. **(C)** Section 2, Objective 7
   The part should be kept cool, if time allows, but should never be placed on ice.

4. **(A)** Section 2, Objective 5
   The pulse and nerve function (sensation and movement) distal to the injury should be checked both before and after splinting. In this case, it is the pedal pulse that is distal to the injury.

5. **(C)** Section 2, Objective 7
   The injury must be splinted while avoiding reintroducing the bone ends into the wound. This may result in additional injury and contamination of the wound.

6. **(B)** Section 1, Objective 9
   This patient has received a significant injury. The initial assessment must ensure that the patient has an adequate airway and breathing.

7. **(B)** Section 2, Objective 1
   The point of impact is at the knee. Any injury to the knee would be due to direct force. The hip was not directly impacted by the dashboard; the force was transmitted through the femur to the hip.

8. **(C)** Section 1, Objective 2
   The epidermis is the outermost layer of the skin. An injury that involves only the epidermis is superficial.

9. **(B)** Section 1, Objective 11
   Using the rule of nines, the anterior chest accounts for 9%, and the anterior surface of a single arm would be 4.5% for a total of 13.5%.

10. **(D)** Section 1, Objective 12
    Although these injuries are abrasions, they are like burns in that a large area of skin has been damaged.

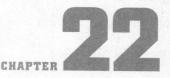

CHAPTER 22

Injuries to the Head and Spine

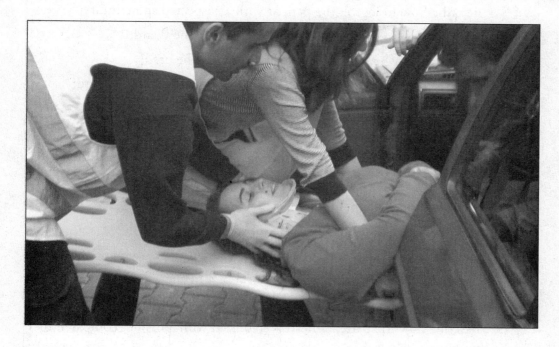

OBJECTIVES

This chapter and the review questions will help readers determine if they are able to

1. state the components of the nervous system;

2. list the functions of the central nervous system;

3. define the structure of the skeletal system as it relates to the nervous system;

4. relate mechanism of injury to potential injuries of the head and spine;

5. describe the implications of not properly caring for potential spine injuries;

6. state the signs and symptoms of a potential spine injury;

7. describe the method of determining if the responsive patient may have a spine injury;

8. relate the airway emergency medical care techniques to the patient with a suspected spine injury;

9. describe how to stabilize the cervical spine immobilization device;

10. discuss indications for sizing and using cervical spine immobilization;

11. establish the relationship between airway management and the patient with head and spine injuries;

12. describe a method for sizing a cervical spine immobilization device;

13. describe how to logroll the patient with a suspected spine injury;

14. describe how to secure the patient to a long spine board;

15. list instances when a short spine board should be used;

16. describe how to immobilize the patient using a short spine board;

17. describe the indications for the use of rapid extrication;

18. list the steps in performing rapid extrication;

19. state the circumstances when a helmet should be left on the patient;

20. discuss the circumstances when a helmet should be removed;

21. identify different types of helmets;

22. describe the unique characteristics of sports helmets;

23. explain the preferred methods to remove a helmet;

24. discuss alternative methods for removal of a helmet;

25. describe how the patient's head is stabilized to remove the helmet;

26. describe how the patient's head is stabilized with a helmet compared to without a helmet.

The nervous system consists of the **central** (brain) and **peripheral** (motor and sensory) systems. The **cranium** and the **spinal column** protect these systems. The spine is made up of 33 vertebrae: 7 cervical, 12 thoracic, 5 lumbar, 5 sacral, and 4 coccyx.

INJURIES TO THE SPINE

Injuries to the spine can be compression, flexion, extension, lateral bending or distraction type. Any injury of the nervous system will be evidenced by some dysfunction in mental status, ability to move, or sensation. Injuries to the vertebrae should be suspected when there is mechanism of injury with tenderness, deformity, pain with movement, loss of sensation, or the ability to move. High cord injuries can disrupt the patient's ability to breathe and respiratory arrest should be anticipated with possible neck injuries.

When spine injuries are suspected, patients should be manually immobilized, then have cervical collars applied and be logrolled onto a spine board. If the patient is in a sitting position, then a short board or Kendrick-type device should be used to immobilize him or her as much as possible before lowering onto a long board. If the patient is critical or the scene is hazardous, the patient can be moved urgently without the short board device using the rapid extrication technique.

INJURIES TO THE HEAD

Injuries to the head can bleed severely. Gentle pressure should be applied to control the bleeding but care should be given in the event there is a skull fracture associated with the wound. Injury to the brain should be suspected with any head injury. Changes in mental status and/or fluid coming from the ears or nose and/or unequal pupils are indicators of head injury.

Helmets should be removed if you are unable to assess the patient with the helmet in place, the helmet does not fit properly, or you are unable to immobilize the patient with the helmet in place.

When immobilizing infants, children, elderly, or any other individual who might not fit onto the board uniformly or has misshapen spines, it should be padded to maintain in-line and neutral positioning.

Scenario 1

A patient walks up to you at the scene of a motor vehicle collision, says he was in one of the vehicles, and complains of neck pain. How should you treat this person?

SOLUTION

Immediately provide manual cervical immobilization, apply a cervical collar, and do a standing board maneuver to get this person onto a backboard and immobilized.

Scenario 2

You are called to assist with an unresponsive man who was pulled from a shallow pool. Besides beginning to resuscitate this patient, what do you think may have happened before he became unresponsive?

SOLUTION

The EMT should always suspect head and neck injuries in unconscious patients, particularly in shallow pools, as there might have been a diving accident prior to the patient becoming unresponsive.

Scenario 3

You are preparing to immobilize a child to a long board. What special consideration do you need to address in children and spinal immobilization?

SOLUTION

Because the head is proportionately larger in many children, you should check positioning on the board to maintain neutral and in-line position and be prepared to pad the child's shoulders to prevent hyperflexion of the neck.

Review Questions

EXERCISES

The exercises in this review are designed to help reinforce your knowledge of the objectives for this chapter. If you find it difficult to meet any of the objectives stated, go back and review those materials again.

1. List the primary functions of each part of the central nervous system in the table below. (Objectives 1 and 2)

Structure	Function
Cerebral Hemispheres	
Cerebellum	
Brain Stem	
Spinal Cord	

2. Complete the table below to describe indications of a spinal injury. (Objectives 4–7)

Assessment	Indications of Spinal Injury
Mechanisms of Injury	
Patient Complaints	
Physical Assessment Findings	

3. The manual maneuver used to open the airway of a patient with suspected spinal injury is the _____ maneuver. (Objective 11)

4. Describe the circumstances under which you should use rapid extrication and the circumstances when you should use a short spinal immobilization device. (Objectives 12 and 17)

_____

_____

_____

_____

5. What are the considerations in deciding to remove a helmet or leave it in place in the patient with suspected head or spine injuries? (Objectives 18–20)

_____

_____

_____

MULTIPLE-CHOICE QUESTIONS

1. A patient has jumped from a second-story balcony and initially landed on his feet. What type of spinal fracture is most likely?
   (A) compression
   (B) distraction
   (C) flexion
   (D) extension

2. A face striking the windshield of a car is likely to cause what type of spinal injury?
   (A) compression
   (B) distraction
   (C) flexion
   (D) extension

3. Which of the following mechanisms is most consistent with the potential for spinal injury?
   (A) motor vehicle collision into a stationary object at 15 miles per hour with a restrained occupant
   (B) gunshot wound just below (distal to) the knee.
   (C) fall from the top step of a 4-foot stepladder, landing head-first on a concrete patio
   (D) being tackled in a game of football

4. Breathing may be impaired if the spine is injured at the level of the _____ vertebrae.
   (A) cervical
   (B) thoracic
   (C) lumbar
   (D) sacral

5. Your patient was the unrestrained driver of a vehicle that struck a large tree at 45 miles per hour. He is unresponsive to painful stimuli, has rapid, weak pulses, and shallow ventilations. Which of the following actions is in the patient's best interest?
   (A) Quickly apply a cervical collar and short spinal immobilization device, remove the patient onto a long backboard, secure him to the board, load him in the ambulance, and then begin assessment and treatment en route to the hospital.
   (B) Quickly apply oxygen, while maintaining manual stabilization of the cervical spine, apply a cervical collar, and rapidly but carefully remove the patient onto a long backboard.
   (C) Apply oxygen, complete a detailed physical examination including vital signs, and then rapidly extricate the patient onto a long backboard.
   (D) Immediately pull the patient from the vehicle onto the ground while stabilizing the head and neck as much as possible with your forearms.

6. Which of the following is part of the central nervous system?
   (A) skull
   (B) spinal cord
   (C) vertebrae
   (D) all of the above

7. Manual immobilization must be maintained in the spine-injured patient until the
   (A) cervical collar is in place.
   (B) patient is placed on the backboard.
   (C) head blocks are in place.
   (D) patient is completely secured to the spine board.

8. Once placed on the spine board, the order in which the straps should be applied is
   (A) torso, feet, head.
   (B) feet, torso, head.
   (C) head, torso, feet.
   (D) head, feet, torso.

9. Signs and symptoms of a possible injury to the spinal cord include
   (A) loss of feeling in the arms or legs.
   (B) inability to move the arms or legs.
   (C) pain over the spine.
   (D) all of the above

10. Your patient is a motorcyclist who struck the side of a car and was ejected. Which of the following would be a reason to remove her helmet?
    (A) The helmet interferes with airway management.
    (B) The helmet prevents proper immobilization of the spine.
    (C) The helmet interferes with assessment of an injury.
    (D) All of the above.

ANSWERS TO REVIEW QUESTIONS

Exercises

1.

Structure	Function
Cerebral Hemispheres	Higher brain functions such as consciousness, thought, memory, language, and emotion.
Cerebellum	Fine-tunes coordination.
Brain Stem	Vegetative functions such as control of breathing and heart rate.
Spinal Cord	Transmits nerve impulses between the brain and the body.

2.

Assessment	Indications of Spinal Injury
Mechanisms of Injury	Motor vehicle collisions with significant impact; occupants ejected from a vehicle; substantial direct blows to the head, face, or spine; falls from a height
Patient Complaints	Tenderness or pain of the spine; numbness, weakness, tingling, or paralysis of any of the extremities
Physical Assessment Findings	Tenderness or deformity of the spine; weakness or paralysis of the extremities

3. The manual maneuver used to open the airway of a patient with suspected spinal injury is the **jaw thrust** maneuver.

4. Rapid extrication is used for patients involved in motor vehicle collisions who are unstable (signs of shock, impaired airway or ventilations). Rapid extrication may also be used if the patient is stable but preventing access to an unstable patient. Otherwise, a short spinal immobilization device should be used to extricate patients who have potential spinal injuries from vehicles.

5. This decision requires judgment on the part of the EMT. If the helmet does not interfere with airway management, proper immobilization, or assessment of injuries, it should be left in place.

Multiple-Choice Answers

1. **(A)** Objective 4

   Compression occurs when the lower part of the body comes to a stop, but the weight of the upper body continues downward, applying pressure to the vertebrae.

2. **(D)** Objective 4

   Extension refers to excessive backward motion of the head and neck.

3. **(C)** Objective 4

   While it is sometimes difficult to determine how much force was applied to a patient, the most concerning mechanism listed—one which unquestionably requires spinal immobilization—is a fall from a height with a direct blow to the head.

4. **(A)** Objective 3

   The nerves that allow contraction of the muscles of respiration arise from the cervical level of the spine.

5. **(B)** Objective 17

   This patient is unstable and must be rapidly extricated from the vehicle, yet proper technique must be used by placing the patient onto a long backboard for removal from the vehicle. If the cervical spine can be adequately manually immobilized and the patient is critical, the cervical collar can be applied after the patient is removed from the vehicle.

6. **(B)** Objective 3

   The skull and vertebrae provide protection to the structures of the central nervous system: the brain and the spinal cord.

7. **(D)** Objective 3

   The spine is treated as a single structure. If any part of it is not immobilized, the cervical spine is not immobilized.

8. **(A)** Objective 8

   The head should be secured last to ensure that patient movement is contained before the head is finally secured. By securing the head last, the EMT ensures that the patient is completely secured before manual immobilization is released.

9. **(D)** Objective 6

   Signs and symptoms of an injury to the cord are related to the area damaged. Injury to the cervical spine can cause respiratory arrest by disrupting the nerves that control breathing. Further down the cord, injury can disrupt nervous communication with the internal organs or the extremities, causing loss of function and sensation.

10. **(D)** Objective 19

There is some controversy as to whether helmets should be removed in the field. This includes sports and motorcycle helmets. In general, the standard of care is that if the helmet can be included in the immobilization of the patient and the EMT can complete the assessment with clear access to the airway, the helmet can remain in place. On the other hand, if the helmet needs to be removed to gain access to the airway or to immobilize or assess the injuries, the helmet should be removed.

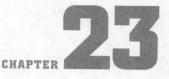
Infants and Children

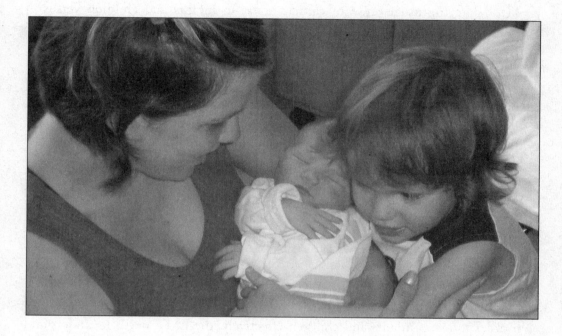

OBJECTIVES

This chapter and the review questions will help readers determine if they are able to

1. identify the developmental considerations for the following age groups:

   - infants
   - toddlers
   - preschool
   - school age
   - adolescents

2. describe the differences in anatomy and physiology of the infant, child, and adult patient;

3. differentiate the response of the ill or injured infant or child (age specific) from that of an adult;

4. indicate various causes of respiratory emergencies;

5. differentiate between respiratory distress and respiratory failure;

6. list the steps in the management of foreign body airway obstruction;

7. summarize emergency medical care strategies for respiratory distress and respiratory failure;

8. identify the signs and symptoms of shock (hypoperfusion) in the infant and child patient;

9. describe the methods of determining end organ perfusion in the infant and child patient;

10. state the usual cause of cardiac arrest in infants and children versus adults;

11. list the common causes of seizures in the infant and child patient;

12. describe the management of seizures in the infant and child patient;

13. differentiate between the injury patterns in adults, infants, and children;

14. discuss the field management of the infant and child trauma patient;

15. summarize the indicators of possible child abuse and neglect;

16. describe the medical legal responsibilities in suspected child abuse;

17. recognize the need for EMT debriefing following a difficult infant or child transport.

DEVELOPMENTAL PHASES

In order to assess infants and children effectively, the EMT needs to understand the developmental phases. These are broken down into birth to 1 year (newborn), 1 to 3 years (toddlers), 3 to 6 years (preschool), 6 to 12 years (school age), and 12 to 18 years (adolescent). The way infants and children respond to the EMT changes at each of these phases. Determining the mental status of a child too young to speak will depend on your assessment of his or her activity level. There are physical differences to remember as well. The smaller, shorter airways and proportionately larger head and tongue of the infant create airway obstruction possibilities different from those of adults.

The equipment used to manage these patients is important to review as well. Nasal or oral airways are not to be used during initial artificial ventilations. Special backboards and other immobilization devices should be used, or the ones you have will need to be adapted to the size and shape of these patients.

In assessing the breathing of infants and children, look for signs of increased respiratory effort: nasal flaring, stridor, or crowing; sternal or intercostal retractions; and grunting or respiratory rates outside of normal limits. In small children, prolonged respiratory distress can lead to respiratory fatigue leaving the child too tired to breathe. When performing detailed physical exams, it is recommended to begin with the trunk before the head.

PROBLEMS IN INFANTS AND CHILDREN

✔ Seizures in children are often febrile. In these cases, clothing should be removed to allow the child to release as much heat as possible.

✔ Poisonings are a common pediatric event. Identify and bring the substance to the hospital if possible and contact medical control for specific treatments like activated charcoal.

✔ Hypoperfusion or shock in children is seldom a cardiac problem. Most often it is secondary to dehydration so be alert for histories of diarrhea, vomiting, or inadequate feeding. Vital signs associated with small children may be confusing. While the respirations may be rapid and weak the pulse rate may actually be bradycardic when the infant is in trouble.

✔ Sudden infant death syndrome (SIDS) may happen to infants in their first year of life. There are many possible causes that are not clearly understood. You should try to resuscitate unless there are signs of rigor mortis.

Trauma

Trauma is the number one cause of death in infants and children with blunt injuries being most common. In assessing for traumatic injuries anticipate patterns different from adults. Infants and small children lead with their heads so head injuries are frequent. The skeleton is soft and pliable so there may be significant internal injuries without obvious external injuries. Infants and children are more susceptible to environmental injuries, too. Infants' total body surface area is proportionately larger than the adult so they lose heat more rapidly and burns subject them to more fluid loss and loss of ability to regulate body temperature.

Abuse

Injuries and stories that do not add up and injuries that would seem to require more energy than the child could generate on his or her own should be suspected of abuse and *must* be reported. Central nervous system injuries are most lethal as is the case of "shaken baby syndrome."

Special Needs Children

Special needs children are just that. Premature babies and children with heart disease or neurologic or neuromuscular disease may have special needs for the EMT to address. It is a good policy to know as much as you can about these infants and children in your service area and what they might need from you. Caring for sick and injured children is one of the hardest things the EMT will have to do. If things go badly, you should be prepared to talk about it and even access critical incident stress management teams.

Scenario 1

You are called to the scene for a sick child. The mother hands you a 3-month-old male child lying limp in your hands. The breathing is shallow and rapid and the pulse is weak and slow. The infant's color is dusky. What do you think is happening and what can you do for him?

SOLUTION

This infant is showing signs and symptoms of shock. High flow oxygen, conserve body heat, and consider bag-valve mask ventilations. Rapid transport to the hospital is important for fluid resuscitation.

Scenario 2

What history could explain the patient's condition?

SOLUTION

Fever with vomiting and/or diarrhea and poor feeding would be consistent with the patient's condition.

Scenario 3

You are on the scene with an apparent SIDS victim. The child is pale, pulseless, and nonbreathing but does not have rigor mortis. What should you do here?

SOLUTION

Begin resuscitation and transport as soon as possible. Also consider that the family is your patient, too, and they are likely going to need understanding and attention.

Review Questions

EXERCISES

The exercises in this review are designed to help reinforce your knowledge of the objectives for this chapter. If you find it difficult to meet any of the objectives stated, go back and review those materials again.

1. Complete the table below to describe the developmental characteristics of each age group. (Objective 1)

	Age	Developmental Characteristics and Considerations in Management
Infants		
Toddlers		
Preschoolers		
School-Age Children		
Adolescents		

2. Describe how children are different from adults in anatomy and physiology. (Objective 2)

Airway:

_____

_____

_____

Skeletal structure:

_____

_____

Abdomen and abdominal organs:

_____

_____

3. Describe the signs and symptoms and emergency medical care of each of the following. (Objectives 3–7)

	Signs and Symptoms	Emergency Medical Care
Partial Airway Obstruction		
Complete Airway Obstruction		
Respiratory Distress		
Respiratory Arrest		

4. List three ways of assessing perfusion status in the child that are unreliable or not able to be checked in adults. (Objective 8)

_____

_____

_____

5. The most common cause of cardiac arrest in infants and children is

_____. (Objectives 9 and 10)

6. List five causes of seizures in children. (Objective 11)

_____

_____

_____

_____

_____

7. The most important consideration in management of the child with a seizure is management of _____. (Objective 12)

8. List at least four indications of possible child abuse. (Objectives 13–15)

_____

_____

_____

_____

MULTIPLE-CHOICE QUESTIONS

1. You are caring for an injured child who expresses concern over disfigurement from her injury. This child is most likely in which of the following age groups?
   (A) infant
   (B) toddler
   (C) preschool
   (D) school-age

2. A child in the _____ age group should be treated as if he or she is an adult.
   (A) toddler
   (B) preschool
   (C) school-age
   (D) adolescent

3. The potential for airway obstruction is compounded in infants and children by
   (A) smaller airways easily blocked by secretions.
   (B) a proportionately larger tongue.
   (C) a large head causing hyperextension when supine.
   (D) all of the above

4. For obstructed airways, abdominal thrusts are eliminated in children
   (A) less than 1 year old.
   (B) 1 to 3 years old.
   (C) 1 to 8 years old.
   (D) 6 to 12 years old.

5. Delivering oxygen to newborns should be accomplished by
   (A) strapping an adult mask to the infant upside down.
   (B) using a newborn oxygen mask.
   (C) using the blow-by oxygen method.
   (D) nasal cannula.

6. Partial upper airway obstruction is indicated by
   (A) stridor on inspiration.
   (B) absence of breath sounds on the affected side.
   (C) wheezing on exhalation.
   (D) lying down.

7. Respiratory distress is indicated by
   (A) nasal flaring.
   (B) sternal or intercostal retraction.
   (C) wheezing.
   (D) all of the above

8. Typical pediatric doses for activated charcoal are between
   (A) 6 to 12.5 gms.
   (B) 12.5 to 25 gms.
   (C) 25 to 50 gms.
   (D) 50 to 75 gms.

9. True or False: Sudden infant death syndrome affects children up to age 3.
   (A) True
   (B) False

10. True or False: Cardiac problems are also a frequent cause of shock in infants and children.
    (A) True
    (B) False

ANSWERS TO REVIEW QUESTIONS
Exercises

	Age	Developmental Characteristics and Considerations in Management
Infants	Birth to 1 year	Minimal stranger anxiety but do not like to be separated from parents; make sure your stethoscope and hands are warm before touching the child; assess the head last
Toddlers	1 to 3 years	Do not like to be touched, have clothing removed, or be separated from parents; may be afraid of needles or believe that illness or injury is punishment for bad behavior
Preschoolers	3 to 6 years	Similar to toddlers; may be afraid of blood, pain, and permanent injury; begins to be modest
School-Age Children	6 to 12 years	May be afraid of blood, pain, permanent injury, and disfigurement
Adolescents	12 to 18 years	Treat as adults; assess privately, away from parents and peers

2. **Airway:** The airways are small and easily obstructed, the tongue is relatively large, and hyperextension of the neck may lead to airway obstruction. Infants are nose breathers and the nasal passages must be kept clear. Can compensate well initially for respiratory problems, but fatigue quickly, leading to respiratory failure.

Skeletal structure: The bones are not fully calcified and are thinner and more flexible. Fractures require more force, so internal injuries can occur without fractures.

Abdomen and abdominal organs: The abdominal organs are relatively large and protrude, while the abdominal muscles are weak and provide less protection.

3.

	Signs and Symptoms	Emergency Medical Care
Partial Airway Obstruction	Child is alert, in sitting position; may have stridor, crowing, or noisy breathing; peripheral perfusion is good	Allow position of comfort; attempt to provide oxygen, but do not agitate the child; transport
Complete Airway Obstruction	Cannot cry, speak, or cough; altered mental status, cyanosis.	Use chest thrusts and back blows to clear the airway of an infant; use abdominal thrusts to clear the airway of a child
Respiratory Distress	May have stridor, wheezing, grunting, retractions, cyanosis, and become fatigued	Provide oxygen and assist ventilations as necessary; be prepared for respiratory failure; transport
Respiratory Arrest	Altered mental status, cyanosis; shallow, ineffective, or absent breathing	Assist ventilations with a bag-valve mask; appropriate airway maneuvers and devices; transport

4. Capillary refill, ask about wet diapers, check for tears when the child (especially an infant) cries.

5. The most common cause of cardiac arrest in infants and children is respiratory failure.

6. Fever, infection, poisoning, hypoxia, head injury.

7. The most important consideration in management of the child with a seizure is management of the airway (and ventilation).

8. Multiple bruises and injuries in various stages of healing, injury inconsistent with mechanism described, repeated calls to the same address, untreated burns, parents seem unconcerned, conflicting versions of what happened, the child is afraid to discuss what happened.

Multiple-Choice Answers

1. **(D)** Objective 1
   Children begin to fear disfigurement when they reach school age. This continues into adolescence.

2. **(D)** Objective 2
   The adolescent is between childhood and adulthood but will be most cooperative if treated as an adult.

3. **(D)** Objective 2
   All of these structural differences can lead to increased potential for airway obstruction in infants and children.

4. **(A)** Objective 2
   The fragile abdominal organs and poor abdominal protection in the infant make abdominal thrusts dangerous in the infant, so chest thrusts are used.

5. **(C)** Objective 2
   The flow of oxygen directly from oxygen delivery devices is too great for newborns. It is better to increase the oxygen content of the air around the newborn by providing "blow-by" oxygen.

6. **(A)** Objective 7
   Upper airway obstruction causes stridor as air flows through the restricted airway. Absent breath sounds and wheezing indicate lower airway obstruction. The child with an airway problem prefers to sit up, not lie down.

7. **(D)** Objective 7
   These are all signs of respiratory distress that must not be missed in assessment of infants and children.

8. **(B)** Objective 7
   The dose of activated charcoal is approximately 1 gram per kilogram, with a minimum of 12.5 grams.

9. **(B)** Objective 1
   SIDS affects infants up to 1 year of age.

10. **(B)** Objective 10
    Primary cardiac problems are unusual in children. Shock is more likely to be caused by trauma, loss of fluids through vomiting or diarrhea, poisoning, and respiratory problems.

Ambulance Operations

 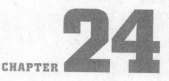

CHAPTER 24

Section 1—Always Ready

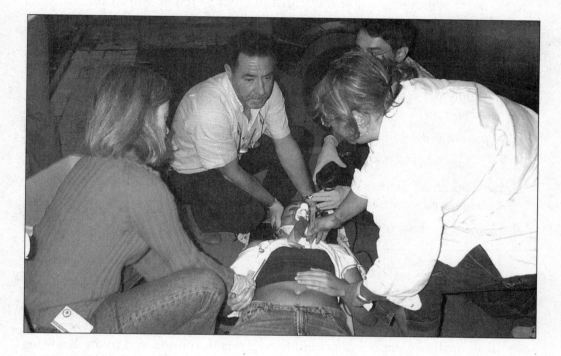

OBJECTIVES

This chapter and the review questions will help readers determine if they are able to

1. discuss the medical and nonmedical equipment needed to respond to a call;

2. list the phases of an ambulance call;

3. describe the general provisions of state laws relating to the operation of the ambulance and privileges in any or all of the following categories;

- speed
- warning lights
- sirens
- right-of-way
- parking
- turning

4. list the contributing factors to unsafe driving conditions;

5. describe the considerations that should be given to:
   - requests for escorts
   - following an escort vehicle
   - intersections

6. discuss "Due Regard for Safety of All Others" while operating an emergency vehicle;

7. state what information is essential in order to respond to a call;

8. discuss various situations that may affect response to a call;

9. differentiate between the various methods of moving the patient to the unit based upon injury or illness;

10. apply the components of the essential patient information in a written report;

11. summarize the importance of preparing the unit for the next response;

12. identify what is essential for completion of a call;

13. distinguish among the terms cleaning, disinfection, high-level disinfection, and sterilization;

14. describe how to clean or disinfect items following patient care.

Ambulance operations include getting ready for the call. This entails checking out all of your equipment (the gear on the ambulance and your personal equipment), daily inspections of your vehicle including fuel, fluids, lights, etc., and tests on all medical equipment including oxygen tank volume, and so on. Knowing how your communications system and dispatch work is also part of learning your ambulance operations systems.

Safe driving of emergency vehicles is a major concern. Intersections are the most frequent place collisions of emergency vehicles occur so training to prevent these events is important. Emergency vehicle operations include recommended driving courses and work practices that encourage alert driving. The use of seat belts and child seats for all passengers and crew is mandatory. Positioning the unit is also important. Uphill from hazards and 100 feet from wreckage are examples of planning for vehicle placement.

Post-run critiques and going over your vehicle and equipment again to make sure you are ready for the next call bring the ambulance operations full circle. Ambulance operations also include understanding procedures for interface with aeromedical transports.

Section 2—Gaining Access

OBJECTIVES

This chapter and the review questions will help readers determine if they are able to

1. describe the purpose of extrication;

2. discuss the role of the EMT in extrication;

3. identify what equipment for personal safety is required for the EMT;

4. define the fundamental components of extrication;

5. state the steps that should be taken to protect the patient during extrication;

6. evaluate various methods of gaining access to the patient;

7. distinguish between simple and complex access.

Gaining access to patients can be simple or complex. The role of the EMT is to get to the patient and care for him or her. If gaining access to the patient requires special tools and the training to use them, the EMT may have to stand by until rescue technicians gain access to the patient.

The EMT arriving on the scene will need to make an assessment as to the difficulty of gaining access. If it requires special technicians and equipment, the earlier that notification is made, the sooner it will be there to get the job done and get the EMT to the patient. It is important that scene safety be determined first and that the EMT has the PPE equal to the situation. In vehicular events this includes turnout gear, including coat, boots, helmet with eye protection, and gloves.

Remembering to "try before you pry" is always important, as in many cases, opening a door is simpler than it may initially appear. Working within the limits of your training and resources and knowing how to access the skilled personnel and equipment you need is of the utmost importance in all rescue situations.

Section 3—Hazards, Casualties, and Disasters

OBJECTIVES

This chapter and the review questions will help readers determine if they are able to

1. explain the EMT role during a call involving hazardous materials;
2. describe what the EMT should do if there is a reason to believe that there is a hazard at the scene;
3. describe the actions the EMT should take to ensure bystander safety;
4. state the role the EMT should perform until appropriately trained personnel arrive at the scene of a hazardous materials situation;
5. break down the steps to approaching a hazardous situation;
6. discuss the various environmental hazards that affect EMS;
7. describe the criteria for a multiple-casualty situation;
8. evaluate the role of the EMT in a multiple-casualty situation;
9. summarize the basic components of basic triage;
10. define the role of the EMT in a disaster operation;
11. describe the basic concepts of incident management;
12. explain the methods for preventing contamination of self, equipment, and facilities;
13. review the local mass-casualty incident plan.

The most important thing for the EMT to remember about hazardous materials is to stay out of it. Patients exposed to hazardous materials should be decontaminated and brought to the EMT for care.

Information on hazardous materials can be obtained from the DOT orange book, *Hazardous Materials, The Emergency Response Handbook*, National Fire Protection Administration (NFPA), and OSHA.

Incident Management Systems include the elements of incident command to manage resources and large incidents. Triage will be a large part of EMS at major incidents.

Scenario 1

You arrive on the scene of a motor vehicle collision and the victims are trapped inside the vehicles. Fire and police are on the scene. What should you expect to do?

SOLUTION

The first thing fire personnel should accomplish is to make the scene safe and gain access for EMS. Once that is done, you may be called on to give aid to the patient while extrication is accomplished.

Scenario 2

You are performing triage at a multiple-casualty event. A patient presents with no pulse and is not breathing. How do you classify this patient?

SOLUTION

This patient would be Code Black or considered dead. In multiple-casualty situations, the EMT should not spend time doing CPR on traumatic arrest victims. New trauma protocols call for recognizing traumatic arrest patients as being dead.

Review Questions

EXERCISES

The exercises in this review are designed to help reinforce your knowledge of the objectives for this chapter. If you find it difficult to meet any of the objectives stated, go back and review those materials again.

Section 1—Always Ready

1. Match each action below with the phase of an ambulance call in which it should be performed. (Objectives 1 and 2)
   (A) Preparation for the call
   (B) Dispatch
   (C) En route to scene
   (D) Arrival at scene
   (E) En route to receiving facility
   (F) Post-run

   _____ Cleaning and disinfection

   _____ Radio report to hospital

   _____ Determine the need for additional resources

   _____ Comply with traffic laws

   _____ Obtain location and nature of call

   _____ Vehicle inspection

2. List at least four considerations in safe emergency vehicle operations. (Objectives 3–6)

_____

_____

_____

_____

Section 2—Gaining Access

1. In what ways should you attempt to access a patient who is in a vehicle before using extrication tools? (Objectives 1–6)

_____

_____

_____

2. What is the difference between simple and complex access in extrication? (Objective 7)

_____

_____

_____

Section 3—Hazards, Casualties, and Disasters

1. You are responding to a motor vehicle collision involving a tanker truck. The bystander who called in the collision reports that a substance is leaking from the truck. You are the first to arrive on scene. Describe the actions you will take. (Objectives 1–5)

_____

_____

_____

_____

2. You have arrived on the scene of a multiple vehicle collision with fire and have been assigned to the triage sector. Match each of the following patient descriptions with their triage priority. Each letter may be used more than once. (Objectives 6–9)
   (A) Highest priority
   (B) Second priority
   (C) Lowest priority

   _____ 19-year-old female with open fractures of both lower legs.

   _____ 7-year-old male who is pulseless and apneic

   _____ 65-year-old female who is responsive only to painful stimuli

   _____ 15-year-old male who cannot move his lower extremities

   _____ 30-year-old female with abrasions and contusions to the face and upper extremities

   _____ 50-year-old male making gurgling sounds due blood in the airway

MULTIPLE-CHOICE QUESTIONS

1. Most collisions involving ambulances occur
   (A) on interstates.
   (B) with oncoming traffic.
   (C) at intersections.
   (D) on two-lane roads.

2. True or False: It is not advisable for the EMT providing patient care to wear a seat belt.
   (A) True
   (B) False

3. True or False: The use of an emergency vehicle escort is highly recommended when transporting critical patients.
   (A) True
   (B) False

4. Which of the following is the EMT's primary role when managing a scene in which a patient is entrapped in a vehicle?
   (A) patient care
   (B) hazard control
   (C) control of bystanders
   (D) use of extrication tools

5. You are inside a vehicle providing care to an entrapped patient. Which of the following pieces of personal protection equipment is required?
   (A) helmet
   (B) safety glasses or goggles
   (C) structural firefighting or bunker gear
   (D) all of the above

6. You are the first to arrive on the scene of a school bus that has collided with a tractor-trailer on a stretch of rural interstate highway. Of the following, what should you do first?
   (A) begin triage
   (B) free any entrapped victims
   (C) establish incident command
   (D) assess the need for additional resources

7. Which of the following provides information on hazardous materials?
   (A) NFPA 704 labels
   (B) U.S. DOT-approved placards
   (C) material safety data sheets
   (D) all of the above

8. As you approach the scene of a motor vehicle collision you can see that a tanker truck is on its side. Which of the following should you do?
   (A) Park down-wind from the truck.
   (B) Immediately remove patients and bystanders from the area.
   (C) Use binoculars to read the placard on the truck.
   (D) Check the truck's bill of lading.

9. EMTs should be trained to the _____ level for hazardous materials.
   (A) awareness
   (B) operations
   (C) technician
   (D) specialist

10. Which of the following best describes the EMT's role at the scene of a hazardous materials incident?
    (A) actively decontaminates patients in the warm zone
    (B) enters the hot zone to remove patients for decontamination and treatment
    (C) stays in the cold zone to receive patients after they are decontaminated
    (D) provides patient care in the warm zone

ANSWERS TO REVIEW QUESTIONS

Exercises

SECTION 1—ALWAYS READY

1. (F) **Post-run:** Cleaning and disinfection
   (E) **En route:** Radio report to hospital
   (D) **Arrival at scene:** Determine the need for additional resources
   (C) **En route to scene:** Comply with traffic laws
   (B) **Dispatch:** Obtain location and nature of call
   (A) **Preparation for the call:** Vehicle inspection

2. Attend an emergency vehicle operations class, stay mentally and physically fit, wear seat belts, be alert to changes in the weather and road conditions, use judgment in the use of sirens and warning lights, maintain a safe following distance, and use due regard for the safety of others.

SECTION 2—GAINING ACCESS

1. Open the doors, or have the patient unlock the doors or roll down the windows.

2. Simple access does not require specialized tools; complex access requires specialized tools.

SECTION 3—HAZARDS, CASUALTIES, AND DISASTERS

1. Approach the scene from an up-wind, uphill direction and get only close enough to read the placard with binoculars. Reference the DOT *Hazardous Materials* guide. Further actions depend upon the information in the guide.

2. (B) **Second priority:** 19-year-old female with open fractures of both lower legs.
   (C) **Lowest priority:** 7-year-old male who is pulseless and apneic
   (A) **Highest priority:** 65-year-old female who is responsive only to painful stimuli
   (B) **Second priority:** 15-year-old male who cannot move his lower extremities
   (A) **Highest priority:** 30-year-old female with abrasions and contusions to the face and upper extremities
   (A) **Highest priority:** 50-year-old male making gurgling sounds due to blood in the airway

Multiple-Choice Answers

1. **(C)** Section 1, Objective 4
Most ambulance collisions occur at intersections in daylight hours during good weather. Always exercise extreme caution when approaching intersections, even if you have the right of way.

2. **(B)** Section 1, Objective 3
The EMT should wear a seatbelt even while providing patient care.

3. **(B)** Section 1, Objective 5
The use of an escort is never recommended because drivers do not anticipate a second emergency vehicle after yielding to the first.

4. **(B)** Section 2, Objective 2
The EMT must provide patient care, but only after taking measures to ensure his or her own safety.

5. **(D)** Section 2, Objective 3
Extrication carries a high risk of injury if proper protective equipment is not worn. All of the items listed must be worn by the EMT who enters the vehicle to care for a patient during extrication.

6. **(D)** Section 3, Objective 8
Care to victims will be delayed unless additional resources are dispatched immediately.

7. **(D)** Section 3, Objective 2
Depending on the location of a hazardous materials incident, any of these sources can provide information about the hazardous materials. Placards are used in transportation of hazardous materials, NFPA 704 labels are used on fixed storage structures, and material data safety sheets are maintained on-site where the material is used.

8. **(C)** Section 3, Objective 2
The scene should be approached from an up-wind, uphill direction and the EMT should only get as close as necessary to read the placard with binoculars.

9. **(A)** Section 3, Objective 2
At a minimum, EMTs should be trained to the awareness level. However, for EMTs employed in fire departments or certain industrial settings, a higher level of training may be required by the employer.

10. **(C)** Section 3, Objective 1
The EMT's primary role at a hazardous materials incident is patient care, which is provided in the cold zone.

Final Exams

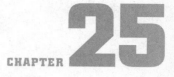

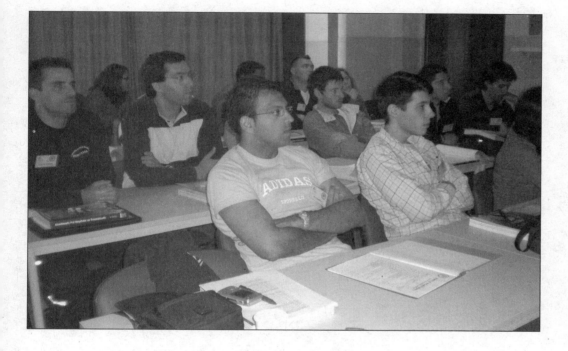

This chapter contains two practice examinations that will help you prepare for test day. Each exam contains 100 multiple-choice questions, which you must answer within two hours. Be sure to review the test-taking strategies outlined in the first chapter before taking these practice exams.

For maximum benefit, it is strongly recommended that you take each practice examination in one sitting as if it were the actual test. Remember to read each question carefully before choosing your answers. Select the choice you believe to be the correct answer and mark your answers on the appropriate answer sheet.

The answers to the test questions and their explanations appear at the end of each practice exam. An overall score of 70 percent is considered passing (in other words, you will need at least 70 correct answers). Remember that although the EMT exam is designed to determine whether or not an individual has the **minimum** basic knowledge required to become a certified EMT, nobody wants to "just pass." To be an effective EMT and to fully serve your community you should be familiar with all of the topics covered in this book. If you do not pass the exam, you may retake it after 14 days.

Good luck!

Answer Sheet

EXAM 1

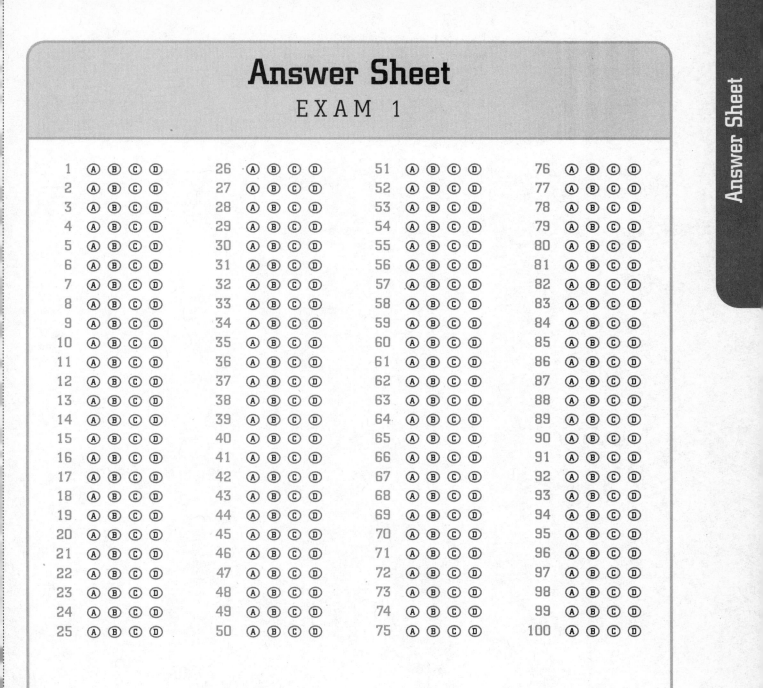

Exam 1

1. EMTs are trained using a National Standard Curriculum that is published by the
   (A) U.S. Department of Homeland Security (DHS).
   (B) U.S. Department of Defense (DOD).
   (C) U.S. Department of Health and Human Services (HHS).
   (D) National Highway Traffic Safety Administration (NHTSA).

2. Which of the following best describes the purpose of quality improvement programs?
   (A) Ensure that no mistakes occur in emergency medical care.
   (B) Detect patterns of care that can be addressed through continuing education or changes in the system.
   (C) Detect individual provider's mistakes so that disciplinary action can be taken.
   (D) Allow the state licensing agency to revoke the licenses of incompetent EMS providers.

3. You are responding to a call for a sick person. Upon arrival there is no bleeding noted, and the patient is not coughing or vomiting. Which of the following items should be used for personal protection against communicable disease?
   (A) gloves
   (B) eye protection
   (C) face mask
   (D) all of the above

4. The regulations for training of EMTs and defining their scope of practice are determined at the _____ level of government.
   (A) federal
   (B) state
   (C) regional
   (D) local

5. A father standing over his dying child shouts, "No, take me!" This is an example of which stage of grief?
   (A) denial
   (B) anger
   (C) bargaining
   (D) depression

6. Your patient is a 25-year-old male who has just learned that his mother has died. He is screaming, crying, and punching the wall. Which of the following statements would best meet the patient's needs?
   - (A) "You need to settle down. Your actions aren't helping anything."
   - (B) "I'm very sorry that your mother died. Is there someone I can call for you?"
   - (C) "If you continue to behave this way, I will have no choice but to call the police."
   - (D) "We can't stay here all day. If you want to go to the hospital, we need to do it now."

7. In which of the following situations would it be appropriate to call for a critical incident stress debriefing?
   - (A) Your partner seems to be experiencing "burn out" and cannot get along with anyone.
   - (B) An aero-medical helicopter carrying crew members with whom your service interacts regularly crashes, killing all aboard.
   - (C) You are distraught after receiving disciplinary action from your supervisor and fear you may lose your job.
   - (D) You just marked in-service from a call in which you found a 75-year-old male with terminal cancer had died in his sleep.

8. Which of the following is the best way to minimize conflicts between your work life and family life?
   - (A) Avoid discussing work with your family.
   - (B) Discuss aspects of your work in a way that does not cause your family undue concern.
   - (C) Only share with your family those aspects of your work that are most disturbing to you.
   - (D) Only share with your family aspects of your work in which you can laugh about the calls you have been on.

9. You are the first to arrive on the scene of a farmer who is trapped in a grain silo. Which of the following should you do?
   - (A) Stage at the scene and await rescue personnel, even if they are several minutes away.
   - (B) Enter the silo from the top to rappel down to the patient's level.
   - (C) Find neighboring farmers who are willing to enter the silo to rescue the patient.
   - (D) Inform the family that it is not possible for the farmer to have survived the incident.

10. You are responding to a report of a person shot at a bar. What information is most important that you ask the dispatcher?
    - (A) whether there are additional patients
    - (B) what type of gun was used
    - (C) whether law enforcement can advise if the scene is safe
    - (D) if the patient is conscious or unconscious

11. You are continuing on the call described in the previous question. Just before arriving at the scene dispatch informs you that law enforcement has not arrived, but the caller advises that the perpetrator is no longer on the scene and the patient is not breathing. Which of the following should you do?
    (A) Park in front of the bar and wait for law enforcement before entering.
    (B) Enter the scene and begin patient care.
    (C) Park a block or two away and shut off your lights and siren while awaiting law enforcement to secure the scene.
    (D) Circle the block until you see law enforcement arrive.

12. When lifting a heavy object the EMT should
    (A) avoid reaching overhead.
    (B) twist at the waist.
    (C) bend at the waist.
    (D) avoid using the legs.

13. You are on-scene at the residence of a woman whose husband beat her with his fists and hit her several times in the head with a telephone receiver. She responds only to painful stimuli and has active bleeding from a number of lacerations on the head and face. Objects and furniture in the room are in disarray from the struggle. Which of the following best describes how you should approach the patient?
    (A) The patient is your only concern. Move whatever you must to gain easy access to the patient.
    (B) The patient is your priority. Provide treatment but do not disturb things more than necessary. Make a note of anything you move.
    (C) You are obligated to assist law enforcement in collecting evidence, even if it delays patient care.
    (D) Do not approach the patient until law enforcement has collected evidence.

14. Your patient is a hiker who became lost and fell down into a ravine. The best device for getting the patient out of the ravine is a
    (A) stair chair.
    (B) basket stretcher.
    (C) long backboard.
    (D) wheeled stretcher.

15. Ensuring that you obtain quality continuing education and submit documentation for renewal of your license or certificate is _____ responsibility.
    (A) your
    (B) your employer's
    (C) your medical director's
    (D) your EMT instructor's

16. Your patient is a 57-year-old female with a history of emphysema. She called 911 because of difficulty breathing. She lives in a third floor apartment with no elevator. Which of the following is the best way to get the patient downstairs?
    (A) Use a stair chair.
    (B) Place the patient supine on the cot.
    (C) Use a scoop stretcher.
    (D) Have the patient walk.

17. Which of the following is an example of online medical control?
    (A) radio communication with a physician at the receiving hospital
    (B) protocols
    (C) an audit and review of ambulance calls conducted by the medical director
    (D) radio communication with dispatch

18. You arrive on the scene of a reported sick person in a park. The patient is a 25-year-old male who is acting strangely and cannot answer your questions appropriately. He is pale and sweating profusely. He denies that he is sick and wants you to leave him alone. Which of the following is the best course of action?
    (A) Do not make further contact with the patient until law enforcement arrives.
    (B) Ask the patient for a relative's phone number so you can obtain consent to treat him.
    (C) Treat him under the doctrine of implied consent.
    (D) Do not treat the patient unless he can be convinced to give expressed consent.

19. You are transferring the care of a patient with chest pain to staff in the emergency department. One of the nurses asks why you did not administer oxygen to the patient and states she is going to report you for negligence. The patient is later released from the hospital after the physician determined the patient's pain was not due to a heart problem. Which of the following best explains whether or not you can be found negligent in your care of the patient?
    (A) You may be negligent because you breached your duty to respond.
    (B) You are negligent because you failed to act as a reasonable person with similar training would have acted.
    (C) You are not negligent because no harm was caused to the patient by your omission of care.
    (D) You are not negligent because no monetary amount can be placed on the harm caused to the patient.

20. You are transporting an elderly female who states she cannot remember how she fractured her arm. You notice that she has both old and new bruises on her back and legs. The patient's daughter-in-law states that the patient is "senile" and that she frequently runs into things and falls down. Which of the following best describes your obligation to the patient?
    (A) There is not sufficient evidence to prove abuse. Therefore, you can be sued for reporting suspected abuse.
    (B) You have no legal obligation to report suspected abuse, but you do have an ethical obligation to inform the hospital staff of your suspicions.
    (C) You have both a legal and an ethical obligation to report your suspicions to the local agency that investigates reports of elder abuse.
    (D) You may have a legal obligation, but there is no ethical obligation to report this situation.

21. You are transporting a 32-year-old male who was ejected from his motorcycle when he hit the side of a car that pulled out in front of him. He was not wearing a helmet and appears to have severe head and internal injuries. It seems almost certain he will die. His driver's license indicates he is an organ donor. Which of the following statements is most accurate concerning this situation?
    (A) Provide the care you would give to any patient in this condition and inform the receiving facility that the patient is an organ donor.
    (B) Provide the care you would give to any patient in this condition, but the internal injuries rule out the possibility of organ donation.
    (C) Treat the patient extremely aggressively and inform the receiving facility that the patient is an organ donor.
    (D) Go through the motions of providing care, but the patient will not survive and his organs cannot be used.

22. Your patient has a deformity about 2 inches above his right wrist, on the same side as the thumb. In writing your report you should describe this injury as
    (A) distal to the wrist on the medial side.
    (B) proximal to the wrist on the medial side.
    (C) distal to the wrist on the lateral side.
    (D) proximal to the wrist on the lateral side.

23. Which of the following best describes the relationship between the esophagus and trachea?
    (A) The esophagus is anterior to the trachea.
    (B) The esophagus is posterior to the trachea.
    (C) The trachea is superior to the esophagus.
    (D) The esophagus is inferior to the trachea.

24. The arteries that can be found on either side of the larynx in the anterior neck are the _____ arteries.
    (A) carotid
    (B) jugular
    (C) vertebral
    (D) brachial

25. Your patient tells you that her platelet count is low. You should be concerned that
    (A) her blood is not carrying enough oxygen.
    (B) she is at risk for infection.
    (C) her blood may not clot properly.
    (D) she cannot sustain an adequate blood glucose level.

26. Your patient has a blue–black discoloration over his right cheekbone. In your report you would refer to this injury as a(n)
    (A) abrasion over the mandible.
    (B) avulsion over the orbit.
    (C) contusion over the zygoma.
    (D) hematoma over the maxilla.

27. Your patient has a deformity of the spine between the shoulder blades. The injury is at the level of the _____ spine.
    (A) cervical
    (B) thoracic
    (C) lumbar
    (D) sacral

28. Your patient has a deformity with bone protruding from the mid-thigh. This is described as an open fracture of the
    (A) hip.
    (B) femur.
    (C) tibia.
    (D) fibula.

29. Oxygen, nutrients, and wastes are exchanged between the cells of the body at the level of the
    (A) arteries.
    (B) arterioles.
    (C) capillaries.
    (D) venules.

30. The roof of the mouth is formed by the
    (A) turbinates.
    (B) uvula.
    (C) palate.
    (D) thyroid cartilage.

31. Deoxygenated blood from the body returns to the _____ of the heart via the _____.
    (A) right atrium; vena cava
    (B) left atrium; vena cava
    (C) right atrium; pulmonary vein
    (D) left atrium; pulmonary artery

32. Which of the following is a function of white blood cells?
    (A) blood clotting
    (B) carrying oxygen
    (C) carrying carbon dioxide
    (D) fighting infection

33. The blood pressure in the arteries during contraction of the heart is known as the
    (A) pulse pressure.
    (B) systolic blood pressure.
    (C) perfusion pressure.
    (D) diastolic blood pressure.

34. The back of the head is referred to anatomically as the _____ region.
    (A) occipital
    (B) parietal
    (C) temporal
    (D) cranial

35. Which of the following is a characteristic of skeletal muscle?
    (A) smooth in appearance under the microscope
    (B) functions involuntarily
    (C) controls the diameter of blood vessels
    (D) attaches to bone via tendons

36. Your patient is a 55-year-old male complaining of chest pain and shortness of breath. You should assess his pulse at the _____ artery.
    (A) carotid
    (B) brachial
    (C) radial
    (D) femoral

37. In newborns, the pulse should be obtained at the _____ artery.
    (A) carotid
    (B) brachial
    (C) radial
    (D) femoral

38. You just listened to your patient's breath sounds bilaterally in the upper lobes at the mid-clavicular line. You did not hear breath sounds on the right. You should document that
    (A) breath sounds are absent on the right side.
    (B) breath sounds are present, but unequal.
    (C) breath sounds are clear on the left, but not on the right.
    (D) you subsequently listened to breath sounds bilaterally at the bases in the mid-axillary line.

39. The first step in an initial assessment is evaluation of the patient's
    (A) mental status.
    (B) airway.
    (C) circulation.
    (D) breathing.

40. You have just arrived on the scene of a call for a sick person. The patient, a 50-year-old female, opens the door when you knock. Which of the following should be documented about her mental status?
    (A) alert
    (B) responds to verbal stimuli
    (C) oriented times three
    (D) confused

41. You are called to the scene of a patient who was struck in the head with a baseball bat. The patient is not moving or speaking but when you touch the injured area he moves and cries out. The patient's level of consciousness is described as
    (A) unresponsive.
    (B) obtunded.
    (C) responsive to painful stimuli.
    (D) disoriented.

42. In which of the following adult patients should the EMT begin positive pressure ventilation with a bag-valve mask device?
    (A) responds to painful stimuli; ventilatory rate of 12
    (B) responds to verbal stimuli; ventilatory rate of 20
    (C) unresponsive; ventilatory rate of 12
    (D) responds to painful stimuli; ventilatory rate of 8

43. Which of the following best describes the proper measurement of a flexible suction catheter for oral suctioning?
    (A) from the corner of the mouth, around the ear, to the sternal notch
    (B) from the center of the chin to the angle of the mandible
    (C) from the nare to the corner of the mouth on the same side
    (D) from the corner of the mouth to the earlobe

44. Your patient is a 6-month-old infant who is unresponsive, limp, and cyanotic. His mother states that he choked while eating peaches. You cannot visualize anything in the airway and your attempt to ventilate him is unsuccessful. What should you do next?
    (A) perform five back blows followed by five chest thrusts, inspect the mouth, attempt to ventilate
    (B) perform chest thrusts until the foreign material is dislodged, attempt to ventilate
    (C) perform abdominal thrusts until the foreign material is dislodged, attempt to ventilate
    (D) perform 30 chest compressions at a rate of 100/minute using the landmarks for CPR

45. In an unresponsive patient, the EMT should assess the _____ pulse.
    (A) femoral
    (B) brachial
    (C) radial
    (D) carotid

46. Which of the following statements about capillary refill is most accurate?
    (A) may not be useful in assessing adult patients
    (B) is most useful in pediatric patients
    (C) is used to assess perfusion when a radial pulse is not present
    (D) is not useful in any age group

47. You arrive on the scene of a motor vehicle collision to find a 14-month-old female still restrained in her car seat. The patient is stable, but the crash is significant and you recognize the need for spinal immobilization. Which of the following methods is best for immobilizing this patient?
    (A) Immobilize the patient in the car seat.
    (B) Remove the patient from the car seat using a short spinal immobilization device.
    (C) Tip the car seat backward and remove the patient onto a long backboard, maintaining alignment of spine.
    (D) Use a vest-type extrication device to remove the patient from the car seat.

48. Your patient is a 20-year-old female with a stab wound to the right upper chest, just below the clavicle. She is conscious but obviously having difficulty breathing. Her respirations are fast and shallow, her skin is pale and clammy, and she has a weak, rapid radial pulse. There is moderate bleeding from the wound. Which of the following best describes the sequence of treatment of this patient?
    (A) Cover the wound with an occlusive dressing, apply firm direct pressure over the dressing, perform a rapid trauma assessment, immobilize the spine, and apply oxygen.
    (B) Apply high-flow oxygen, check the breath sounds on both sides, take vital signs, apply a wet dressing to the wound, and prepare for transport.
    (C) Cover the wound with an occlusive dressing sealed on three sides, apply high-flow oxygen, perform a rapid trauma assessment, and prepare for transport.
    (D) Assist ventilations with a bag-valve mask and supplemental oxygen, control bleeding from the wound, perform a focused physical exam, and prepare for transport.

49. Your patient is a 33-year-old male who was injured while using a chain saw. He has an 8-inch laceration to the medial left thigh, 9 inches proximal to the knee, with heavy bleeding. Which of the following should be attempted first?
    (A) a circumferential pressure dressing
    (B) a tourniquet
    (C) direct pressure
    (D) manual compression of the femoral artery

50. All of the following are indications for spinal immobilization EXCEPT
    (A) when the patient complains of neck or back pain.
    (B) if the mechanism of injury suggests spine injuries.
    (C) all falls and motor vehicle collisions.
    (D) when the patient is found unconscious with no witnesses.

51. Your patient works at a meat-processing plant where he was accidentally slashed across the abdomen with a sharp knife. He has loops of intestine protruding from a 5-inch wound across his abdomen. He responds to your voice by opening his eyes, is pale and diaphoretic, has shallow respirations at about 24 per minute, and a weak, rapid radial pulse greater than 100 per minute. Which of the following should you do first?
    (A) manually stabilize the cervical spine
    (B) control bleeding from the wound
    (C) complete your assessment to check for other injuries
    (D) apply high-flow oxygen

52. Your patient is a 3-year-old male who fell onto a garden tool. He has a laceration to the abdomen through which a loop of intestine is protruding. He is crying loudly and has good skin color and capillary refill. How should you treat this wound?
    (A) Apply a sterile dressing moistened with saline, cover the dressing with foil or plastic, and secure in place.
    (B) Apply a dry, sterile dressing and tape in place.
    (C) Apply an occlusive dressing, such as petroleum gauze, and secure with a bandage encircling the abdomen.
    (D) Place a moist, sterile dressing over the wound and apply a cold pack.

53. Your patient is a 30-year-old male in good health who was injured when he was thrown from a bull in a rodeo event. You should be concerned about his ventilatory rate if it is
    (A) 12 per minute.
    (B) 18 per minute.
    (C) 20 per minute.
    (D) 24 per minute.

54. Your patient is a 20-year-old female who was struck by a vehicle at approximately 20 miles per hour as she crossed the street. She had no loss of consciousness. She has an open fracture of her right lower leg. Your initial assessment reveals that she is breathing 20 times per minute and has a radial pulse at a rate of about 80. You should first
    (A) complete a full spinal immobilization.
    (B) apply oxygen by nonrebreather mask at a rate of 12 liters per minute.
    (C) complete a detailed physical examination.
    (D) splint the lower extremity injury.

55. Which of the following patients has a significant mechanism of injury?
    (A) A 25-year-old male vehicle driver whose passenger is dead on the scene.
    (B) An 85-year-old female who fell when she tripped on a throw rug in her kitchen.
    (C) A 12-year-old male with a stab wound to his forearm.
    (D) A 30-year-old female vehicle driver who was unrestrained in a 20 miles per hour collision.

56. You have performed a rapid trauma assessment on your patient, which revealed that he has a single gunshot wound to his left anterior chest with no exit wound. The patient responds to verbal stimuli. Which of the following is the correct classification and transport decision for this patient?
    (A) critical; consider immediate transport before further assessment or treatment
    (B) critical; a more detailed assessment is needed before moving the patient
    (C) noncritical; a more detailed assessment should be performed before moving the patient
    (D) noncritical; the patient should be immobilized and further assessment should be done during transport

57. You are called to assist a patient who has cut his finger while cutting open a box. Bleeding is easily controlled with direct pressure. This patient should be considered
    (A) critical; transport immediately.
    (B) critical; perform an assessment focused on the injury and the mechanism of that injury.
    (C) noncritical; perform an assessment focused on the injury and the mechanism of that injury.
    (D) noncritical; transport immediately.

58. Your patient is a 12-month-old whose head and neck were burned when he pulled a cup of hot coffee off of a table. The percentage of body surface area burned according to the Rule of Nines is
    (A) 4.5%.
    (B) 9%.
    (C) 18%.
    (D) 24%.

59. Your patient is a 40-year-old male who sustained burns to his anterior chest and entire right arm when he poured charcoal lighter onto hot coals in his barbeque grill. The burned areas are red, moist, and blistered. Which of the following best describes the severity and body surface area of the burns?
    (A) superficial; 18%
    (B) full thickness; 27%
    (C) partial thickness; 36%
    (D) partial thickness; 27%

60. Your patient is a 90-year-old female who received partial thickness burns to her lower abdomen and the anterior lower extremities when she spilled boiling water on herself. This injury is classified as a _____ burn.
    (A) minor
    (B) moderate
    (C) significant
    (D) critical

61. Injuries to the spinal cord at the _____ level may impair respirations.
    (A) cervical
    (B) thoracic
    (C) lumbar
    (D) sacral

62. Your patient is an industrial worker who had a dry powdered chemical spilled on him. This situation is best managed by first
    (A) flushing the skin with copious amounts of water.
    (B) wiping the skin with a damp wash cloth.
    (C) brushing away as much of the powder as possible.
    (D) coating the skin with vegetable or mineral oil.

63. Diabetes is caused by a problem with the
    (A) liver.
    (B) gall bladder.
    (C) spleen.
    (D) pancreas.

64. Which of the following medications is carried on a BLS ambulance?
    (A) albuterol
    (B) epinephrine
    (C) nitroglycerin
    (D) activated charcoal

65. The medication an EMT may administer in the case of overdose or oral poisoning is
    (A) activated charcoal.
    (B) nitroglycerin.
    (C) epinephrine.
    (D) syrup of ipecac.

66. Your patient is a 35-year-old female with a history of diabetes. She is confused and her husband states she has not felt well since the evening before. Of the following, which is the most important information for the EMT to obtain?
    (A) whether there is a family history of diabetes
    (B) whether the patient has been urinating frequently
    (C) the name of the patient's physician
    (D) whether the patient checks her blood glucose level daily

67. Your patient states she thinks she is having an allergic reaction to shellfish. Which of the following is your first concern?
    (A) whether there is a history of allergy to shellfish
    (B) obtaining the patient's pulse rate
    (C) assessing the patient's airway
    (D) checking the skin for hives or rashes

68. When you perspire, heat is lost from your body via
    (A) radiation.
    (B) conduction.
    (C) convection.
    (D) evaporation.

69. Which of the following statements concerning a patient's dangerous, disturbing, or inappropriate behavior is most accurate?
    (A) It is strictly a law enforcement issue.
    (B) It is a medical issue that may require the assistance of law enforcement.
    (C) It is a private matter between the patient and his or her family.
    (D) It is strictly a medical issue and contacting law enforcement is a violation of the patient's rights.

70. Your patient is a 55-year-old female complaining of difficulty breathing. She states that it is hard to catch her breath. Which of the following should you do first?
(A) Use a head-tilt chin-lift to ensure an open airway.
(B) Assume the airway is open and continue with the initial assessment.
(C) Assume the initial assessment is complete and obtain a focused history.
(D) Assist the patient with her metered-dose inhaler.

71. Your patient is a 7-months pregnant female who tripped on a curb and twisted her ankle. Bystanders are insisting that the patient lie flat. During your assessment you find that the patient's respirations are 20, heart rate is 90, and blood pressure is 78/50. The most likely explanation for this is
(A) the patient has experienced more severe injuries from the fall than initially thought.
(B) these are normal vital signs at this stage of pregnancy.
(C) the patient's position is allowing the uterus to prevent adequate blood return to the heart.
(D) the fall resulted in placenta previa and the patient has internal bleeding.

72. Your patient is a 30-year-old female who is 8 months pregnant. She states that she is having regular contractions and feels the need to have a bowel movement. You should advise the patient that
(A) she must remove her undergarments so you can check for crowning.
(B) there is plenty of time to get to the hospital since preterm deliveries take longer.
(C) she needs to empty her bowels before you transport her to the hospital.
(D) she is in false labor because she has not yet reached full term.

73. You are called to a residence for an 18-year-old female who appears pregnant and states she is in labor. Which of the following should you determine first?
(A) how far apart the contractions are
(B) whether the baby is crowning
(C) whether the mother had regular prenatal care
(D) what hospital the patient wants to go to

74. Your patient is a 78-year-old female in a nursing home. The nursing staff called because the patient, who normally is oriented to person, place, and time, does not recognize her caregivers and is confused about where she is and what day it is. Which of the following best describes the level of concern you should have for this patient's condition?
(A) This is of low concern because loss of memory is a normal part of aging.
(B) This is of low concern. It is probably a stroke, but nothing can be done about it and the patient is stable.
(C) This is of significant concern because the changes can be caused by a number of medical problems that may be reversible.
(D) This is of significant concern, but once these changes occur they are irreversible.

75. The most common cause of seizures in children is
    (A) head injury.
    (B) diabetes.
    (C) fever.
    (D) allergic reactions.

76. All of the following statements concerning nitroglycerin are true EXCEPT that it is
    (A) carried in tablet form on BLS ambulances.
    (B) available as tablet or spray.
    (C) administered under the tongue.
    (D) used to dilate the coronary arteries.

77. Your patient is a 60-year-old male with a history of emphysema and chronic bronchitis. He is sitting at the kitchen table, leaning forward on his elbows. You notice a metered-dose inhaler lying on the table. His head is bobbing, his eyes are closed, and he does not acknowledge your presence. His face and nail beds are cyanotic, and his skin is diaphoretic. His respiratory rate is 44 and shallow, but you do not hear wheezing. He has an irregular radial pulse of about 88. Which of the following is the first action you should take?
    (A) administer high-flow oxygen by nonrebreather mask
    (B) assist the patient with his Ventolin inhaler
    (C) assist the patient's ventilations with a bag-valve mask
    (D) lie the patient supine and insert a nonvisualized airway such as a CombiTube, LMA, or King LT

78. Your patient is a 25-year-old male who complains of a sudden onset of shortness of breath while playing a video game. He denies other complaints. He has no history of asthma or any other chronic conditions, takes no medications, and has no allergies. He appears to be having difficulty breathing, with a respiratory rate of 26 per minute, although there is no cyanosis. His Pulse Ox is 93% on room air. Upon auscultating the breath sounds you are unable to hear breath sounds in the upper lobe of the right lung. Otherwise, breath sounds are clear. The most likely explanation for this is
    (A) spontaneous pneumothorax.
    (B) pulmonary embolism.
    (C) acute pulmonary edema.
    (D) hyperventilation syndrome.

79. Your patient is an obese 55-year-old female with a history of diabetes and smoking. She is complaining of pain in her upper back between the shoulder blades, shortness of breath, and nausea. The symptoms began about 45 minutes ago as she was driving home from the grocery store. She is alert and anxious. Her skin is slightly pale, moist, and cool. Her blood pressure is 150/88, pulse is 84 with an occasional irregular beat, and respirations are 20 with adequate depth. You hear fine crackles in the bases of both lungs. Which of the following problems is most likely?
    (A) spontaneous pneumothorax
    (B) hyperventilation syndrome
    (C) acute coronary syndrome
    (D) pneumonia

80. Your patient is a 58-year-old male found "down" in his office by a coworker who last saw the patient a half an hour earlier. The patient has a history of diabetes, but additional history is unavailable. On your arrival, the patient is pulseless and apneic, but no one is doing CPR. You should immediately
    (A) perform 5 cycles of CPR at a ratio of 30 compressions to 2 breaths.
    (B) get a history to determine exactly how long the patient has been down.
    (C) apply the AED.
    (D) check the blood glucose level.

81. You are caring for an adult patient in cardiac arrest. After 2 minutes of CPR initially, you attach the AED pads and allow the AED to analyze the rhythm. A shock is advised and delivered. You should immediately
    (A) analyze the rhythm again.
    (B) check the carotid pulse.
    (C) deliver a second shock.
    (D) begin CPR.

82. You have attached an AED to an adult patient. The AED gives a "No shock advised" message. You should immediately
    (A) reanalyze the rhythm to ensure there is really no shock advised.
    (B) override the AED to deliver a shock.
    (C) begin CPR.
    (D) check with medical control about the advisability of continuing resuscitative efforts.

83. Your patient is a 72-year-old diabetic who presents with a sudden onset of facial drooping and difficulty speaking. You have checked the blood glucose level and it is 100 mg/dL. You should suspect that the
    (A) patient's blood glucose level is too low and administer oral glucose.
    (B) patient's blood glucose level is too high.
    (C) patient is having a stroke and assess for arm drift.
    (D) patient is having a seizure.

84. Your patient is a 59-year-old male who complained of a sudden onset of a severe headache. On your arrival the patient responds to painful stimuli only. The respirations are 20, pulse is 52, strong and regular, and the blood pressure is 182/102. You should treat the patient as if he is suffering from a
    (A) stroke.
    (B) seizure.
    (C) cardiac emergency.
    (D) diabetic emergency.

85. Your patient is suffering from a severe anaphylactic reaction. You assist him in administering epinephrine via his prescribed auto-injector because epinephrine will cause
    (A) vasodilation and bronchodilation.
    (B) vasoconstriction and bronchoconstriction.
    (C) vasoconstriction and bronchodilation.
    (D) vasodilation and bronchoconstriction.

86. You have administered epinephrine to a patient with an anaphylactic reaction, which has greatly reduced his signs and symptoms. The patient does not wish to be transported to the hospital. You should advise the patient that
    (A) he can call 911 again if his symptoms reappear.
    (B) he should follow up with his physician if his symptoms are not entirely gone in 24 hours.
    (C) he should take some Benadryl (diphenhydramine) to alleviate his rash and hives.
    (D) the effects of epinephrine are very short and the reappearance of his symptoms may be life threatening.

87. Your patient is a 19-year-old male who was bitten by a snake just above his ankle. He is complaining of weakness, nausea, and pain at the site of envenomation. Which of the following is most appropriate in the care of this patient?
    (A) Administer epinephrine by auto-injector.
    (B) Get as complete a description of the snake as possible.
    (C) Elevate the leg on pillows during transport.
    (D) Apply ice to the area of envenomation.

88. You respond to a college dorm for a report of a "sick person." Your patient is a 20-year-old female who is prone on the bed and unresponsive to painful stimuli. There is a strong odor of alcohol about the patient. Which of the following statements about this situation is most accurate?
    (A) This is a potentially life-threatening situation and you should transport the patient to the hospital.
    (B) You should advise the patient's roommate to observe the patient carefully for the next couple of hours.
    (C) You should advise the patient's roommate to allow the patient to "sleep it off."
    (D) This is a matter for law enforcement and you should contact the university police department.

89. Your patient is an 82-year-old female complaining of intermittent, "crampy" abdominal pain, along with nausea and constipation. On your examination, the patient is unable to localize the pain. Which of the following statements about this situation is most accurate?
    (A) These findings indicate a mild disorder that does not require emergency treatment.
    (B) The patient most likely has a mild disorder, but should be transported for evaluation.
    (C) These findings are common in the elderly and a laxative should be suggested to relieve the discomfort.
    (D) The patient has a potentially life-threatening condition and must be transported to the emergency department for evaluation.

90. Your patient is a 72-year-old female who lives in an older apartment building with no air conditioning. The high temperatures have been above 90° Fahrenheit for 5 days. The patient's daughter called when she found the patient with a decreased level of consciousness and a temperature in the apartment of 94°. Which of the following should you do first?
    (A) Remove the patient from the apartment.
    (B) Remove the patient's clothes.
    (C) Apply cold packs to the neck, armpits, and groin.
    (D) Give the patient plenty of plain, cool water to drink.

91. You are staged on the scene of a water-rescue attempt. An 8-year-old male fell through the ice while ice skating and has been submerged for 20 minutes. When the patient is removed from the water, you should immediately
    (A) ask the parents to identify their child for the medical examiner.
    (B) assess the patient's airway, breathing, and circulation and begin CPR if no pulse is found within 5 seconds.
    (C) assess the patient's airway, breathing, and circulation and begin CPR if no pulse is found within 10 seconds.
    (D) begin active rewarming of the patient before assuming that the patient is in cardiac arrest.

92. Your patient complains of feeling sad, worthless, and hopeless. He is tearful as he explains to you that he cannot sleep or eat and that no one understands how he feels. This is most consistent with
    (A) depression.
    (B) anxiety.
    (C) bipolar disorder.
    (D) schizophrenia.

93. Your patient is a 34-year-old female who called 911 because she attempted suicide by cutting her wrists. The lacerations are superficial and you have controlled the bleeding. Which of the following statements about this situation is most accurate?
    (A) The patient is obviously just trying to get attention because she called 911 herself and the wounds are superficial.
    (B) Now that the patient has gotten the attention she is seeking, it is unlikely that she will attempt suicide in the future.
    (C) You should treat this as a serious suicide attempt, empathize with the patient to gain her trust, and transport.
    (D) You should transport, but remain impersonal and give as little attention to the patient as possible to demonstrate that attempting suicide is not a way to get attention.

94. All of the following are characteristic of hyperglycemia EXCEPT
    (A) warm, flushed, dry skin.
    (B) rapid onset of an altered level of consciousness.
    (C) extreme thirst and hunger.
    (D) fruity odor to the breath that may be confused with alcohol consumption.

95. Your patient is a 48-year-old male who became lost while hiking in the woods in below-freezing temperatures. He was found by a neighbor, who called 911. You find the patient sitting on a fallen tree about one-quarter of a mile into the woods. The patient's chief complaint is that both of his feet are numb. He has no other complaints and denies both trauma and a history of medical problems. It is not possible to get your vehicle any closer to the patient, and you will not be able to bring the ambulance stretcher to the patient. Which of the following should you do?
    (A) Determine whether the patient has superficial cold injury to the feet or deep cold injury. If it is deep cold injury, it is safe to have the patient walk to the ambulance.
    (B) Determine whether the patient has superficial cold injury to the feet or deep cold injury. If it is superficial cold injury, the patient can walk to the ambulance.
    (C) Start rewarming the feet, immobilize the patient on a long backboard, and carry him to the ambulance, asking assistance from the neighbor, if necessary.
    (D) Utilize a basket-type stretcher to carry the patient to the ambulance, calling for additional help if necessary.

96. Under which circumstances of complicated childbirth would the EMT place a gloved hand in the vagina to attempt to push the infant several inches back into the birth canal?
    (A) prolapsed umbilical cord
    (B) umbilical cord is around the infant's neck
    (C) placenta previa
    (D) breech birth with head undelivered

97. You are triaging patients at a mass casualty incident and you are presented with an ambulatory patient with an obvious fracture of the right forearm. He should be classified as
    (A) red.
    (B) yellow.
    (C) green.
    (D) black.

98. You are triaging patients at a mass casualty incident. You are presented with a patient who has an open wound to the right anterior chest and is having difficulty breathing. This patient should be classified as
    (A) red.
    (B) yellow.
    (C) green.
    (D) black.

99. You are responding to a motor vehicle collision involving a tanker truck. You have identified a placard on the back of the tanker. You should reference it with which of the following resources?
    (A) DOT Emergency Response Guidebook
    (B) NFPA 704 Manual
    (C) CHEMTREC
    (D) local fire department personnel

100. When correcting an error on an EMS form, the EMT should
    (A) draw a line through the mistake, write the word "error," and initial the correction.
    (B) use white-out, making sure to do so on all copies.
    (C) tear up the report and start over.
    (D) completely mark out the error with ink and initial it.

If there is still time remaining, you may review your answers.

Answer Key

EXAM 1

1.	D	26.	C	51.	B	76.	A
2.	B	27.	B	52.	A	77.	C
3.	A	28.	B	53.	D	78.	A
4.	B	29.	C	54.	B	79.	C
5.	C	30.	C	55.	A	80.	A
6.	B	31.	A	56.	A	81.	D
7.	B	32.	D	57.	C	82.	C
8.	B	33.	B	58.	C	83.	C
9.	A	34.	A	59.	D	84.	A
10.	C	35.	D	60.	D	85.	C
11.	C	36.	C	61.	A	86.	D
12.	A	37.	B	62.	C	87.	B
13.	B	38.	D	63.	D	88.	A
14.	B	39.	B	64.	D	89.	D
15.	A	40.	A	65.	A	90.	A
16.	A	41.	C	66.	B	91.	C
17.	A	42.	D	67.	C	92.	A
18.	C	43.	D	68.	D	93.	C
19.	C	44.	D	69.	B	94.	B
20.	C	45.	D	70.	B	95.	D
21.	A	46.	B	71.	C	96.	A
22.	D	47.	A	72.	A	97.	C
23.	B	48.	C	73.	A	98.	A
24.	A	49.	C	74.	C	99.	A
25.	C	50.	C	75.	C	100.	A

ANSWERS TO EXAM 1

1. **(D)** Chapter 2, Objective 1
All levels of National Standard Curricula for EMS are published by NHTSA.

2. **(B)** Chapter 2, Objective 5
Quality improvement programs are system-wide efforts to detect problems that are addressed through education or changes in the system. It is not intended to single out individuals for punishment taken.

3. **(A)** Chapter 2, Objective 3
Gloves are adequate in this case.

4. **(B)** Chapter 2, Objective 7
EMTs' training and scope of practice are determined by the state in which they are certified or licensed.

5. **(C)** Chapter 3, Objective 2
This is an example of bargaining. The father is expressing willingness to die in order to save his child.

6. **(B)** Chapter 3, Objective 3
The anger will pass, but would be aggravated by any of the other statements.

7. **(B)** Chapter 3, Objective 5
CISD is intended for management of unusually stressful acute incidents that affect EMS personnel.

8. **(B)** Chapter 3, Objective 4
It is important that you discuss your work with family and friends, but not to unduly concern them with graphic or disturbing details.

9. **(A)** Chapter 3, Objective 10
Only trained rescuers should attempt this rescue. Grain silos pose a number of hazards.

10. **(C)** Chapter 3, Objective 7
All of the other information is secondary to determining whether the scene is safe.

11. **(C)** Chapter 3, Objective 10
Park a block or two away and shut off your lights and sirens while awaiting law enforcement to secure the scene. The caller's information may be inaccurate, the perpetrator may return to the scene, or others at the scene may be violent.

12. **(A)** Chapter 7, Objectives 1 and 2
This is the only sound principle of body mechanics. The EMT should never reach overhead or twist or bend at the waist, but should use the muscles of the legs.

13. **(B)** Chapter 3, Objective 10
Medical care of the patient is your first priority, but it is also in the patient's interest that you do not jeopardize the police investigation.

14. **(B)** Chapter 7, Objective 12
This is the type of situation for which basket-type stretchers are designed.

15. **(A)** Chapter 2, Objective 7
Continuing education and licensure or certification are a personal responsibility.

16. **(A)** Chapter 7, Objective 6
This is the type of situation for which stair chairs are designed. A patient with difficulty breathing must not be placed in a supine position.

17. **(A)** Chapter 2, Objective 6
Online medical control involves voice contact with a physician.

18. **(C)** Chapter 4, Objective 3
Because of the person's behavior, confusion, and physical signs and symptoms, it is clear that he is sick and needs immediate treatment, but is not capable of giving consent.

19. **(C)** Chapter 4, Objective 7
Because there was no harm to the patient, negligence cannot be established.

20. **(C)** Chapter 4, Objective 12
You have both a legal and an ethical obligation to report a reasonable suspicion of abuse. Most states have laws to protect individuals who report abuse in good faith, even if it turns out that the patient was not abused.

21. **(A)** Chapter 4, Objective 10
All patients, regardless of potential for survival or organ donor status should receive the same level of care, but the hospital should be notified that the patient is an organ donor.

22. **(D)** Chapter 4, Objectives 1 and 2
In the anatomical position, the deformity described is on the lateral side, proximal to the thumb.

23. **(B)** Chapter 5, Objectives 1 and 2
The esophagus lies posterior to, or behind, the trachea, which is palpable in the anterior neck.

24. **(A)** Chapter 5, Objectives 1 and 2
The carotid arteries can be found in the anterior neck on either side of the laryngeal prominence.

25. **(C)** Chapter 5, Objective 2
Platelets are important to forming blood clots.

26. **(C)** Chapter 5, Objective 1
The blue–black discoloration describes a contusion and the location is the zygoma.

27. **(B)** Chapter 5, Objectives 1 and 2
The thoracic vertebrae form the posterior portion of the chest, or thorax.

28. **(B)** Chapter 5, Objective 2
The femur is the large bone found in the thigh.

29. **(C)** Chapter 5, Objective 2
Capillaries are microscopic vessels one cell-layer thick to permit exchange of materials between cells.

30. **(C)** Chapter 5, Objective 2
The palate forms part of the floor of the skull and the roof of the mouth.

31. **(A)** Chapter 5, Objective 2
The vena cava is the large vein that transports blood from the venous system to the right atrium of the heart.

32. **(D)** Chapter 5, Objective 2
There are several types of white blood cells, which all play a role in the immune system.

33. **(B)** Chapter 6, Objective 20
Systolic blood pressure is the maximum blood pressure exerted against the walls of the arteries as a result of blood being pumped through the arteries when the heart contracts.

34. **(A)** Chapter 5, Objective 2
The back of the skull is made up of the occipital bone. The region of the head associated with it is called the occipital region.

35. **(D)** Chapter 5, Objective 2
This is the only characteristic of skeletal muscle listed. The other characteristics describe smooth, or involuntary muscle.

36. **(C)** Chapter 6, Objective 6
If the patient is able to complain, he is awake and you will assess the radial artery.

37. **(B)** Chapter 6, Objective 6
The easiest and most reliable pulse to palpate in newborns is the brachial pulse in the upper arm.

38. **(D)** Chapter 6, Objective 3
Even though breath sounds are absent in one lobe of the lung, there may still be breath sounds in the other lobes, which you cannot describe unless you listen to them.

39. **(B)** Chapter 9, Section 2, Objectives 4, 6, and 12
The steps of an initial assessment include ABCD: checking the airway, assessing breathing, checking circulation, and then checking for disability, which refers to mental and neurological status.

40. **(A)** Chapter 9, Section 2, Objective 1
The patient is alert enough to answer the door, but nothing else can yet be said about her mental status.

41. **(C)** Chapter 9, Section 2, Objective 1
The patient responds to painful stimuli, so is therefore not unresponsive. Obtunded is a confusing term that should be avoided, and the patient must be able to answer questions to determine disorientation.

42. **(D)** Chapter 9, Section 2, Objective 6
Even though the patient in Choice (C) is unresponsive, assistance with ventilation is indicated when the spontaneous rate is 8 or less, or 30 or more per minute. However, depth of respirations must also be considered in making the decision to assist ventilations.

43. **(D)** Chapter 8, Objective 8
The approximate depth of the oropharynx, to which oral suctioning is limited, is determined by measuring the distance from the corner of the mouth to the earlobe.

44. **(D)** Chapter 8, Objective 3
According the 2005 American Heart Association guidelines for complete airway obstruction in an infant, you should perform 30 chest compressions, as you would in CPR.

45. **(D)** Chapter 9, Section 2, Objective 12
The carotid pulse is the quickest and most reliable way to determine the presence of a pulse in an unresponsive patient.

46. **(B)** Chapter 9, Section 2, Objective 18
Capillary refill is a reliable way of assessing perfusion in pediatric patients, but by itself, is considered unreliable in adults. However, there are times when capillary refill time can add to the information you have about perfusion status in an adult.

47. **(A)** Chapter 22, Objective 8
Immobilizing the patient in the car seat allows for the least possibility of spinal movement and provides a secure way of immobilizing the spine.

48. **(C)** Chapter 20, Objective 3
While choices (A) and (C) may seem similar, sealing the wound by applying direct pressure may lead to a tension pneumothorax. Additionally, there is nothing in the scenario to indicate the need for spinal immobilization, which will delay transport of a patient who has an obvious problem with ventilation.

49. **(C)** Chapter 20, Objective 3
Direct pressure is always the first attempt to control bleeding in civilian settings. Military considerations may differ.

50. **(C)** Chapter 22, Objective 6
Not *every* fall and motor vehicle collision calls for the patient to be immobilized.

51. **(B)** Chapter 20, Objective 3
The major threat to life is continued bleeding from the wound. The patient is already in shock and you must prevent ongoing blood loss.

52. **(A)** Chapter 20, Objective 3

A sterile, saline-moistened dressing will prevent the exposed organ from drying out or being further contaminated. The foil or plastic prevents the bandage from drying out and becoming contaminated. A circumferential bandage may compromise the circulation to the organ. The organ should be kept warm, not cold, and a dry dressing may adhere to the organ.

53. **(D)** Chapter 9, Section 2, Objective 6

The normal adult ventilatory rate is between 12 and 20 per minute. A rate of 24 is elevated above normal and may indicate chest injury or shock.

54. **(B)** Chapter 19, Objective 6

Your patient is at risk for developing shock, based on the mechanism of injury. The first action, of those listed, is to apply oxygen.

55. **(A)** Chapter 24, Section 3, Objective 9

The death of an occupant in the same vehicle is a significant mechanism of injury. Penetrating trauma does not constitute a significant mechanism if it is distal to the knee or elbow.

56. **(A)** Chapter 24, Section 3, Objective 9

The patient has penetrating trauma to the chest and a decreased level of responsiveness. He is critical and a more detailed assessment is delayed until you are en route to the hospital.

57. **(C)** Chapter 24, Section 3, Objective 9

This is neither a significant mechanism nor injury. You should do a focused physical assessment and treat the injury. There is no need for immediate transport, as the patient is not critical.

58. **(C)** Chapter 21, Objectives 11–16 and 19

The head and neck of infants and small children are disproportionate in size to their trunks and extremities, making up a larger percentage of total body surface area (18%) than in adults (9%).

59. **(D)** Chapter 21, Objectives 11–17

The anterior chest is 18% of total body surface area, and the arm is 9%, for a total of 27%. The description of the burn is characteristic of partial thickness burns.

60. **(D)** Chapter 21, Objectives 11–17

This is a critical burn due to the patient's age, although it would be considered a moderate burn in a younger person.

61. **(A)** Chapter 8, Objective 1

The nerves that cause the diaphragm to contract arise from the cervical area of the spine.

62. **(C)** Chapter 21, Objective 28

Because some dry powder chemicals react with water in a way that causes heat or increases chemical damage, as much of the powder as possible should be brushed away *before* flushing with copious amounts of water.

63. **(D)** Chapter 15, Objective 1

Diabetes results when the beta cells of the islets of Langerhans in the pancreas cannot produce enough insulin to meet the body's needs.

64. **(D)** Chapter 14, Objective 41

While albuterol, epinephrine, and nitroglycerin are drugs with which the EMT can assist the patient who has the drug prescribed to him or her, these drugs are not carried on the ambulance.

65. **(A)** Chapter 16, Section 2, Objective 6

Activated charcoal is indicated in many poisonings by ingestion because it binds many substances to its surface so that poisons are not absorbed as they travel through the gastrointestinal system. Syrup of ipecac is no longer recommended in most cases, and is not used by the EMT.

66. **(B)** Chapter 15, Objective 1

Given the onset of the patient's illness, the most useful information is determining if the patient has other signs and symptoms of a diabetic emergency, such as frequent urination.

67. **(C)** Chapter 16, Section 1, Objective 1

The airway may swell in severe allergic reactions, posing a threat to life.

68. **(D)** Chapter 17, Objective 1

When liquids evaporate, they take heat from the body with them.

69. **(B)** Chapter 18, Objective 1

Patients with a behavioral emergency must receive a medical evaluation, but the assistance of law enforcement may be needed if the patient is violent, uncooperative, or the ability to consent to or refuse care is in question.

70. **(B)** Chapter 9, Section 2, Objective 6

Since the patient is talking, the airway is open, but you still need to assess the breathing, circulation, and mental status to complete the initial assessment.

71. **(C)** Chapter 19, Objective 5

The blood pressure is not normal for any stage of pregnancy, but the mechanism of injury is minor. It is common for the pregnant uterus to obstruct the return of blood to the heart by compressing the vena cava when the pregnant female is in a supine position. Placenta previa is a condition in which the placenta implants near or over the cervix.

72. **(A)** Chapter 19, Objective 4

The patient is experiencing symptoms of imminent delivery and may deliver despite being less than full term. Premature babies are smaller and delivery may occur quickly. Allowing the patient to use the bathroom may result in delivery of the infant into the toilet.

73. **(A)** Chapter 19, Objective 4

Determining how far apart the contractions are allows you to make a decision about whether you need to check for crowning.

74. **(C)** Chapter 18, Objectives 1–3
A number of reversible medical causes can result in an acute onset of behavioral changes. Some of these conditions may be life threatening and the patient must be evaluated.

75. **(C)** Chapter 23, Objective 11
A fever that increases quickly can cause seizures in susceptible children. The other conditions listed are not common causes of seizures in children.

76. **(A)** Chapter 14, Objective 4
The EMT may assist a patient in taking his or her prescribed nitroglycerin to relieve chest pain by dilating the arteries that supply the heart muscle, but nitroglycerin is not carried on the BLS ambulance.

77. **(C)** Chapter 13, Objectives 2 and 5
This patient is in respiratory failure and needs immediate ventilatory assistance. It should be noted that the heart rate may not be significantly elevated, as many patients with COPD have a heart condition for which they take medicines that prevent the heart rate from increasing when it normally would.

78. **(A)** Chapter 13, Objective 2
These signs and symptoms, when taken altogether, are most consistent with spontaneous pneumothorax.

79. **(C)** Chapter 14, Objective 7
Both female gender and diabetes are associated with atypical presentation of acute coronary syndrome, including pain that occurs between the shoulder blades.

80. **(A)** Chapter 14, Objective 10
It is likely that the patient has been down longer than 4 to 5 minutes. Therefore, CPR is required to provide the heart with nutrients and oxygen to increase the likelihood that defibrillation, if needed, will be successful. The patient may have a low blood glucose level, but perfusing the heart and brain are the first priorities.

81. **(D)** Chapter 14, Objective 31
According to the 2005 American Heart Association guidelines for resuscitation, CPR should be performed for 2 minutes after a shock is delivered.

82. **(C)** Chapter 14, Objective 12
This reliably indicates that the patient is not in a shockable rhythm. You should continue CPR. The AED has advised "No shock."

83. **(C)** Chapter 15, Objective 5
The patient's blood glucose level is in the normal range. The patient's age and history of diabetes increase the risk of stroke. This presentation would be very atypical for a seizure.

84. **(A)** Chapter 15, Objective 5

The sudden, severe headache, decreased level of consciousness, and slow pulse accompanied by increased blood pressure all indicate a hemorrhagic stroke with increased intracranial pressure.

85. **(C)** Chapter 16, Section 1, Objective 5

Epinephrine affects alpha$_1$ receptors in the smooth muscle of blood vessels, causing them to constrict and increase blood pressure; it also affects beta$_2$ receptors in the smooth muscle of the bronchioles, causing them to dilate.

86. **(D)** Chapter 16, Section 1, Objective 5

While epinephrine is effective in treating anaphylaxis, its effects last only about 10 minutes. The patient may need additional epinephrine, as well as other medications, and must be transported.

87. **(B)** Chapter 16, Section 2, Objective 7

The patient is showing signs of toxicity (not anaphylaxis). Antivenins are specific, so knowing the type of snake that bit the patient is very important. Elevating the leg may speed the absorption of venom into the blood stream. Ice may increase local tissue necrosis (death).

88. **(A)** Chapter 16, Section 2, Objective 7

Alcohol poisoning is epidemic on college campuses. Alcohol may continue to be absorbed from the gastrointestinal tract for up to 2 hours after the patient's last drink. Therefore, the blood alcohol level, which is obviously already high, can continue to rise. Alcohol is a central nervous system depressant and death can occur from acute alcohol poisoning. Additionally, the patient's unresponsiveness and intoxication put her at risk for vomiting and aspiration of stomach contents.

89. **(D)** Chapter 9, Section 4, Objective 2

The elderly can have significantly decreased sensitivity to pain. Additionally, this pain is indicative of stretching of a hollow organ, such as the intestine. The elderly are prone to bowel obstruction, which, if untreated, leads to death. The severity of pain is not necessarily an indicator of the severity of the condition causing it.

90. **(A)** Chapter 17, Objective 5

While removing the patient's clothing and actively cooling her are indicated, neither will do any good unless she is first removed from the environment. Even though the patient is dehydrated, her decreased level of consciousness is a contraindication to giving anything by mouth.

91. **(C)** Chapter 17, Objective 6

Survival after submersion in cold water for more than 30 minutes has been reported. Resuscitative measures are indicated. Because the patient is hypothermic, you must check for a pulse for at least 10 seconds, as the heart rate can be very slow in hypothermia. Active rewarming is not done in the prehospital setting.

92. **(A)** Chapter 18, Objective 6
These complaints are all associated with depression.

93. **(C)** Chapter 18, Objective 4
Despite the apparent ambivalence about committing suicide, the patient obviously is in emotional distress for which she does not perceive another way of getting help. Many patients who are successful in suicide have made previous attempts. It is the EMT's professional obligation to be empathetic to the patient.

94. **(B)** Chapter 15, Objective 1
Hyperglycemic emergencies develop over several hours to days.

95. **(D)** Chapter 17, Objective 2
Whether the patient has superficial or deep cold injury, it is not advisable to allow him to walk unless there is no other way of getting him to help. A basket-type stretcher is designed for carrying the patient over rough terrain, while a long backboard is not.

96. **(A)** Chapter 19, Objective 14
If the umbilical cord is the presenting part, the EMT should attempt to push the baby's head up and away from the cord so that it is not compressed. In a breech delivery, the EMT may use a gloved hand to form a "V" around the baby's nose in case he or she starts to breathe before the head is delivered.

97. **(C)** Chapter 24, Section 3, Objective 9
This patient is a "walking wounded" and has a low priority for care.

98. **(A)** Chapter 24, Section 3, Objective 9
This patient is critical, yet may survive with immediate care.

99. **(A)** Chapter 24, Section 3, Objective 2
The DOT Emergency Response Guidebook is a reference for the placards found on highway transportation vehicles carrying hazardous materials.

100. **(A)** Chapter 10, Objective 5
The only acceptable way to make a correction to a run sheet is to draw a single line through the incorrect information, write the word "error," and initial the correction.

Answer Sheet

EXAM 2

1	Ⓐ Ⓑ Ⓒ Ⓓ	26	Ⓐ Ⓑ Ⓒ Ⓓ	51	Ⓐ Ⓑ Ⓒ Ⓓ	76	Ⓐ Ⓑ Ⓒ Ⓓ
2	Ⓐ Ⓑ Ⓒ Ⓓ	27	Ⓐ Ⓑ Ⓒ Ⓓ	52	Ⓐ Ⓑ Ⓒ Ⓓ	77	Ⓐ Ⓑ Ⓒ Ⓓ
3	Ⓐ Ⓑ Ⓒ Ⓓ	28	Ⓐ Ⓑ Ⓒ Ⓓ	53	Ⓐ Ⓑ Ⓒ Ⓓ	78	Ⓐ Ⓑ Ⓒ Ⓓ
4	Ⓐ Ⓑ Ⓒ Ⓓ	29	Ⓐ Ⓑ Ⓒ Ⓓ	54	Ⓐ Ⓑ Ⓒ Ⓓ	79	Ⓐ Ⓑ Ⓒ Ⓓ
5	Ⓐ Ⓑ Ⓒ Ⓓ	30	Ⓐ Ⓑ Ⓒ Ⓓ	55	Ⓐ Ⓑ Ⓒ Ⓓ	80	Ⓐ Ⓑ Ⓒ Ⓓ
6	Ⓐ Ⓑ Ⓒ Ⓓ	31	Ⓐ Ⓑ Ⓒ Ⓓ	56	Ⓐ Ⓑ Ⓒ Ⓓ	81	Ⓐ Ⓑ Ⓒ Ⓓ
7	Ⓐ Ⓑ Ⓒ Ⓓ	32	Ⓐ Ⓑ Ⓒ Ⓓ	57	Ⓐ Ⓑ Ⓒ Ⓓ	82	Ⓐ Ⓑ Ⓒ Ⓓ
8	Ⓐ Ⓑ Ⓒ Ⓓ	33	Ⓐ Ⓑ Ⓒ Ⓓ	58	Ⓐ Ⓑ Ⓒ Ⓓ	83	Ⓐ Ⓑ Ⓒ Ⓓ
9	Ⓐ Ⓑ Ⓒ Ⓓ	34	Ⓐ Ⓑ Ⓒ Ⓓ	59	Ⓐ Ⓑ Ⓒ Ⓓ	84	Ⓐ Ⓑ Ⓒ Ⓓ
10	Ⓐ Ⓑ Ⓒ Ⓓ	35	Ⓐ Ⓑ Ⓒ Ⓓ	60	Ⓐ Ⓑ Ⓒ Ⓓ	85	Ⓐ Ⓑ Ⓒ Ⓓ
11	Ⓐ Ⓑ Ⓒ Ⓓ	36	Ⓐ Ⓑ Ⓒ Ⓓ	61	Ⓐ Ⓑ Ⓒ Ⓓ	86	Ⓐ Ⓑ Ⓒ Ⓓ
12	Ⓐ Ⓑ Ⓒ Ⓓ	37	Ⓐ Ⓑ Ⓒ Ⓓ	62	Ⓐ Ⓑ Ⓒ Ⓓ	87	Ⓐ Ⓑ Ⓒ Ⓓ
13	Ⓐ Ⓑ Ⓒ Ⓓ	38	Ⓐ Ⓑ Ⓒ Ⓓ	63	Ⓐ Ⓑ Ⓒ Ⓓ	88	Ⓐ Ⓑ Ⓒ Ⓓ
14	Ⓐ Ⓑ Ⓒ Ⓓ	39	Ⓐ Ⓑ Ⓒ Ⓓ	64	Ⓐ Ⓑ Ⓒ Ⓓ	89	Ⓐ Ⓑ Ⓒ Ⓓ
15	Ⓐ Ⓑ Ⓒ Ⓓ	40	Ⓐ Ⓑ Ⓒ Ⓓ	65	Ⓐ Ⓑ Ⓒ Ⓓ	90	Ⓐ Ⓑ Ⓒ Ⓓ
16	Ⓐ Ⓑ Ⓒ Ⓓ	41	Ⓐ Ⓑ Ⓒ Ⓓ	66	Ⓐ Ⓑ Ⓒ Ⓓ	91	Ⓐ Ⓑ Ⓒ Ⓓ
17	Ⓐ Ⓑ Ⓒ Ⓓ	42	Ⓐ Ⓑ Ⓒ Ⓓ	67	Ⓐ Ⓑ Ⓒ Ⓓ	92	Ⓐ Ⓑ Ⓒ Ⓓ
18	Ⓐ Ⓑ Ⓒ Ⓓ	43	Ⓐ Ⓑ Ⓒ Ⓓ	68	Ⓐ Ⓑ Ⓒ Ⓓ	93	Ⓐ Ⓑ Ⓒ Ⓓ
19	Ⓐ Ⓑ Ⓒ Ⓓ	44	Ⓐ Ⓑ Ⓒ Ⓓ	69	Ⓐ Ⓑ Ⓒ Ⓓ	94	Ⓐ Ⓑ Ⓒ Ⓓ
20	Ⓐ Ⓑ Ⓒ Ⓓ	45	Ⓐ Ⓑ Ⓒ Ⓓ	70	Ⓐ Ⓑ Ⓒ Ⓓ	95	Ⓐ Ⓑ Ⓒ Ⓓ
21	Ⓐ Ⓑ Ⓒ Ⓓ	46	Ⓐ Ⓑ Ⓒ Ⓓ	71	Ⓐ Ⓑ Ⓒ Ⓓ	96	Ⓐ Ⓑ Ⓒ Ⓓ
22	Ⓐ Ⓑ Ⓒ Ⓓ	47	Ⓐ Ⓑ Ⓒ Ⓓ	72	Ⓐ Ⓑ Ⓒ Ⓓ	97	Ⓐ Ⓑ Ⓒ Ⓓ
23	Ⓐ Ⓑ Ⓒ Ⓓ	48	Ⓐ Ⓑ Ⓒ Ⓓ	73	Ⓐ Ⓑ Ⓒ Ⓓ	98	Ⓐ Ⓑ Ⓒ Ⓓ
24	Ⓐ Ⓑ Ⓒ Ⓓ	49	Ⓐ Ⓑ Ⓒ Ⓓ	74	Ⓐ Ⓑ Ⓒ Ⓓ	99	Ⓐ Ⓑ Ⓒ Ⓓ
25	Ⓐ Ⓑ Ⓒ Ⓓ	50	Ⓐ Ⓑ Ⓒ Ⓓ	75	Ⓐ Ⓑ Ⓒ Ⓓ	100	Ⓐ Ⓑ Ⓒ Ⓓ

Exam 2

1. The component of an EMS system that consists of a system of internal and external reviews and audits to ensure the highest possible level of care is known as
   (A) continuous quality improvement.
   (B) online medical direction.
   (C) accreditation.
   (D) ambulance certification.

2. You are preparing to load a patient in cardiac arrest into your ambulance. The patient's wife asks, "Is he going to be okay?" Which of the following is the most appropriate answer?
   (A) "Ma'am, that's not for me to say. I'm only an EMT."
   (B) "We are doing everything we can, but your husband's condition is critical."
   (C) "Everything is okay. I don't want you to worry."
   (D) "I don't have time to answer your questions right now. It is important that we get going to the hospital."

3. All of the following are recommended ways of dealing with EMS work stress EXCEPT
   (A) gathering with coworkers after work to relax over beer or cocktails.
   (B) engaging in a regular exercise routine.
   (C) reducing the intake of fats, simple sugars, and caffeine.
   (D) talking with family and coworkers about work stress.

4. An EMT's scope of practice is determined by
   (A) the National Standard Curriculum.
   (B) state laws.
   (C) the EMT's training program.
   (D) the EMT's employer.

5. Legally, for a "do not resuscitate" (DNR) order to be honored by an EMT, all of the following are required EXCEPT
   (A) the signature of the patient or legal guardian.
   (B) the signature of the patient's physician.
   (C) an EMS system protocol for honoring DNRs.
   (D) that at least two consenting family members must be present.

6. Handheld radios transmitting at 1 to 5 watts with limited range are considered
   (A) base stations.
   (B) portable radios.
   (C) repeaters.
   (D) mobile radios.

7. Your patient is a 29-year-old male who is unresponsive following a motor vehicle collision. Which of the following statements regarding consent is true?
   (A) You must have the patient's expressed consent.
   (B) You may treat the patient according to implied consent.
   (C) You must have a family member's consent.
   (D) You must obtain consent from medical control.

8. Which of the following statements regarding consent is not true?
   (A) A competent patient must be informed of the risks if he or she refuses treatment and/or transport.
   (B) A competent patient must be informed of what care will be provided, and any risks associated with it.
   (C) Competent patients aged 16 years and older can refuse care and transportation, even if they have a concerning illness or injury.
   (D) A patient who extends his or her arm toward you when seeing you hold a blood pressure cuff is offering a type of consent.

9. Which of the following statements regarding consent for treatment of minors is true?
   (A) Minors can refuse care, but cannot consent to care.
   (B) Parents can refuse care for a minor, even when there is a possible life threat.
   (C) Pregnant minors can give consent for their own care.
   (D) A minor is any patient under the age of 21 years.

10. You are dropping off a patient at the emergency department when you receive another call. The patient has not yet been triaged and assigned a bed. A nurse's aid says she will stay with the patient until a nurse can triage the patient. Which of the following statements is most accurate concerning this situation?
    (A) This is abandonment, even if no harm comes to the patient.
    (B) If the patient's condition deteriorates, it will be considered abandonment.
    (C) This is negligence, even if no harm comes to the patient.
    (D) If the patient's condition deteriorates, it will be considered negligence.

11. You are caring for a patient who appears to be "faking" unconsciousness. Your partner says loudly to him, "Open up your eyes or I'm going to stick a big tube down your nose and it's going to hurt." This is an example of
    (A) battery.
    (B) assault.
    (C) negligence.
    (D) slander.

12. Which of the following does not legally establish a duty to respond for the licensed or certified EMT?
    (A) You are on duty and being paid and are dispatched on a call.
    (B) You are at an out-of-state football game and a spectator near you collapses.
    (C) You are driving to work and stop to provide care to a man who was injured when he crashed his bicycle.
    (D) You are on duty while volunteering and are dispatched on a call.

13. Which of the following would be a violation of patient confidentiality?
    (A) Releasing records to the patient's attorney with the patient's written consent.
    (B) Discussing the patient with other providers involved in the patient's care.
    (C) Releasing records to an attorney who is suing the patient.
    (D) Testifying to the patient's condition in court.

14. You are transporting a critically injured patient who does not have health care insurance. The nurses at the nearest trauma center complain when you bring uninsured patients to them. As a result, you bypass the trauma center and take the patient to an emergency department 10 minutes farther away. The legislation violated in this situation is
    (A) EMTALA.
    (B) HIPAA.
    (C) the Ryan White Act.
    (D) the Good Samaritan Law.

15. A move to be used when there is a danger to the patient and rescuers is _____ move.
    (A) an urgent
    (B) an emergency
    (C) a nonurgent
    (D) a routine

16. Rapid extrication is an example of _____ move.
    (A) an urgent
    (B) an emergency
    (C) a nonurgent
    (D) a routine

17. The bone that makes up the "wing" of the pelvis on each side is the
    (A) ilium.
    (B) ischium.
    (C) coccyx.
    (D) pubis.

18. With your patient in the anatomical position, the bone of the forearm on the medial side is the
    (A) radius.
    (B) ulna.
    (C) humerus.
    (D) scapula.

19. The medial malleolus is the distal end of the
    (A) tibia.
    (B) fibula.
    (C) patella.
    (D) femur.

20. Your patient was found lying face-down. In your report you should describe this position as
    (A) supine.
    (B) lateral recumbent.
    (C) Fowler's.
    (D) prone.

21. The primary function of insulin is to
    (A) increase the blood glucose level by breaking down stored carbohydrates in the liver.
    (B) decrease the blood glucose level by making it easier for glucose to enter cells.
    (C) increase the blood glucose level by causing the breakdown of stored fat in the body.
    (D) decrease the blood glucose level by helping the body eliminate excess glucose through the kidneys.

22. In normal individuals, the stimulus to inhale is
    (A) increased carbon dioxide in the blood.
    (B) decreased oxygen in the blood.
    (C) decreased carbon dioxide in the blood.
    (D) increased oxygen in the blood.

23. Which of the following statements is true with regard to the beginning of inspiration?
    (A) The diaphragm is lower than in the resting state.
    (B) The size of the chest cavity is smaller than in the resting state.
    (C) The pressure inside the lungs is higher than in the resting state.
    (D) The ribs assume a lower position than in the resting state.

24. You have assessed the pulse on the top of the foot in a patient who has an injured lower extremity, and found it present. You should document the presence of the pulse in the _____ artery.
    (A) popliteal
    (B) posterior tibial
    (C) dorsalis pedis
    (D) brachial

25. The leaf-shaped flap of tissue that covers the opening of the larynx during swallowing is the
    (A) uvula.
    (B) cricoid cartilage.
    (C) epiglottis.
    (D) thyroid cartilage.

26. The tissue membrane that covers the lungs and lines the chest cavity is called
    (A) pleura.
    (B) peritoneum.
    (C) pericardium.
    (D) pia mater.

27. The trachea
    (A) is located anterior and midline in the neck.
    (B) is located posterior and midline in the neck.
    (C) participates in gas exchange.
    (D) conducts solids and liquids into the digestive tract.

28. The thick, clear, jelly-like substance that fills the eye and gives it shape is the
    (A) aqueous humor.
    (B) cerebrospinal fluid.
    (C) vitreous humor.
    (D) conjunctiva.

29. The deepest layer of skin that consists of fat cells is the
    (A) epidermis.
    (B) dermis.
    (C) subcutaneous.
    (D) facia.

30. With regard to patient assessment, the general impression is
    (A) a determination of what the patient's problem is.
    (B) a determination of whether the patient is critical or noncritical.
    (C) what the patient says is wrong, in his or her own words.
    (D) a determination of whether the patient requires transport.

31. Capillary refill time should be no less than _____ seconds.
    (A) 5
    (B) 4
    (C) 3
    (D) 2

32. When assessing your patient's pupils you notice that the whites of his eyes have a yellow discoloration. This is an indication that the patient is suffering from
    (A) anemia.
    (B) hypoxia.
    (C) carbon monoxide poisoning.
    (D) liver disease.

33. Your patient is complaining of chest pain. Which of the following would be a pertinent negative?
    (A) Patient denies having a headache.
    (B) Patient complains of having a headache.
    (C) Patient denies nausea.
    (D) Patient complains of having nausea.

34. Which of the following is a subjective finding to be documented in the patient care report?
    (A) vital signs
    (B) patient's medications
    (C) patient's age
    (D) chief complaint

35. The focused medical assessment is based on the
    (A) chief complaint.
    (B) patient's medications.
    (C) general impression.
    (D) vital signs.

36. Just as you enter the residence for a report of a child with difficulty breathing you hear a high-pitched "crowing" sound. Given this information you should anticipate that the patient is suffering from
    (A) complete upper airway obstruction.
    (B) partial upper airway obstruction.
    (C) asthma.
    (D) lower respiratory infection.

37. Upon assessment you notice that both of your patient's pupils are constricted. This is most consistent with
    (A) narcotics use.
    (B) traumatic brain injury.
    (C) crack cocaine use.
    (D) severe hypoxia.

38. Your patient has a blood pressure of 72/48. This would be normal if your patient is _____ year(s) old.
    (A) less than 1
    (B) 3 to 5
    (C) 8 to 10
    (D) 12 to 15

39. Your patient is a 3-month-old infant whose pulse is 60 per minute. You should suspect
    (A) blood loss.
    (B) hypoxia.
    (C) dehydration.
    (D) fever.

40. Which of the following results from taking a child's blood pressure with an adult-sized blood pressure cuff?
    (A) difficulty hearing the blood pressure, but an accurate reading
    (B) ability to detect the blood pressure by watching the needle on the gauge bounce without having to listen with a stethoscope
    (C) orthostatic hypotension
    (D) an artificially low reading

41. All of the following can lead to inaccurate pulse oximetry readings EXCEPT
    (A) hypoxia.
    (B) carbon monoxide poisoning.
    (C) nail polish on the patient's nails.
    (D) hypothermia.

42. When assessing pupils, smaller pupils are said to be
    (A) dilated.
    (B) constricted.
    (C) nonreactive.
    (D) unequal.

43. When suctioning, the EMT should
    (A) limit suctioning to 10–15 seconds.
    (B) suction while inserting the suction catheter into the mouth.
    (C) suction while inserting and withdrawing the suction catheter into the mouth.
    (D) rinse the suction catheter with water before inserting it into the airway.

44. A rigid suction catheter (Yankeur or "tonsil tip") is measured from the
    (A) corner of the mouth to the earlobe.
    (B) nare to the earlobe.
    (C) center of the chin to the angle of the jaw.
    (D) center of the chin to the tip of the nose.

45. The proper rate of bag-valve mask ventilation for an adult with a pulse is _____ ventilations per minute.
    (A) 6 to 10
    (B) 10 to 12
    (C) 12 to 16
    (D) 16 to 20

46. The purpose of the Sellick maneuver is to
    (A) prevent gastric distention during artificial ventilation.
    (B) relieve an obstructed airway.
    (C) decrease an abnormally fast heart rate.
    (D) restore circulation in a pulseless extremity.

47. A nasopharyngeal airway is properly measured from the
    (A) corner of the mouth to the earlobe.
    (B) corner of the mouth to the sternal notch.
    (C) nare to the earlobe.
    (D) nare to the sternal notch.

48. The manual airway maneuver that is used in patients with suspected cervical spine trauma is the
    (A) cross-finger technique.
    (B) head-tilt chin-lift maneuver.
    (C) jaw-thrust maneuver.
    (D) sniffing position.

49. Because of the larger size of a small child's or infant's head, which of the following modifications should be made in airway management?
    (A) Use greater flexion of the neck.
    (B) Use greater hyperextension of the neck.
    (C) Place a folded towel under the head.
    (D) Place a folded towel under the shoulders.

50. Your patient is a 35-year-old female whose sister called 911 because she witnessed the patient overdose on her anti-anxiety medication. On your arrival, the patient is very drowsy. She wakes up when you speak loudly and shake her shoulder, but immediately falls asleep again. Her respirations are 12 per minute, pulse is 76 per minute, and blood pressure is 118/72. Which of the following is most appropriate?
    (A) Apply oxygen and place the patient in the left lateral recumbent position for transport.
    (B) Initiate bag-valve mask ventilations with supplemental oxygen, place the patient supine, and immobilize her on a long backboard.
    (C) Apply oxygen and place supine for transport.
    (D) Apply oxygen and place in semi-Fowler's (head-elevated) position for transport.

51. The EMT can administer nitroglycerin by which of the following routes?
    (A) metered-dose inhalation
    (B) sublingual
    (C) oral
    (D) all of the above

52. Your patient states he has a history of emphysema. This is a type of
    (A) infection in the lungs.
    (B) heart failure, leading to fluid build-up in the lungs.
    (C) chronic obstructive lung disease.
    (D) allergy that leads to anaphylactic reactions.

53. You are presented with an unresponsive 50-year-old male. He is pale and breathing rapidly. You hear gurgling noises with each breath. Once you open the airway, your next step will be to
    (A) place him in the recovery position.
    (B) administer oxygen with a nonrebreather mask.
    (C) suction the patient's airway.
    (D) ventilate the patient using a bag-valve mask.

54. Your patient is complaining of chest pain and has several medications. Of the following medications, which should you assist him or her with in this situation?
    (A) epinephrine auto-injector
    (B) albuterol metered-dose inhaler
    (C) nitroglycerin metered-dose spray
    (D) oral glucose

55. Which of the following is a contraindication for nitroglycerin?
    (A) The patient took Cialis the day before.
    (B) The patient's systolic blood pressure is over 150 mmHg.
    (C) The patient complains of difficulty breathing.
    (D) All of the above.

56. Your patient is a 55-year-old male complaining of chest pain, shortness of breath, and nausea. He is alert with pale, clammy skin. His blood pressure is 134/90, pulse is 88 with occasional irregular beats, and respirations are 16. Which of the following is the most appropriate position for transport?
    (A) supine with head elevated 6 to 10 inches
    (B) sitting on the stretcher in a position of comfort
    (C) recovery position
    (D) Trendelenberg position

57. You just delivered a full-term infant who is limp and not crying, but has a pulse over 100 per minute. Your first action should be to
    (A) perform chest compressions for 2 minutes.
    (B) provide "blow-by" oxygen.
    (C) vigorously dry the baby with a towel.
    (D) begin bag-valve mask ventilations.

58. You just delivered a full-term infant who is limp, cyanotic, and pulseless. Your first action should be to
    (A) apply the AED.
    (B) wrap the baby in blankets to keep him or her warm.
    (C) begin CPR.
    (D) provide "blow-by" oxygen.

59. A 22-year-old female who is 7 months pregnant with her first child presents with a complaint of headache and blurred vision. Physical examination shows swelling of the face and extremities, a blood pressure of 148/90, heart rate of 90, and respirations of 24. You should
    (A) place the patient on her left side, provide high-flow oxygen, and transport with the patient compartment lights dimmed and avoid the use of emergency lights and siren.
    (B) place the patient in the Trendelenberg position for transport, provide oxygen by nasal cannula, and avoid the use of emergency lights and siren.
    (C) place the patient in a sitting position, provide high-flow oxygen, and transport with emergency lights and siren.
    (D) place the patient on her left side, provide high-flow oxygen, and transport with emergency lights and siren.

60. A 22-year-old female who is 7 months pregnant with her first child presents with a complaint of headache and blurred vision. Physical examination shows swelling of the face and extremities, a blood pressure of 148/90, heart rate of 90, and respirations of 24. The most likely cause is
    (A) abruptio placentae.
    (B) preeclampsia.
    (C) premature labor.
    (D) uterine rupture.

61. Your patient is an 80-year-old female with a severe nosebleed that she has been unable to control on her own. The most effective prehospital treatment of this patient is to
    (A) pinch the nostrils and have the patient tilt her head back.
    (B) apply ice to the forehead.
    (C) pinch the nostrils and have the patient lean slightly forward.
    (D) pack the nostrils with gauze.

62. A 9-year-old male is choking on a piece of hard candy. He is coughing weakly and having severe difficulty speaking. You should
    (A) lay the patient across your lap and give alternating sequences of five back blows and five chest thrusts.
    (B) position yourself behind the patient, reach around his torso, and provide sequences of five abdominal thrusts.
    (C) lay the patient on the floor, straddle his lower body, and give sequences of five chest thrusts.
    (D) lay the patient supine and perform 2 minutes of chest compressions.

63. Your patient is a 3-year-old male who has ingested an entire 24-tablet bottle of "baby aspirin" about 15 minutes ago. Prehospital treatment of this child includes
    (A) administration of 15 grams of activated charcoal.
    (B) administering nothing by mouth.
    (C) administration of 30 mL of syrup of ipecac.
    (D) encouraging the patient to drink copious amounts of milk or water.

64. Your patient is a 58-year-old female who called 911 because she had a sudden onset of slurred speech, facial droop, and weakness on one side. When you arrive, the patient has no complaints or signs of illness. Which of the following is most likely?
    (A) This is a behavioral emergency and the patient is just seeking attention.
    (B) The patient has had a transient ischemic attack (TIA).
    (C) The patient is having a stroke.
    (D) The patient had a seizure, but it has resolved.

65. You are on the scene of a young adult male with bizarre, aggressive behavior. He is pale and sweating profusely. Law enforcement has restrained him and is getting ready to put him in the back of a squad car. You should
    (A) assume this is a behavioral emergency and mark back in service since the situation is under control.
    (B) indicate to one of the officers that the patient's behavior could be due to a medical problem and you would like to assess him.
    (C) advise the officers that they need to transport the patient to the emergency department for evaluation.
    (D) insist that the officers remove the restraints so you can assess and treat the patient.

66. Automatic external defibrillators should be placed on
    (A) patients complaining of chest pain.
    (B) unresponsive patients.
    (C) patients without pulse and respirations.
    (D) patients with a history of previous cardiac arrest.

67. The type of stroke that occurs due to the formation of a blood clot in an artery in the brain is known as _____ stroke.
    (A) a transient
    (B) a thrombotic
    (C) an embolic
    (D) a hemorrhagic

68. A prehospital stroke screen includes all of the following EXCEPT
    (A) checking for facial droop.
    (B) checking for arm drift.
    (C) checking for problems with speech.
    (D) checking for difficulty walking.

69. A seizure that lasts more than 5 minutes, or multiple seizures without a period of consciousness in between is called
    (A) petit mal epilepsy.
    (B) a complex seizure.
    (C) status epilepticus.
    (D) a grand mal seizure.

70. Your patient has been stung by a wasp. She has swelling and redness at the site. She is concerned because her mother has had severe allergic reactions to wasp stings. The patient carries an epinephrine auto-injector because of an allergy to nuts. You should
    (A) treat the localized reaction to the wasp sting by scraping away the stinger.
    (B) advise the patient to use her auto-injector to prevent an anaphylactic reaction.
    (C) apply high-flow oxygen by nonrebreather mask to prevent an anaphylactic reaction.
    (D) apply a constricting band above the site of the sting to prevent absorption of the wasp venom.

71. Which of the following is a source of carbon monoxide poisoning?
    (A) sewer gas
    (B) industrial farm sites with large amounts of animal waste
    (C) a faulty fireplace
    (D) aerosol propellants

72. Your patient was released from the hospital a month ago after having a heart attack. She called 911 today because she has been experiencing shortness of breath, especially when she lies down to sleep, and she has swelling in her ankles and feet. She is alert, her skin is pale and clammy, her blood pressure is 168/100, pulse is 100 and irregular, and respirations are 24. She has jugular venous distension and you can hear fine crackles in her lungs. The most likely explanation for this is
    (A) congestive heart failure.
    (B) chronic obstructive pulmonary disease.
    (C) pulmonary embolism.
    (D) pneumonia.

73. A 22-year-old male is threatening to jump from a 10th-floor balcony. Your first priority is to
    (A) gain the patient's trust.
    (B) determine if the patient has a history of mental illness.
    (C) determine if drugs are involved.
    (D) look for anything the patient might use as a weapon.

74. Which of the following is a contraindication to the use of an automatic external defibrillator (AED)?
    (A) The patient has a nitroglycerin patch on the chest.
    (B) The patient has an automated implanted cardioverter/defibrillator (AICD).
    (C) The patient takes a drug such as Viagra or Cialis for erectile dysfunction.
    (D) The patient has a weak carotid pulse, but no palpable blood pressure.

75. When you arrive on the scene for a report of chest pain, the patient's wife tells you that the patient lost consciousness just as you were parking in front of the residence. You confirm that the patient is pulseless and apneic. You should then
    (A) perform 2 minutes of CPR, then apply the automatic external defibrillator (AED).
    (B) immediately apply the automatic external defibrillator (AED).
    (C) perform 2 minutes of CPR, request ALS intercept, and insert an advanced airway device.
    (D) provide ventilations for 2 minutes with high-flow oxygen, then apply the automatic external defibrillator (AED).

76. Which of the following is true of a biphasic defibrillator?
    (A) It is more effective, but delivers less energy and causes less damage to the heart.
    (B) It is more effective for the patient, but poses a greater risk to the EMT.
    (C) It is more effective, but delivers more energy and causes more damage to the heart.
    (D) Its effectiveness and safety are about the same as a monophasic defibrillator, but they are cheaper and smaller.

77. The pain associated with an acute cardiac emergency is commonly located or radiates to all of the following areas EXCEPT the
    (A) upper abdomen.
    (B) neck.
    (C) inside of the arm.
    (D) groin.

78. Which of the following medications is indicated for use by patients having acute respiratory difficulty due to asthma or COPD?
    (A) atropine
    (B) advair
    (C) albuterol
    (D) acetylcysteine

79. Which of the following medications is part of the EMT's prehospital treatment of patients with an acute anaphylactic reaction?
    (A) diphenhydramine (Benadryl)
    (B) albuterol
    (C) epinephrine
    (D) prednisone

80. In a patient with diabetes, too little _____ is produced by the pancreas.
    (A) glucagon
    (B) insulin
    (C) glucose
    (D) bile

81. You just assisted a patient in taking nitroglycerin when she suddenly complains of light-headedness and a headache. You should
    (A) check the patient's blood pressure.
    (B) ask the patient about her chest pain.
    (C) explain that this is a side effect of nitroglycerin.
    (D) all of the above

82. A 25-year-old man has been working in an extremely hot area of a steel mill. He has been working all day wearing heavy protective gear over his clothing. He is weak, dizzy, pale, and diaphoretic. He is likely suffering from
    (A) heat cramps.
    (B) heat exhaustion.
    (C) heat stroke.
    (D) heat collapse.

83. Your patient was the unrestrained driver of a vehicle involved in a frontal collision at 45 miles per hour. There is about 2 feet of "crush" to the front of the vehicle. The dash beneath the steering wheel is broken. The windshield is not "starred" or broken. You should have a high index of suspicion for
    (A) cervical spine injury.
    (B) hip dislocation.
    (C) ankle fractures.
    (D) all of the above

84. You are on the scene of a young male patient who was not wearing a helmet when he crashed his motorcycle. He is unresponsive with shallow, irregular respirations, a heart rate of 50, and a blood pressure of 152/92. The most likely cause of these findings is that the
    (A) patient has a traumatic brain injury with increasing intracranial pressure.
    (B) patient has a skull fracture.
    (C) patient has severe internal injuries and blood loss.
    (D) patient suffered a seizure, causing the motorcycle crash.

85. Your patient is a 5-year-old girl who was restrained by a lap belt in a frontal impact collision, but not in a child booster seat. Your highest index of suspicion should be for
    (A) cervical spine injury.
    (B) fractured femurs.
    (C) internal abdominal injuries.
    (D) rib fractures.

86. A person who jumps from a height and lands on his or her feet should be suspected of having injuries to the
    (A) femur.
    (B) calcaneus.
    (C) spine.
    (D) all of the above

87. Which of the following is an example of a primary phase blast injury?
    (A) rupture of the intestines
    (B) lacerations from flying debris
    (C) burns
    (D) fractures

88. Which of the following is an example of a low-velocity mechanism of penetrating trauma?
    (A) assault rifle
    (B) handgun
    (C) bomb shrapnel
    (D) knife

89. The best definition of shock is
    (A) significant blood loss.
    (B) hypotension.
    (C) hypoperfusion.
    (D) vasoconstriction.

90. Your patient is a 35-year-old female factory worker, whose hair became entangled in machinery, producing a "scalping" wound. She has lost a significant amount of blood. Her skin is pale and cool, she is restless, and her vital signs are blood pressure, 128/88, heart rate, 104, and respirations, 20. The patient's condition is most accurately described as
    (A) compensated shock.
    (B) decompensated shock.
    (C) impending shock.
    (D) late shock.

91. Your patient is an 8-year-old male with a pencil impaled in his right eye. The proper treatment for this is to
    (A) remove the pencil and place a patch over the right eye.
    (B) stabilize the pencil in place and bandage both eyes.
    (C) stabilize the pencil in place and bandage the right eye.
    (D) remove the pencil and bandage both eyes.

92. Assuming each dressing listed would be taped in place on three sides, which of the following would NOT be an appropriate dressing for an open chest wound?
    (A) the foil wrapper from a package of vaseline gauze
    (B) the plastic wrapper from an oxygen mask
    (C) a 5″ by 9″ absorbent dressing
    (D) a piece of household plastic wrap

93. Your patient is a 45-year-old male who was the unrestrained driver of a vehicle that crashed "head-on" into a tree. He responds to verbal stimuli, has pale, cool, diaphoretic skin, a tender abdomen, and deformities to both thighs. His blood pressure is 90/62, pulse is weak at 112 per minute, and respirations are 24. Which of the following is the best course of action?
    (A) Use a short spinal immobilization device to extricate the patient, perform a detailed physical exam, use traction splints to immobilize the thigh injuries, secure to a long backboard, and transport.
    (B) Apply high-flow oxygen, use rapid extrication to remove the patient from the vehicle. Immobilize the patient on a long backboard and begin transport before performing additional assessment.
    (C) Use an emergency move to remove the patient from the vehicle, apply high-flow oxygen, place the patient on a long backboard, begin transport, and finalize spinal immobilization en route.
    (D) Use rapid extrication to remove the patient from the vehicle, perform a detailed physical exam, obtain a SAMPLE history, immobilize the patient on a long backboard, and transport.

94. Your patient struck his head on the sidewalk after being thrown from his bicycle. When you pinch the patient's shoulder, he reacts with extension of the extremities. This is most accurately described as
    (A) a positive Babinski reflex.
    (B) decerebrate posturing.
    (C) Cushing's triad.
    (D) Glasgow's coma sign.

95. A 16-year-old male dove into the shallow end of a swimming pool, striking his head on the concrete bottom of the pool. You should suspect spinal injury due to
    (A) compression.
    (B) flexion.
    (C) extension.
    (D) distraction.

96. Your patient presents with his right eye extending from its socket, lying on the patient's cheek. You should
    (A) irrigate the empty orbit with sterile saline and gently replace the eye into the socket, and bandage over the eye.
    (B) cover the extruded eye with a moist, sterile dressing, and place an occlusive dressing over the top of it.
    (C) stabilize the eye in place with a bulky, dry, sterile dressing.
    (D) place a paper cup over the eye, bandage it in place, covering the unaffected eye, as well.

97. Which of the following weapons of mass destruction would result in muscle twitching, copious oral secretions, abdominal cramps, vomiting, diarrhea, and excessive tearing of the eyes?
    (A) cyanide
    (B) vesicant
    (C) nerve agent
    (D) biological agent

98. In a hazardous materials incident the EMT provides patient care in the
    (A) hot zone.
    (B) warm zone.
    (C) decontamination zone.
    (D) safe zone.

99. The first attempted method of accessing a patient who remains in the vehicle after a collision is to
    (A) use hydraulic spreaders to "pop" the door.
    (B) use a spring-loaded punch to break and remove a window.
    (C) try to open the door.
    (D) cut the "A" posts and roll the roof back.

100. Your long backboard is covered with blood after a trauma call. After cleaning the board, you should use
    (A) low-level disinfection.
    (B) intermediate-level disinfection.
    (C) high-level disinfection.
    (D) sterilization.

Answer Key

EXAM 2

1.	A	26.	A	51.	B	76.	A
2.	B	27.	A	52.	C	77.	D
3.	A	28.	C	53.	C	78.	C
4.	B	29.	C	54.	C	79.	C
5.	D	30.	B	55.	A	80.	B
6.	B	31.	D	56.	B	81.	D
7.	B	32.	D	57.	C	82.	B
8.	C	33.	C	58.	C	83.	D
9.	C	34.	D	59.	A	84.	A
10.	A	35.	A	60.	B	85.	C
11.	B	36.	B	61.	C	86.	D
12.	B	37.	A	62.	B	87.	A
13.	C	38.	A	63.	A	88.	D
14.	A	39.	B	64.	B	89.	C
15.	B	40.	D	65.	B	90.	A
16.	A	41.	A	66.	C	91.	B
17.	A	42.	B	67.	B	92.	C
18.	B	43.	A	68.	D	93.	B
19.	A	44.	A	69.	C	94.	B
20.	D	45.	B	70.	A	95.	A
21.	B	46.	A	71.	C	96.	D
22.	A	47.	C	72.	A	97.	C
23.	A	48.	C	73.	D	98.	D
24.	C	49.	D	74.	D	99.	C
25.	C	50.	A	75.	B	100.	B

Exam 2

ANSWERS TO EXAM 2

1. **(A)** Chapter 2, Objective 1
   Continuous quality improvement is an ongoing evaluation of the EMS system to improve the quality of care provided.

2. **(B)** Chapter 3, Objective 3
   The EMT must be honest with the patient's family and not provide false hope.

3. **(A)** Chapter 3, Objective 5
   The use of alcohol to relax is not a recommended way to reduce stress.

4. **(B)** Chapter 2, Objective 7
   Although there are national guidelines, regulations that determine an EMT's exact scope of practice are determined at the state level.

5. **(D)** Chapter 4, Objective 2
   Having consenting family members present is not a requirement for honoring a DNR.

6. **(B)** Chapter 10, Objective 1
   Handheld radios are called portable radios. The radios mounted in vehicles are called mobile radios.

7. **(B)** Chapter 4, Objective 4
   Unresponsive patients are treated under the doctrine of implied consent.

8. **(C)** Chapter 4, Objective 5
   To be considered an adult, except in unusual circumstances, a person must be at least 18 years old.

9. **(C)** Chapter 4, Objective 5
   Pregnancy is one of the conditions in which a minor is considered emancipated.

10. **(A)** Chapter 4, Objective 7
    Terminating patient care without turning care over to an equally or higher trained provider, whether or not harm results, is abandonment.

11. **(B)** Chapter 4, Objective 7
    Placing a person in fear of bodily harm is assault.

12. **(B)** Chapter 4, Objective 8
    Legal duty to respond applies to the EMT only in the state in which he or she is licensed or certified.

13. **(C)** Chapter 4, Objective 9
    Unless the records are subpoenaed to be released to the opposing attorney or the patient gives written consent, the EMT may not share the patient's information.

14. **(A)** Chapter 4, Objective 7
EMTALA is the Emergency Medical Treatment and Active Labor Act, which prevents patients in need of immediate care from being denied care or "dumped" on other facilities.

15. **(B)** Chapter 7, Objective 11
Only when the patient or providers are in immediate danger of harm, such as imminent fire, explosion, or traffic hazard, is an emergency move used.

16. **(A)** Chapter 7, Objective 11
Rapid extrication is an urgent move, since the patient is first assessed and immediate life-threatening conditions are addressed before moving.

17. **(A)** Chapter 5, Objective 1
The ilium is the largest and uppermost pelvic bone. It is distinct for its "wings," which flare out on either side of the spine.

18. **(B)** Chapter 5, Objective 1
The ulna is on the medial or little finger side of the forearm.

19. **(A)** Chapter 5, Objective 1
The tibia makes up the medial malleolus.

20. **(D)** Chapter 5, Objective 1
Lying face down is prone; on the back is supine.

21. **(B)** Chapter 15, Objective 1
Insulin allows glucose to enter cells readily, removing it from the bloodstream.

22. **(A)** Chapter 8, Objective 2
Chemoreceptors in the aorta and carotid arteries detect both oxygen and carbon dioxide levels, but the primary stimulus to breathe in healthy individuals is increased carbon dioxide.

23. **(A)** Chapter 8, Objective 2
When the diaphragm contracts, it moves downward, increasing the size of the chest cavity, causing lower intrathoracic pressure, which causes air to move from the higher atmospheric pressure into the lungs to equalize the pressure.

24. **(C)** Chapter 6, Objective 5
The dorsalis pedis, or pedal, pulse is the pulse on the top of the feet.

25. **(C)** Chapter 8, Objective 1
The epiglottis is the leaf-shaped tissue that protects the airway.

26. **(A)** Chapter 8, Objective 1
The pleura covers the lungs and lines the chest wall.

27. **(A)** Chapter 8, Objective 1
The trachea is located anterior and midline in the neck.

28. **(C)** Chapter 5, Objective 2
The vitreous humor is the substance that fills the eye.

29. **(C)** Chapter 21, Section 1, Objective 2
The subcutaneous layer is the third or deepest layer of the skin.

30. **(B)** Chapter 9, Section 2, Objective 1
The general impression is a determination of the urgency with which the EMT must proceed, but is not an exact determination of the problem.

31. **(D)** Chapter 6, Objective 5
Capillary refill time should be no less than two seconds.

32. **(D)** Chapter 9, Section 2, Objective 15
Yellow pigments collect in the tissues when the liver cannot effectively break down the contents of old red blood cells.

33. **(C)** Chapter 14, Objective 2
Nausea is commonly expected with chest pain, but not present in this case, making it a pertinent negative.

34. **(D)** Chapter 11, Objective 1
What the patient says or complains of is subjective. What the EMT observes for himself or herself is objective.

35. **(A)** Chapter 9, Section 4, Objective 1
The chief complaint guides the focused medical assessment.

36. **(B)** Chapter 13, Objective 2
"Crowing" sounds are associated with stridor, which occurs as airflow through the upper airway is restricted.

37. **(A)** Chapter 6, Objective 16
Constricted pupils are consistent with the use of many narcotics, but not typical of the other choices provided.

38. **(A)** Chapter 6, Objective 19
This blood pressure is considered normal only in the infant age group.

39. **(B)** Chapter 23, Objective 2
Bradycardia in this age group is most commonly due to hypoxia. The other conditions listed most typically cause an increase in heart rate.

40. **(D)** Chapter 6, Objective 19
A cuff that is too wide results in a falsely low reading.

41. **(A)** Chapter 13, Objective 5
Pulse oximetry is designed to detect hypoxia.

42. **(B)** Chapter 6, Objective 15
Smaller pupils are said to be constricted.

43. **(A)** Chapter 8, Objective 8
Suction is applied only as the catheter is withdrawn, for no more than 15 seconds. The catheter should be rinsed after suctioning.

44. **(A)** Chapter 8, Objective 8
Measure from the corner of the mouth to the earlobe.

45. **(B)** Chapter 8, Objective 12
The proper rate for bag-valve mask ventilations in an adult is 10 to 12 per minute.

46. **(A)** Chapter 8, Objective 12
The Sellick maneuver consists of pressing the cricoid cartilage posteriorly to obstruct the esophagus during ventilation to prevent gastric distention.

47. **(C)** Chapter 8, Objective 18
A nasopharyngeal airway is measured from the nare to earlobe.

48. **(C)** Chapter 8, Objective 6
The jaw-thrust maneuver allows the airway to be opened without movement of the cervical spine.

49. **(D)** Chapter 22, Objective 8
A folded towel under the shoulders aligns the child's torso and head, preventing flexion of the neck.

50. **(A)** Chapter 16, Section 2, Objective 5
The patient's respirations are adequate and she is responsive to pain. However, if she vomits, as may occur with overdoses, her decreased level of responsiveness may leave her unable to protect her airway.

51. **(B)** Chapter 14, Objective 41
The only acceptable method for prehospital administration of nitroglycerin is sublingual.

52. **(C)** Chapter 13, Objective 2
Emphysema is one of the chronic obstructive pulmonary (lung) diseases.

53. **(C)** Chapter 13, Objective 2
The gurgling indicates fluid in the airway. The patient must be immediately suctioned to prevent aspiration.

54. **(C)** Chapter 14, Objective 41
Although the EMT may administer or assist with all of these medications, only nitroglycerin is indicated for chest pain.

55. **(A)** Chapter 14, Objective 41
The use of drugs like Levitra, Viagra, and Cialis can result in a profound drop in blood pressure when nitroglycerin is administered.

56. **(B)** Chapter 13, Objective 5
Patients with cardiac and respiratory problems who are alert and have an adequate blood pressure should be allowed to assume a position of comfort, which typically is sitting up.

57. **(C)** Chapter 19, Objective 8
Often, tactile stimulation is all that is needed to stimulate the newborn to breathe.

58. **(C)** Chapter 19, Objective 13
CPR is started in infants with a heart rate less than 60.

59. **(A)** Chapter 19, Objective 3

The patient is presenting with signs and symptoms of preeclampsia, or toxemia of pregnancy. Stimulation such as unnecessary movement, lights, or noise may cause a seizure in preeclamptic patients. Even with her high blood pressure, the patient is placed in left lateral recumbent position to prevent supine hypotensive syndrome.

60. **(B)** Chapter 19, Objective 3

These are signs and symptoms of preeclampsia.

61. **(C)** Chapter 20, Objective 3

Pinching the nostrils will control an anterior nose bleed. The head is tilted forward to prevent the patient from swallowing or aspirating blood. Swallowing blood may result in vomiting.

62. **(B)** Chapter 13, Objective 10

The Heimlich maneuver is used in patients in this age group who are conscious with a severe airway obstruction.

63. **(A)** Chapter 16, Section 2, Objective 6

Only activated charcoal should be given, on the advice of medical control.

64. **(B)** Chapter 15, Objective 1

A TIA presents as a stroke, but resolves, usually within an hour.

65. **(B)** Chapter 15, Objective 1

Many medical conditions can lead to bizarre behavior. The patient may have a potentially life-threatening cause of the behavior, such as hypoglycemia, and needs to be evaluated. However, even if the cause of the patient's behavior is medical, he may still pose a threat and the restraints should not be removed at this point.

66. **(C)** Chapter 14, Objective 22

Automatic external defibrillators are only applied to patients who are unresponsive, pulseless, and apneic.

67. **(B)** Chapter 15, Objective 1

When a blood clot forms in a blood vessel it is called a thrombus. It would not be an embolus unless a blood clot in another part of the body broke loose and traveled to the circulation of the brain.

68. **(D)** Chapter 15, Objective 1

If there is any indication that a patient has weakness or paralysis, he or she should not be allowed to walk, and the way the patient walks will not give the EMT additional information about whether the patient is having a stroke.

69. **(C)** Chapter 15, Objective 1

Status epilepticus.

70. **(A)** Chapter 16, Objective 4

The patient is experiencing a localized reaction. Although it could progress to anaphylaxis, neither oxygen nor epinephrine is given to prevent this from occurring. Wasp stings are treated in the prehospital setting by scraping away the stinger, if it remains at the site of the sting.

71. **(C)** Chapter 24, Section 3, Objective 2
Carbon monoxide is a product of incomplete combustion of carbon-containing fuels, such as wood, coal, natural gas, and petroleum products.

72. **(A)** Chapter 13, Objective 2
Because the patient has been getting progressively worse over the month, this is not an acute coronary problem. The patient's signs and symptoms are "classic" for congestive heart failure, which has likely occurred because her heart muscle was damaged by her recent heart attack.

73. **(D)** Chapter 18, Objective 4
Although the patient is suicidal, it does not rule out the possibility that the patient may be violent toward others.

74. **(D)** Chapter 14, Objective 12
The AED is only applied to pulseless patients. None of the other conditions are contraindications, although the nitroglycerin patch should be removed before using the AED.

75. **(B)** Chapter 14, Objective 17
The patient has been "down" less than 4 minutes. The greatest chance for successful defibrillation in this patient is to defibrillate, if indicated, as quickly as possible.

76. **(A)** Chapter 14, Objective 21
A biphasic defibrillator is more effective, delivers less energy, and causes less damage to the heart.

77. **(D)** Chapter 14, Objective 2
The groin is not a typical location or point of radiation for cardiac pain.

78. **(C)** Chapter 13, Objective 8
Although these drugs have similar names and all may be used by patients with respiratory problems, only albuterol, which relaxes bronchial smooth muscle, is indicated in acute respiratory distress.

79. **(C)** Chapter 12, Objective 3
All of these medications may be used by ALS personnel in the treatment of anaphylaxis, but only epinephrine is in the EMT's scope of practice.

80. **(B)** Chapter 15, Objective 1
Insulin is not produced or is produced insufficiently in diabetes.

81. **(D)** Chapter 14, Objective 5
Nitroglycerin relieves chest pain by dilating the coronary arteries. However, it is not specific to just the coronary arteries, and may result in headache and hypotension.

82. **(B)** Chapter 17, Objective 4
The complaints of weakness and dizziness and the patient's pale, diaphoretic skin are most consistent with heat exhaustion.

83. **(D)** Chapter 9, Section 1, Objective 5
All of these injuries should be suspected with this mechanism of injury.

84. **(A)** Chapter 22, Objective 4
When the brain swells inside the skull, the body attempts to maintain blood flow through the increased pressure by increasing the blood pressure. In response, the heart rate drops. Irregular, slow, or shallow breathing occurs when the brainstem is injured or compressed.

85. **(C)** Chapter 9, Section 1, Objective 4
Adult lap belts do not fit children properly, often coming to rest across the abdomen. When the body's forward motion is suddenly stopped by the seatbelt, it may result in injuries to the abdomen and lumbar spine.

86. **(D)** Chapter 9, Section 1, Objective 4
Energy travels in a straight line through the body and can injure any structure in its path.

87. **(A)** Chapter 9, Section 1, Objective 4
The blast wave causes sudden compression and decompression of gas or air-filled structures, resulting in injury to the sinuses, lungs, and gastrointestinal tract.

88. **(D)** Chapter 9, Section 1, Objective 4
Knife wounds are "low" velocity penetration injuries.

89. **(C)** Chapter 20, Objective 9
Shock is a state of hypoperfusion of the tissues, resulting in the inability of the tissue to meet its metabolic needs.

90. **(A)** Chapter 20, Objective 9
The patient's blood pressure is within normal range because of the vasoconstriction causing the pale, cool skin, and the increase in heart rate. This describes the "compensated shock" state.

91. **(B)** Chapter 21, Section 1, Objective 26
The impaled object is stabilized in place. Since the eyes move together, the uninjured eye is bandaged to prevent movement of the injured eye.

92. **(C)** Chapter 21, Section 1, Objective 10
The dressing material must be capable of forming an airtight seal. The absorbent dressing is porous and cannot form a seal.

93. **(B)** Chapter 9, Section 3, Objective 2
The patient is critical and unstable. He must be rapidly removed from the vehicle and immobilized before transport. However, transport must not be further delayed by detailed assessment on the scene.

94. **(B)** Chapter 22, Objective 7
Decerebrate posturing is illustrated by the extension of the extremities when stimulated.

95. **(A)** Chapter 22, Objective 4
The weight of the body compresses the vertebrae in the neck as it continues in its downward trajectory.

96. **(D)** Chapter 21, Objective 21
The eye should not be replaced in the orbit. The proper care is to protect it with a paper cup or similar device and to bandage the unaffected eye as well, since the eyes move together.

97. **(C)** Chapter 24, Section 3, Objective 2
These are the signs and symptoms that occur when a nerve agent prevents the breakdown of the neurotransmitter acetylcholine at the nerve ends.

98. **(D)** Chapter 24, Section 3, Objective 4
The EMT cares for patients in the cold, or safe, zone.

99. **(C)** Chapter 24, Section 2, Objective 4
It is very often possible, and much quicker, to try to open the doors.

100. **(B)** Chapter 24, Section 1, Objective 14
Intermediate-level disinfection is needed because of the visible blood on the board. However, since the backboard does not come into contact with mucus membranes and is not used invasively, higher-level disinfection or sterilization is not needed.

Glossary

A

Abandonment. Termination of patient-provider relationship without assuring continuing care at a level equal to or greater than that provided prior to termination.

Abdomen. The portion of the body between the diaphragm and the pelvis.

Abortion. Spontaneous or intentional termination of pregnancy prior to the twentieth week of pregnancy.

Abrasion. An open soft tissue injury caused by scraping away the superficial layers of skin.

Acceleration. The rate of increasing speed.

Acute. Rapid onset, severe, and short in duration.

Advanced EMT. An individual trained according to the DOT curriculum for intermediate life support, which includes a limited amount of advanced skills.

Advanced Life Support (ALS). Patient care given in the hospital or by paramedics in the field, which includes the use of defibrillators, intravenous and drug therapy, and advanced airway interventions.

Alkali. A strong base.

Allergic reaction. A hypersensitivity to a substance that results in potentially life-threatening reactions.

Allied Health. Referring to health care providers other than physicians, including nurses, technicians, therapists, EMT-Bs, EMT-Is, and EMT-Ps.

Alpha radiation. The lowest level of nuclear radiation that can be stopped by a sheet of paper.

Alveoli. Air sacs in the lungs at the end of the bronchioles that take carbon dioxide from the pulmonary capillaries in exchange for oxygen.

Alzheimer's disease. A progressive degenerative disease that attacks the brain, impairing memory, thinking, and behavior.

Amniotic fluid. Fluid in the amniotic sac that surrounds and protects the developing fetus.

Amniotic sac. Membranes that contain the amniotic fluid, surrounding and protecting the developing fetus.

Amputation. Partial or complete severing of a part of the body.

Anaphylaxis. Severe allergic reaction that can be rapidly fatal.

Anatomy. The study of living body structures.

Aneurysm. Bulging area of a weakened blood vessel.

Antibiotics. Medications given to combat bacterial infections.

Antidote. Substance given to counteract the effects of another substance.

Anxiety. A feeling of apprehension, uneasiness, or dread.

APGAR scoring. Numerical system used to describe a newborn's condition by evaluating appearance, pulse, grimace, activity, and color.

Apnea. Absence of breathing.

Arachnoid membrane. Middle layer of meninges that surround the brain.

Arteriosclerosis. A thickening and hardening of the veins and arteries that limits their flexibility.

Asphyxia. Increasing carbon dioxide and decreasing oxygen levels caused by cessation of, or insufficient, breathing that ultimately results in death.

Aspiration. Foreign bodies, solid or liquid, drawn into and obstructing the airway and lungs.

Assault. A violent physical attack; places a person in fear of bodily harm.

Atherosclerosis. The most common form of arteriosclerosis in which fatty deposits collect on the insides of medium to large arteries, narrowing them and limiting blood flow.

Auscultation. Listening to sounds made by internal organs.

Autonomic nervous system. The part of the nervous system that controls involuntary body functions.

Avulsion. An open soft tissue injury where tissue is gouged or torn away completely or leaving a flap of skin.

Axial loading. Extreme compression of the cervical vertebrae.

B

Bacteria. Small, independent living organisms that can cause infections or assist in body functions.

Ballistics. Study of the motion of projectiles and their effects on the objects they strike.

Battery. The unlawful touching of a person without that person's consent.

Battle's sign. Discoloration behind the ears that can indicate basilar skull fractures.

Beta radiation. Medium nuclear radiation that can be blocked by clothing or the outer layers of the skin.

Bile. Greenish yellow fluid secreted by the liver and stored in the gallbladder that aids in the digestion of fats.

Bradycardia. Heart rates below 60.

Bronchi. Branches of the trachea leading into the lungs.

Bronchioles. Smaller extensions of the bronchi leading to the alveoli.

Burnout. Losing interest in one's job following constant unresolved stress.

C

Capillary. Microscopic blood vessels that connect small arteries to veins.

Capillary refill. An assessment of the circulatory system that measures the time it takes for the capillaries to refill with blood after compression.

Cardiogenic shock. Shock caused by failure of the heart to act as a pump.

Cardiovascular disease. Disease that affects the heart and/or the blood vessels.

Cavity. Hollow spaces in the body (i.e., chest and abdomen) that contain the body's organs.

Cell. The basic unit of life, which makes up and is specific to every body tissue.

Cerebrospinal fluid. Clear fluid surrounding the brain and spinal cord, providing cushioning and nutrition.

Cerebrovascular accident (CVA). Death of brain tissue caused by either blockage of a blood vessel or rupture of a blood vessel.

Cerebrum. Largest part of the brain, divided into two hemispheres and responsible for consciousness and higher mental functions such as thought, memory, and emotions.

Cheyne-Stokes respirations. A respiratory pattern common in brain-injured patients in which the rate and volume of respirations increase then abruptly subside and begin again, repeating the cycle.

Chronic. Of continuing or long duration.

Chronic Obstructive Pulmonary Disease (COPD). Diseases that impair breathing that include asthma, emphysema, and chronic bronchitis.

Circumferential. Encircling or going all the way around something.

Civil law. Law dealing with noncriminal issues.

Coma. A state of unconsciousness.

Command post. A fixed location set up to coordinate efforts of multiple companies and/or agencies operating at a large event.

Compensated shock. The body's compensation for blood loss that involves constriction of blood vessels and increasing the heart rate to maintain adequate circulation.

Computer-aided Dispatch (CAD). Enhanced dispatch systems that have the capability of storing information on addresses and occupants and helping to manage response capabilities.

Concussion. A brain injury that is typified by a momentary loss of consciousness.

Conduction. Moving electrons, heat, or energy through a medium. For example, water is a good conductor, while air is a poor conductor.

Consent. Permission to treat.

Contrecoup. Something occurring on the opposite side; a blow to the forehead causing injury to the rear of the brain.

Contusion. A closed soft tissue injury in which the skin is unbroken but underlying tissues are damaged.

Convection. Transferring heat through air or water currents.

Cranium. The boxlike part of the skull that houses and protects the brain.

Crepitation. A grating or crackling sensation associated with subcutaneous emphysema or bone endings rubbing together.

Cricothyroid membrane. A thin membrane located between the cricoid and thyroid cartilages.

Criminal law. Laws dealing with crimes against society.

Critical incident. An event that carries the potential for strong, potentially damaging emotional impact.

Critical Incident Stress Management. A plan to provide support from peers and professionals in the event of exposure to critical incident stress.

Croup. Viral infection common in children that causes swelling of the upper airways and is characterized by a barklike cough.

Crowning. Presentation of the baby's head in the vaginal opening that signifies imminent birth.

Cyanosis. Bluish color to the skin caused by hypoxia.

D

Deceleration. The rate at which something that is moving comes to a stop.

Decompensated shock. Failure of the compensation mechanism in which the blood vessels dilate causing the blood pressure to drop precipitously and making circulation inadequate.

Decorticate posturing. Posturing in which an unresponsive patient's arms are flexed with clenched fists and the legs extended. This posturing is typical of patients with brain injury above the upper brain stem.

Defibrillation. The process of using an electrical charge to cease disorganized electrical activity in the heart allowing organized electrical activity to restart.

Dehydration. Loss of body fluids through elimination or evaporation (sweating).

Delirium. Acute alteration in mental functioning.

Delirium tremens (DTs). Body tremors and hallucinations suffered by alcoholics when blood alcohol drops too low.

Delusion. False belief held despite evidence to the contrary.

Dementia. Frequently progressive and irreversible deterioration of mental status.

Depression. An overpowering feeling of hopelessness.

Dermis. The second layer of skin that produces the epidermis and contains the blood vessels and nerve endings.

Diabetes mellitus. Condition in which the pancreas either fails to secrete insulin or secretes insulin erratically, causing the patient to be unable to utilize sugar as fuel to cellular metabolism.

Dialysis. A mechanical process used in place of failed kidneys to filter impurities out of the blood.

Diastole. The relaxation phase of the heart's contraction cycle.

Diastolic. The bottom number in blood pressure readings representing the pressure in the vessels between contractions.

Direct medical control. Medical direction given directly to field personnel via radio or phone.

Disentanglement. The process of removing a vehicle from a trapped occupant.

Dislocation. Disruption of the proper position of the bones in a joint.

Dispatch. The center that receives requests for service and the exchange of information with the responding units.

Dura mater. The outermost layer of meninges that covers and protects the brain.

Durable power of attorney. Legal designation of responsibility to one person for another.

Dyspnea. Difficulty breathing.

E

Ecchymosis. Bruising.

Ectopic pregnancy. A fetus developing outside the uterus.

Elderly. Patients over 65 years of age.

Emboli. A clot or other particle that lodges in a blood vessel.

Emergency medical dispatcher. Dispatcher who is trained following the DOT curriculum for dispatchers.

Emergency medical responder. Commonly called "first responders," these providers perform basic life support focused on scene work without transport training.

Emergency medical services. The prehospital emergency care delivery system.

Emergency Medical Technician (EMT). An individual trained according to the DOT curriculum for basic life support.

Epidermis. The outermost layer of skin.

Epidural hematoma. A pool of blood that accumulates between the dura and the cranium.

Epigastrum. The abdominal area directly below the sternum.

Epiglottis. Leaf-shaped muscle that covers either the trachea or esophagus depending on whether one is swallowing or breathing.

Ethics. The rules, standards, or morals that govern the activities of professionals within a society.

Evaporation. The process through which a substance changes from a liquid to a gas.

Expressed consent. The act of an individual actually giving written or verbal consent to a health care professional.

Extrication. Removal of an entrapped person from his or her confinement.

F

Flail chest. Describing two or more ribs broken in two or more places creating a free-floating section of the chest wall.

Fontanelles. Soft areas on an infant's head where the bones of the skull have not yet fused together.

Fracture. Any break in the continuity of the bone.

G

Gag reflex. A reflex that protects the airway from foreign bodies by creating a spasm and cough to clear the airway.

Gamma radiation. The third and strongest level of radiation that requires lead shielding to block.

Genitalia. Reproductive organs.

Geriatrics. The study of the special needs of the elderly.

Glasgow coma scale. A scoring system used to evaluate the neurological status of patients that looks at eye opening, verbal responses, and motor response.

Glottis. Opening between the vocal cords.

Golden hour. The time in which definitive care must be provided following injury for the best chance of survival.

Good Samaritan laws. Laws that provide for protection from liability for good-intentioned individuals providing emergency care.

Grand mal seizures. Seizure activity characterized by tonic clonic muscular contractions.

Greenstick fracture. Common fracture in children that causes bones to bend and fray.

Guarding. Positioning to minimize pain.

H

Hallucination. Seeing or hearing things that are not real.

Hazard zone. The area around an emergency that requires special protective equipment and training and isolation from bystanders.

Heat cramps. Painful muscle spasms associated with exposure to heat and subsequent dehydration.

Heat exhaustion. Weakness, dizziness, and nausea associated with vasodilation secondary to exposure to heat.

Heatstroke. Loss of consciousness due to exposure to heat.

Hematemesis. Vomiting blood.

Hematoma. Blood pooling beneath the skin from broken blood vessels.

Hematuria. Blood in the urine.

Hemoglobin. The part of red blood cells that enables the transport of oxygen and carbon dioxide.

Hemoptysis. Coughing up blood.

Hemothorax. The collapse of a lung due to the accumulation of blood in the chest cavity.

Hyperglycemia. Elevated blood sugar levels.

Hypertension. Elevated blood pressure.

Hyperthermia. Abnormally high body temperature.

Hypoglycemia. Low blood sugar levels.

Hypothermia. Unusually low body temperature.

Hypoxia. The state of low oxygen blood content.

I

Implied consent. The rule that allows for unresponsive patients to be treated with the assumption that they would consent to care if they were able to.

Incident Command System (ICS). The system that provides for command and supervision of all of the functions at an emergency scene.

Incident commander. The individual with ultimate authority and responsibility at an emergency scene.

Incision. A very clean precise laceration made by a sharp instrument.

Indirect medical control. Medical control provided with standard operating procedures.

Informed consent. The provision that in order to give consent or remove treatment a patient must be informed as to their condition and possible complications from nontreatment.

Ingestion. Swallowing a substance entering the body through the digestive tract.

Inhalation. Breathing in a substance entering the body through the respiratory tract.

Injection. Describing a substance entering the body by breaking the skin, such as a sting, bite, or needle.

Inspection. Visual exam of the body.

Insulin. The hormone secreted by the pancreas to facilitate transport of sugar into cells.

Intercostal muscles. The muscles between the ribs that facilitate breathing.

Intracerebral bleeding. Bleeding directly into tissues of the brain.

Intracranial pressure (ICP). Pressure within the skull exerted on the brain.

Intubation. Passing a tube through the vocal cords into the trachea to facilitate ventilation and isolation of the airway from the potential for aspiration.

Involuntary consent. Consent obtained against the wishes of the patient.

Iris. Portion of the eye that contains the pigment that gives the eye its color.

K

Ketoacidosis. Condition created in a diabetic whose insulin production is insufficient to transport sugar out of the blood and into the cells. This accumulated sugar causes the blood to become more acidic. Without sugar making it into the cells to produce energy, the patient will eventually lose consciousness and without treatment, die; also called diabetic coma.

Kinetic energy. The energy of motion.

Kussmaul's respirations. Deep, gulping breaths, common in diabetic emergencies; also called air hunger.

Kyphosis. Exaggerated curvature of the spine; generally causes the patient to appear stooped.

L

Labor. The period of childbirth.

Laceration. An open soft tissue injury characterized by a tear in the skin with jagged borders.

Laryngospasm. Normally a mechanism to protect the airway against aspiration; this spasm of the vocal cords can also block the airway and cause asphyxiation.

Libel. Make false accusations or statements that injure a person's reputation.

Licensure. Verification that a governmental unit has authorized a person to practice a given, regulated profession.

Ligament. Connective tissue connecting bone to bone and holding joints together.

Litigation. The act of filing a lawsuit against another person.

Living will. A document that instructs providers on what type of care the patient wishes and which care the patient refuses. In the event that this patient is unable to give consent, this document is to be honored in place of that consent.

M

Magill forceps. A curved forceps used to position tubes into the airway or to clear foreign bodies from the airway.

Mammalian diving reflex. An ancient reflex that decreases circulation to every area of the body except the brain. This reflex can be stimulated by submersing the face into water.

Maxillary. Referring to the maxilla or jawbone.

Mechanism of injury. The events and physical activity that create injury.

Meconium. Dark green material in the amniotic fluid. It is the product of fetal distress causing the fetus to move its bowel into the fluid. It also refers to the first bowel movement of the newborn.

Mediastinum. Space between the lungs and the sternum and spine.

Medical director. Physician responsible for the training of and protocols for prehospital care providers.

Medulla oblongata. Lower portion of the brain stem responsible for maintaining respirations.

Melena. Black, tarry, especially foul-smelling stool caused by blood decomposing in the lower intestines.

Meninges. Membranes covering and protecting the brain. There are three of them: dura, arachnoid, and pia.

Meningitis. An infection of the meninges, the layers of tissue covering and protecting the brain.

Mesentery. Folds of tissue within the body that support and supply organs with blood.

Midbrain. The portion of the brain that connects the pons and the cerebral hemispheres.

Minute volume. The amount of air inhaled and exhaled in one minute.

N

Nares. The openings in the nose that lead into the airway.

Nasal flaring. Excessive widening of the nares with respirations.

National standard curriculum. The curriculum for prehospital care providers prepared under the direction of the U.S. Department of Transportation.

Negligence. Deviation from standard of care that causes injury.

Neonate. Term used to describe infants from birth to one month old.

O

Organ. Group of tissues with a common function.

Overdose. A drug taken in excess of its intended dose causing a potential threat to life.

P

Packaging. Preparing a patient using stretchers, boards, blankets, pillows, and whatever else is necessary, for safe transport to the hospital.

Palpation. Assessment using the sense of touch.

Palpitation. A sensation that the heart is pounding, or a strong, rapid heartbeat that the patient feels.

Paradoxical movement. Referring to a section of the chest wall that moves in a direction opposite from the direction it should move during respiration. This is caused by two or more ribs being broken in two or more places creating a free-floating section of the chest wall.

Paramedic. An individual trained according to the DOT curriculum for advanced life support.

Parasympathetic nervous system. Part of the nervous system controlling vegetative function.

Parietal pleura. A thin sheath of tissue covering the inside of the chest wall.

Patent. Secure and open; a patent airway is a secure and open airway.

Patient assessment. Examinination of a patient to determine his or her condition.

Percussion. Striking an area or object to elicit a sound or vibration.

Perfusion. Fluid flowing into and out of tissue providing nourishment and removing waste.

Pericardial tamponade. Any fluid accumulating in the sac surrounding the heart that inhibits the contraction of the heart muscle.

Pericardium. Double-layered sac surrounding the heart.

Peripheral vascular resistance. Pressure exerted back against the flow of blood from the heart by the peripheral vascular bed.

Peristalsis. Wavelike muscular contractions of the digestive tract that help to move the food along as it is digested.

Petit mal seizure. Form of seizure activity that may or may not involve a loss of consciousness; may be a twitch of a single extremity or a person may "black out" for a moment.

Physiology. The study of the function of the body and its parts.

Pia mater. Innermost of the three meningeal layers covering and protecting the brain.

Placenta. The organ that is attached to the wall of the uterus and supplies the growing fetus with its blood supply.

Plasma. The fluid portion of the blood that transports the blood cells and platelets.

Pleura. Membranes that line the inside of the chest wall and covering the lungs.

Poison control center. A resource center staffed with trained personnel to give up-to-date information on poisons and the proper response to poisonings.

Poisoning. Taking harmful substances into the body.

Postpartum. The period after the birth of the child.

Prenatal. The time period before the birth of the child. Another term for this period is antepartum.

Primary assessment. Rapid initial assessment designed to identify any immediate life threats.

Professional. A person who exhibits the qualities and conduct characteristic of a practitioner in a given field.

Protocols. Policies and procedures addressing all aspects of an EMS system.

Proximate cause. Legal term that refers to being able to determine that an injury is the result of another person's negligent action or inaction.

Psychosis. Change in personality that prevents a person from behaving normally.

Pulmonary embolism. Blood or other type of clot that lodges in pulmonary blood vessels impairing pulmonary function.

Pulse oximeter. Device that measures oxygen concentration in the blood.

Puncture. Open soft tissue injury typified as a hole punched into or through tissues.

Q

Quality assurance (QA). Process that evaluates service performance for compliance to protocols and measures outcomes.

R

Radio. An electronic communication device that transmits sound waves and telemetry over distances.

Rales. Also described as "crackles," lung sounds heard on auscultation when fluid accumulates in lungs.

Rebound tenderness. Tenderness noted when gentle pressure is released on palpation of abdomen, signifying peritoneal irritation.

Reciprocity. Certification or licensure granted in recognition of similar licensure or certification granted by another agency.

Repeater. A radio booster designed to amplify a radio signal received by a weaker transmitter.

Rescue. To remove someone from a hazardous or dangerous situation.

Research. Establishing fact through diligent investigation and experimentation.

Resource. Personnel and equipment available to responders.

Respiration. Exchange of gasses between a living organism and its environment.

Retraction. Drawing-in motion as in "sternal or intercostal retractions" seen in infants with difficulty breathing.

Retroperitoneal. Posterior abdominal space containing the kidneys and abdominal descending aorta and inferior vena cava.

Rhonchi. Rattling sounds heard when mucus or fluid is in the upper airways.

S

Safety officer. Specially trained responder who supervises the safety of a scene and the personnel working it.

Scapula. Large, flat, wing-shaped bones forming the posterior part of the shoulders.

Schizophrenia. Mental disorder characterized by disturbances in thought, mood, and behavior.

Sebaceous glands. Sebum (oil)-secreting gland found in the dermis.

Sebum. Fatty oil secreted by the sebaceous glands that keep the skin pliable and waterproof.

Secondary assessment. Detailed history and physical exam that seeks to determine the patient's condition.

Sector. Referring to an area of an incident that has been sectioned off and assigned to a sector officer for management by incident command.

Seizure. Spasm or loss of motor function due to disorderly discharge of neurons in the brain.

Senile dementia. Decline of mental functions common in elderly patients.

Sepsis. Infection in the blood.

Septic shock. Infection in the blood causing vasodilation and hypotension.

Shock. Inadequate tissue perfusion. Different types that describe the underlying cause include hemorrhagic hypovolemia, metabolic or nonhemorrhagic hypovolemia, neurogenic, psychogenic, anaphylactic, and septic.

Size up. A quick assessment of the scene to determine immediate needs.

Slander. Injure a person's reputation by making false statements.

Snoring. Audible noises created by upper airway obstruction.

Staging. Describing a place for equipment and personnel to congregate until they are needed or until the scene is made safe for their entry.

Standing orders. Predetermined orders written by the system medical director for specific patient situations, allowing field personnel to administer care without contacting medical control for orders.

START. An acronym that stands for Simple Triage and Rapid Treatment. The system is designed to triage a large number of patients in a short period of time to enable assembling and utilizing necessary resources.

Status epilepticus. A state in which a patient has multiple and continuous grand mal seizures without regaining consciousness between them.

Sternocleidomastoid muscles. Muscles that attach to the mastoid bones on both sides of the neck and connect to the clavicle and sternum. These muscles serve as accessory muscles to breathing in patients in respiratory distress.

Stimulus. Any provocation that creates a response as in verbal or painful stimulus applied during assessment of a patient.

Stridor. High-pitched crowing sound caused by constriction of the upper airways.

Stroke. Injury to the brain caused by an interruption of blood flow to the brain. Dysfunction is directly relative to the area of the brain involved.

Subcutaneous emphysema. Air trapped in subcutaneous tissues causing a swollen appearance and a crackling sensation when palpated.

Subdural hematoma. Blood accumulating beneath the dura meninges covering the brain.

Subluxation. Incomplete dislocation of a joint that causes deformity while the bone ends are still in contact with one another.

Sudden infant death syndrome (SIDS). Death due to undetermined causes during the first year of life.

Surfactant. Material secreted by cells in the lungs contributing to elastic properties necessary to normal pulmonary function.

Sympathetic nervous system. Part of the autonomic nervous system that allows the body to respond to stress. Sympathetic stimuli cause the heart and respiratory rates to respond to the stress.

Synapse. Space between nerve cells across which chemicals conduct electrical impulses.

Syncope. A momentary loss of consciousness caused by an interruption in blood flow to the brain.

Systole. Contraction of the heart muscle.

Systolic. The top number in blood pressure readings representing the pressure in the vessels during contractions.

T

Tachycardia. Heart rate above 100.

Tachypnea. Rapid breathing.

Tendon. Connective tissue that attaches muscle to bone.

Tension pneumothorax. Condition in which air accumulates in the chest, collapsing one lung and compressing the uninvolved lung and the heart and large blood vessels between the lungs, resulting in increased dyspnea and decreased cardiac output.

Tentorium. Extension of the dura mater that separates the cerebrum from the cerebellum.

Tissue. A group of cells with a common function, such as skin, muscle, or bone.

Tonic phase. Phase of a seizure characterized by contraction of muscles.

Toxins. Poisonous substances.

Tracheal tugging. Retraction of tissues in the neck of a patient attempting to breathe with obstructions of the airway.

Trajectory. The path that a projectile follows.

Transfer of command. The planned process of transferring command from one individual to another in an incident command situation.

Transient ischemic attack (TIA). Temporary interruption of blood flow causing temporary dysfunction relative to the area of the brain involved.

Trauma. Injury caused by a violent intentional or unintentional act.

Trauma center. A hospital that has been designated to treat trauma patients due to its commitment to specialized equipment, personnel, and training.

Traumatic asphyxia. Severe compression injury to the chest causing disruption of the organs in the chest cavity and impairing circulation and breathing.

Triage. Picking, choosing, and sorting patients according to the severity of their condition.

U

Umbilical cord. Cord that contains nerves and blood vessels, connecting the fetus to the placenta and providing blood supply and nutrients to the fetus.

Umbilicus. Also called naval or belly button; a remnant of the umbilical connection to the placenta during fetal development.

Universal precautions. Another term for BSI or Body Substance Isolation referring to precautions responders take to prevent exposure to any body substances.

V

Vallecula. A depression between the epiglottis and the base of the tongue.

Valsalva maneuver. Maneuver used to slow a patient's pulse rate by increasing intra-abdominal and intrathoracic pressure. This can be brought about by forcing exhalation against a closed glottis as in trying to blow up a rigid balloon.

Velocity. The rate of speed at which an object is traveling.

Vertigo. Dizziness and a sense that everything around you is moving.

Virus. Microscopic organisms, smaller than bacteria, that require another living host and are the frequent causes of disease.

Visceral pleura. Pleural lining covering the lungs.

Vitreous humor. Clear watery fluid within the posterior portion of the eye.

W

Wheezing. Audible whistling sound heard in patients suffering from obstruction of the lower airways as in asthma and emphysema.

Appendix

In the preceding text we put together summaries and tools to help you prepare for the EMT written exam. To become a licensed EMT you will also have to pass a practical examination. To assist you with that, we have included the National Registry Practical Skill Sheets that describe how candidates are evaluated and the performance level needed to successfully pass the practical exam. The skill sheets appear courtesy of the

National Registry of Emergency Medical Technicians
Rocco V. Morando Building
6610 Busch Boulevard
P.O. Box 29233
Columbus, Ohio 43229
Telephone: (614) 888-4484
Fax: (614) 888-8920

For more information on registering for the National Registry EMT Examination, contact the Registry at the numbers listed above or visit their Web site at *www.nremt.org*.

AIRWAY, OXYGEN AND VENTILATION SKILLS
UPPER AIRWAY ADJUNCTS AND SUCTION

Start Time: _____

Stop Time: _____ Date: _____

Candidate's Name: _____

Evaluator's Name: _____

OROPHARYNGEAL AIRWAY	Points Possible	Points Awarded
Takes, or verbalizes, body substance isolation precautions	1	
Selects appropriately sized airway	1	
Measures airway	1	
Inserts airway without pushing the tongue posteriorly	1	
Note: The examiner must advise the candidate that the patient is gagging and becoming conscious		
Removes the oropharyngeal airway	1	

SUCTION

	Points Possible	Points Awarded
Note: The examiner must advise the candidate to suction the patient's airway		
Turns on/prepares suction device	1	
Assures presence of mechanical suction	1	
Inserts the suction tip without suction	1	
Applies suction to the oropharynx/nasopharynx	1	

NASOPHARYNGEAL AIRWAY

	Points Possible	Points Awarded
Note: The examiner must advise the candidate to insert a nasopharyngeal airway		
Selects appropriately sized airway	1	
Measures airway	1	
Verbalizes lubrication of the nasal airway	1	
Fully inserts the airway with the bevel facing toward the septum	1	
Total:	13	

Critical Criteria

_____ Did not take, or verbalize, body substance isolation precautions

_____ Did not obtain a patent airway with the oropharyngeal airway

_____ Did not obtain a patent airway with the nasopharyngeal airway

_____ Did not demonstrate an acceptable suction technique

_____ Inserted any adjunct in a manner dangerous to the patient

BAG-VALVE-MASK
APNEIC PATIENT

Start Time: _____

Stop Time: _____   Date: _____

Candidate's Name: _____

Evaluator's Name: _____

	Points Possible	Points Awarded
Takes, or verbalizes, body substance isolation precautions	1	
Voices opening the airway	1	
Voices inserting an airway adjunct	1	
Selects appropriately sized mask	1	
Creates a proper mask-to-face seal	1	
Ventilates patient at proper rate and adequate volume **(The examiner must witness for at least 30 seconds)**	1	
Connects reservoir and oxygen	1	
Adjusts liter flow to 15 liters/minute or greater	1	
The examiner indicates arrival of a second EMT. The second EMT is instructed to ventilate the patient while the candidate controls the mask and the airway		
Voices re-opening the airway	1	
Creates a proper mask-to-face seal	1	
Instructs assistant to resume ventilation at proper rate and adequate volume **(The examiner must witness for at least 30 seconds)**	1	
Total:	11	

Critical Criteria

_____ Did not take, or verbalize, body substance isolation precautions

_____ Did not immediately ventilate the patient

_____ Interrupted ventilations for more than 20 seconds

_____ Did not provide high concentration of oxygen

_____ Did not provide, or direct assistant to provide proper volume/breath or rate
(more than 2 ventilation errors per minute)

_____ Did not allow adequate exhalation

BLEEDING CONTROL/SHOCK MANAGEMENT

Start Time: _____

Stop Time: _____ Date: _____

Candidate's Name: _____

Evaluator's Name:	Points Possible	Points Awarded
Takes, or verbalizes, body substance isolation precautions	1	
Applies direct pressure to the wound	1	
Elevates the extremity	1	
Note: The examiner must now inform the candidate that the wound continues to bleed.		
Applies an additional dressing to the wound	1	
Note: The examiner must now inform the candidate that the wound still continues to bleed. The second dressing does not control the bleeding.		
Locates and applies pressure to appropriate arterial pressure point	1	
Note: The examiner must now inform the candidate that the bleeding is controlled		
Bandages the wound	1	
Note: The examiner must now inform the candidate the patient is now showing signs and symptoms indicative of hypoperfusion		
Properly position the patient	1	
Applies high concentration oxygen	1	
Initiates steps to prevent heat loss from the patient	1	
Indicates the need for immediate transportation	1	
Total:	10	

Critical Criteria

_____ Did not take, or verbalize, body substance isolation precautions

_____ Did not apply high concentration oxygen

_____ Applied a tourniquet before attempting other methods of bleeding control

_____ Did not control hemorrhage in a timely manner

_____ Did not indicate a need for immediate transportation

CARDIAC ARREST MANAGEMENT/AED
WITH BYSTANDER CPR IN PROGRESS

Start Time: _____

Stop Time: _____   Date: _____

Candidate's Name: _____

Evaluator's Name: _____	Points Possible	Points Awarded
ASSESSMENT		
Takes, or verbalizes, body substance isolation precautions	1	
Briefly questions the rescuer about arrest events	1	
Turns on AED power	1	
Attaches AED to the patient	1	
Directs rescuer to stop CPR and ensures all individuals are clear of the patient	1	
Initiates analysis of the rhythm	1	
Delivers shock	1	
Directs resumption of CPR	1	
TRANSITION		
Gathers additional information about the arrest event	1	
Confirms effectiveness of CPR (ventilation and compressions)	1	
INTEGRATION		
Verbalizes or directs insertion of a simple airway adjunct (oral/nasal airway)	1	
Ventilates, or directs ventilation of the patient	1	
Assures high concentration of oxygen is delivered to the patient	1	
Assures adequate CPR continues without unnecessary/prolonged interruption	1	
Continues CPR for 2 minutes	1	
Directs rescuer to stop CPR and ensures all individuals are clear of the patient	1	
Initiates analysis of the rhythm	1	
Delivers shock	1	
Directs resumption of CPR	1	
TRANSPORTATION		
Verbalizes transportation of the patient	1	
Total:	20	

Critical Criteria

_____ Did not take, or verbalize, body substance isolation precautions

_____ Did not evaluate the need for immediate use of the AED

_____ Did not immediately direct initiation/resumption of CPR at appropriate times

_____ Did not assure all individuals were clear of patient before delivering a shock

_____ Did not operate the AED properly or safely (inability to deliver shock)

_____ Prevented the defibrillator from delivering any shock

IMMOBILIZATION SKILLS
JOINT INJURY

Start Time: _____

Stop Time: _____ Date: _____

Candidate's Name: _____

Evaluator's Name: _____

	Points Possible	Points Awarded
Takes, or verbalizes, body substance isolation precautions	1	
Directs application of manual stabilization of the shoulder injury	1	
Assesses motor, sensory and circulatory function in the injured extremity	1	
Note: The examiner acknowledges "motor, sensory and circulatory function are present and normal."		
Selects the proper splinting material	1	
Immobilizes the site of the injury	1	
Immobilizes the bone above the injured joint	1	
Immobilizes the bone below the injured joint	1	
Reassesses motor, sensory and circulatory function in the injured extremity	1	
Note: The examiner acknowledges "motor, sensory and circulatory function are present and normal."		
Total:	8	

Critical Criteria

_____ Did not support the joint so that the joint did not bear distal weight

_____ Did not immobilize the bone above and below the injured site

_____ Did not reassess motor, sensory and circulatory function in the injured extremity before and after splinting

IMMOBILIZATION SKILLS
LONG BONE INJURY

Start Time: _____

Stop Time: _____ Date: _____

Candidate's Name: _____

Evaluator's Name: _____	Points Possible	Points Awarded
Takes, or verbalizes, body substance isolation precautions	1	
Directs application of manual stabilization of the injury	1	
Assesses motor, sensory and circulatory function in the injured extremity	1	
Note: The examiner acknowledges "motor, sensory and circulatory function are present and normal"		
Measures the splint	1	
Applies the splint	1	
Immobilizes the joint above the injury site	1	
Immobilizes the joint below the injury site	1	
Secures the entire injured extremity	1	
Immobilizes the hand/foot in the position of function	1	
Reassesses motor, sensory and circulatory function in the injured extremity	1	
Note: The examiner acknowledges "motor, sensory and circulatory function are present and normal"		
Total	10	

Critical Criteria

_____ Grossly moves the injured extremity

_____ Did not immobilize the joint above and the joint below the injury site

_____ Did not reassess motor, sensory and circulatory function in the injured extremity before and after splinting

IMMOBILIZATION SKILLS
TRACTION SPLINTING

Start Time: _____

Stop Time: _____ Date: _____

Candidate's Name: _____

Evaluator's Name: _____

	Points Possible	Points Awarded
Takes, or verbalizes, body substance isolation precautions	1	
Directs application of manual stabilization of the injured leg	1	
Directs the application of manual traction	1	
Assesses motor, sensory and circulatory function in the injured extremity	1	
Note: The examiner acknowledges "motor, sensory and circulatory function are present and normal"		
Prepares/adjusts splint to the proper length	1	
Positions the splint next to the injured leg	1	
Applies the proximal securing device (e.g..ischial strap)	1	
Applies the distal securing device (e.g..ankle hitch)	1	
Applies mechanical traction	1	
Positions/secures the support straps	1	
Re-evaluates the proximal/distal securing devices	1	
Reassesses motor, sensory and circulatory function in the injured extremity	1	
Note: The examiner acknowledges "motor, sensory and circulatory function are present and normal"		
Note: The examiner must ask the candidate how he/she would prepare the patient for transportation		
Verbalizes securing the torso to the long board to immobilize the hip	1	
Verbalizes securing the splint to the long board to prevent movement of the splint	1	
Total:	14	

Critical Criteria

_____ Loss of traction at any point after it was applied

_____ Did not reassess motor, sensory and circulatory function in the injured extremity before and after splinting

_____ The foot was excessively rotated or extended after splint was applied

_____ Did not secure the ischial strap before taking traction

_____ Final immobilization failed to support the femur or prevent rotation of the injured leg

_____ Secured the leg to the splint before applying mechanical traction

Note: If the Sagar splint or the Kendricks Traction Device is used without elevating the patient's leg, application of manual traction is not necessary. The candidate should be awarded one (1) point as if manual traction were applied.

Note: If the leg is elevated at all, manual traction must be applied before elevating the leg. The ankle hitch may be applied before elevating the leg and used to provide manual traction.

MOUTH TO MASK WITH SUPPLEMENTAL OXYGEN

Start Time: _____

Stop Time: _____ Date: _____

Candidate's Name: _____

Evaluator's Name: _____

	Points Possible	Points Awarded
Takes, or verbalizes, body substance isolation precautions	1	
Connects one-way valve to mask	1	
Opens patient's airway or confirms patient's airway is open (manually or with adjunct)	1	
Establishes and maintains a proper mask to face seal	1	
Ventilates the patient at the proper volume and rate	1	
Connects the mask to high concentration or oxygen	1	
Adjusts flow rate to at least 15 liters per minute	1	
Continues ventilation of the patient at the proper volume and rate	1	
Note: The examiner must witness ventilations for at least 30 seconds		
Total:	8	

Critical Criteria

_____ Did not take, or verbalize, body substance isolation precautions

_____ Did not adjust liter flow to at least 15 liters per minute

_____ Did not provide proper volume per breath
(more than 2 ventilation errors per minute)

_____ Did not ventilate the patient at a rate of 10-12 breaths per minute

_____ Did not allow for complete exhalation

OXYGEN ADMINISTRATION

Start Time: _____

Stop Time: _____ Date: _____

Candidate's Name: _____

Evaluator's Name: _____	Points Possible	Points Awarded
Takes, or verbalizes, body substance isolation precautions	1	
Assembles the regulator to the tank	1	
Opens the tank	1	
Checks for leaks	1	
Checks tank pressure	1	
Attaches non-rebreather mask to oxygen	1	
Prefills reservoir	1	
Adjusts liter flow to 12 liters per minute or greater	1	
Applies and adjusts the mask to the patient's face	1	
Note: The examiner must advise the candidate that the patient is not tolerating the non-rebreather mask. The medical director has ordered you to apply a nasal cannula to the patient.		
Attaches nasal cannula to oxygen	1	
Adjusts liter flow to 6 liters per minute or less	1	
Applies nasal cannula to the patient	1	
Note: The examiner must advise the candidate to discontinue oxygen therapy		
Removes the nasal cannula from the patient	1	
Shuts off the regulator	1	
Relieves the pressure within the regulator	1	
Total:	15	

Critical Criteria

_____ Did not take, or verbalize, body substance isolation precautions

_____ Did not assemble the tank and regulator without leaks

_____ Did not prefill the reservoir bag

_____ Did not adjust the device to the correct liter flow for the non-rebreather mask
(12 liters per minute or greater)

_____ Did not adjust the device to the correct liter flow for the nasal cannula
(6 liters per minute or less)

Patient Assessment/Management - Medical

Start Time: _____

Stop Time: _____ Date: _____

Candidate's Name: _____

Evaluator's Name: _____

		Points Possible	Points Awarded
Takes, or verbalizes, body substance isolation precautions		1	
SCENE SIZE-UP			
Determines the scene is safe		1	
Determines the mechanism of injury/nature of illness		1	
Determines the number of patients		1	
Requests additional help if necessary		1	
Considers stabilization of spine		1	
INITIAL ASSESSMENT			
Verbalizes general impression of the patient		1	
Determines responsiveness/level of consciousness		1	
Determines chief complaint/apparent life threats		1	
Assesses airway and breathing	Assessment	1	
	Indicates appropriate oxygen therapy	1	
	Assures adequate ventilation	1	
Assesses circulation	Assesses/controls major bleeding	1	
	Assesses pulse	1	
	Assesses skin (color, temperature and condition)	1	
Identifies priority patients/makes transport decisions		1	
FOCUSED HISTORY AND PHYSICAL EXAMINATION/RAPID ASSESSMENT			
Signs and symptoms (Assess history of present illness)		1	

Respiratory	Cardiac	Altered Mental Status	Allergic Reaction	Poisoning/ Overdose	Environmental Emergency	Obstetrics	Behavioral
*Onset? *Provokes? *Quality? *Radiates? *Severity? *Time? *Interventions?	*Onset? *Provokes? *Quality? *Radiates? *Severity? *Time? *Interventions?	*Description of the episode. *Onset? *Duration? *Associated Symptoms? *Evidence of Trauma? *Interventions? *Seizures? *Fever?	*History of allergies? *What were you exposed to? *How were you exposed? *Effects? *Progression? *Interventions?	*Substance? When did you ingest/become exposed? *How much did you ingest? *Over what time period? *Interventions? *Estimated weight?	*Source? *Environment? *Duration? *Loss of consciousness? *Effects-general or local?	*Are you pregnant? *How long have you been pregnant? *Pain or contractions? *Bleeding or discharge? *Do you feel the need to push? *Last menstrual period?	*How do you feel? *Determine suicidal tendencies. *Is the patient a threat to self or others? Is there a medical problem? Interventions?

	Points Possible	Points Awarded
Allergies	1	
Medications	1	
Past pertinent history	1	
Last oral intake	1	
Event leading to present illness (rule out trauma)	1	
Performs focused physical examination (assesses affected body part/system or, if indicated, completes rapid assessment)	1	
Vitals (obtains baseline vital signs)	1	
Interventions (obtains medical direction or verbalizes standing order for medication interventions and verbalizes proper additional intervention/treatment)	1	
Transport (re-evaluates the transport decision)	1	
Verbalizes the consideration for completing a detailed physical examination	1	
ONGOING ASSESSMENT (verbalized)		
Repeats initial assessment	1	
Repeats vital signs	1	
Repeats focused assessment regarding patient complaint or injuries	1	
Total:	30	

Critical Criteria

_____ Did not take, or verbalize, body substance isolation precautions when necessary

_____ Did not determine scene safety

_____ Did not obtain medical direction or verbalize standing orders for medical interventions

_____ Did not provide high concentration of oxygen

_____ Did not find or manage problems associated with airway, breathing, hemorrhage or shock (hypoperfusion)

_____ Did not differentiate patient's need for transportation versus continued assessment at the scene

_____ Did detailed or focused history/physical examination before assessing the airway, breathing and circulation

_____ Did not ask questions about the present illness

_____ Administered a dangerous or inappropriate intervention

Patient Assessment/Management - Trauma

Start Time: _____

Stop Time: _____ Date: _____

Candidate's Name: _____

Evaluator's Name: _____

		Points Possible	Points Awarded
Takes, or verbalizes, body substance isolation precautions		1	
SCENE SIZE-UP			
Determines the scene is safe		1	
Determines the mechanism of injury		1	
Determines the number of patients		1	
Requests additional help if necessary		1	
Considers stabilization of spine		1	
INITIAL ASSESSMENT			
Verbalizes general impression of the patient		1	
Determines responsiveness/level of consciousness		1	
Determines chief complaint/apparent life threats		1	
Assesses airway and breathing	Assessment	1	
	Initiates appropriate oxygen therapy	1	
	Assures adequate ventilation	1	
	Injury management	1	
Assesses circulation	Assesses/controls major bleeding	1	
	Assesses pulse	1	
	Assesses skin (color, temperature and conditions)	1	
Identifies priority patients/makes transport decision		1	
FOCUSED HISTORY AND PHYSICAL EXAMINATION/RAPID TRAUMA ASSESSMENT			
Selects appropriate assessment (**focused or rapid assessment**)		1	
Obtains, or directs assistance to obtain, baseline vital signs		1	
Obtains S.A.M.P.L.E. history		1	
DETAILED PHYSICAL EXAMINATION			
Assesses the head	Inspects and palpates the scalp and ears	1	
	Assesses the eyes	1	
	Assesses the facial areas including oral and nasal areas	1	
Assesses the neck	Inspects and palpates the neck	1	
	Assesses for JVD	1	
	Assesses for tracheal deviation	1	
Assesses the chest	Inspects	1	
	Palpates	1	
	Auscultates	1	
Assesses the abdomen/pelvis	Assesses the abdomen	1	
	Assesses the pelvis	1	
	Verbalizes assessment of genitalia/perineum as needed	1	
Assesses the extremities	1 point for each extremity includes inspection, palpation, and assessment of motor, sensory and circulatory function	4	
Assesses the posterior	Assesses thorax	1	
	Assesses lumbar	1	
Manages secondary injuries and wounds appropriately **1 point for appropriate management of the secondary injury/wound**		1	
Verbalizes re-assessment of the vital signs		1	
	Total:	40	

Critical Criteria

_____ Did not take, or verbalize, body substance isolation precautions
_____ Did not determine scene safety
_____ Did not assess for spinal protection
_____ Did not provide for spinal protection when indicated
_____ Did not provide high concentration of oxygen
_____ Did not find, or manage, problems associated with airway, breathing, hemorrhage or shock (hypoperfusion)
_____ Did not differentiate patient's need for transportation versus continued assessment at the scene
_____ Did other detailed physical examination before assessing the airway, breathing and circulation
_____ Did not transport patient within (10) minute time limit

SPINAL IMMOBILIZATION
SEATED PATIENT

Start Time: _____

Stop Time: _____ Date: _____

Candidate's Name: _____

Evaluator's Name: _____

	Points Possible	Points Awarded
Takes, or verbalizes, body substance isolation precautions	1	
Directs assistant to place/maintain head in the neutral in-line position	1	
Directs assistant to maintain manual immobilization of the head	1	
Reassesses motor, sensory and circulatory function in each extremity	1	
Applies appropriately sized extrication collar	1	
Positions the immobilization device behind the patient	1	
Secures the device to the patient's torso	1	
Evaluates torso fixation and adjusts as necessary	1	
Evaluates and pads behind the patient's head as necessary	1	
Secure the patient's head to the device	1	
Verbalizes moving the patient to a long board	1	
Reassesses motor, sensory and circulatory function in each extremity	1	
Total:	**12**	

Critical Criteria

_____ Did not immediately direct, or take, manual immobilization of the head

_____ Released, or ordered release of, manual immobilization before it was maintained mechanically

_____ Patient manipulated, or moved excessively, causing potential spinal compromise

_____ Device moved excessively up, down, left or right on the patient's torso

_____ Head immobilization allows for excessive movement

_____ Torso fixation inhibits chest rise, resulting in respiratory compromise

_____ Upon completion of immobilization, head is not in the neutral position

_____ Did not assess motor, sensory and circulatory function in each extremity after voicing immobilization to the long board

_____ Immobilized head to the board before securing the torso

SPINAL IMMOBILIZATION
SUPINE PATIENT

Start Time: _____

Stop Time: _____ Date: _____

Candidate's Name: _____

Evaluator's Name: _____	Points Possible	Points Awarded
Takes, or verbalizes, body substance isolation precautions	1	
Directs assistant to place/maintain head in the neutral in-line position	1	
Directs assistant to maintain manual immobilization of the head	1	
Reassesses motor, sensory and circulatory function in each extremity	1	
Applies appropriately sized extrication collar	1	
Positions the immobilization device appropriately	1	
Directs movement of the patient onto the device without compromising the integrity of the spine	1	
Applies padding to voids between the torso and the board as necessary	1	
Immobilizes the patient's torso to the device	1	
Evaluates and pads behind the patient's head as necessary	1	
Immobilizes the patient's head to the device	1	
Secures the patient's legs to the device	1	
Secures the patient's arms to the device	1	
Reassesses motor, sensory and circulatory function in each extremity	1	
Total:	14	

Critical Criteria

_____ Did not immediately direct, or take, manual immobilization of the head

_____ Released, or ordered release of, manual immobilization before it was maintained mechanically

_____ Patient manipulated, or moved excessively, causing potential spinal compromise

_____ Patient moves excessively up, down, left or right on the device

_____ Head immobilization allows for excessive movement

_____ Upon completion of immobilization, head is not in the neutral position

_____ Did not assess motor, sensory and circulatory function in each extremity after immobilization to the device

_____ Immobilized head to the board before securing the torso

VENTILATORY MANAGEMENT
DUAL LUMEN DEVICE INSERTION FOLLOWING
AN UNSUCCESSFUL ENDOTRACHEAL INTUBATION ATTEMPT

Start Time: _____

Stop Time: _____ Date: _____

Candidate's Name: _____

Evaluator's Name: _____

	Points Possible	Points Awarded
Continues body substance isolation precautions	1	
Confirms the patient is being properly ventilated with high percentage oxygen	1	
Directs the assistant to pre-oxygenate the patient	1	
Checks/prepares the airway device	1	
Lubricates the distal tip of the device (may be verbalized)	1	
Note: The examiner should remove the OPA and move out of the way when the candidate is prepared to insert the device		
Positions the patient's head properly	1	
Performs a tongue-jaw lift	1	
USES COMBITUBE / **USES THE PTL**		
Inserts device in the mid-line and to the depth so that the printed ring is at the level of the teeth / Inserts the device in the mid-line until the bite block flange is at the level of the teeth	1	
Inflates the pharyngeal cuff with the proper volume and removes the syringe / Secures the strap	1	
Inflates the distal cuff with the proper volume and removes the syringe / Blows into tube #1 to adequately inflate both cuffs	1	
Attaches/directs attachment of BVM to the first (esophageal placement) lumen and ventilates	1	
Confirms placement and ventilation through the correct lumen by observing chest rise, auscultation over the epigastrium and bilaterally over each lung	1	
Note: The examiner states, "You do not see rise and fall of the chest and hear sounds only over epigastrium"		
Attaches/directs attachment of BVM to the second (endotracheal placement) lumen and ventilates	1	
Confirms placement and ventilation through the correct lumen by observing chest rise, auscultation over the epigastrium and bilaterally over each lung	1	
Note: The examiner states, "You see rise and fall off the chest, there are no sounds over the epigastrium and breath sounds are equal over each lung"		
Secures device or confirms that the device remains properly secured	1	
Total:	15	

Critical Criteria

_____ Did not take or verbalize body substance isolation precautions

_____ Did not initiate ventilations within 30 seconds

_____ Interrupted ventilations for more than 30 seconds at any time

_____ Did not pre-oxygenate the patient prior to placement of the dual lumen airway device

_____ Did not provide adequate volume per breath (maximum 2 errors/minute permissable)

_____ Did not ventilate the patient at a rate of 10-12 breaths per minute

_____ Did not insert the dual lumen airway device at a proper depth or at the proper place within 3 attempts

_____ Did not inflate both cuffs properly

_____ **Combitube** - Did not remove the syringe immediately following inflation of each cuff

_____ **PTL** - Did not secure the strap prior to cuff inflation

_____ Did not confirm, by observing chest rise and auscultation over the epigastrium and bilaterally over each lung that the proper lumen of the device was being used to ventilate the patient

Inserted any adjunct in a manner that was dangerous to the patient

VENTILATORY MANAGEMENT
ENDOTRACHEAL INTUBATION

Start Time: _____

Stop Time: _____ Date: _____

Candidate's Name: _____

Evaluator's Name: _____

Note: If a candidate elects to initially ventilate the patient with a BVM attached to a reservoir and oxygen, full credit must be awarded for steps denoted by "**" provided first ventilation is delivered within the initial 30 seconds

	Points Possible	Points Awarded
Takes, or verbalizes, body substance isolation precautions	1	
Opens the airway manually	1	
Elevates the patient's tongue and inserts a simple airway adjunct (oropharyngeal/nasopharyngeal airway)	1	
Note: The examiner must now inform the candidate, "No gag reflex is present and the patient accepts the airway adjunct."		
**Ventilates the patient immediately using a BVM device unattached to oxygen	1	
**Ventilates the patient with room air	1	
Note: The examiner must now inform the candidate that ventilation is being properly performed without difficulty		
Attaches the oxygen reservoir to the BVM	1	
Attaches the BVM to high flow oxygen (15 liter per minute)	1	
Ventilates the patient at the proper volume and rate of 10-12 breaths per minute	1	
Note: After 30 seconds, the examiner must auscultate the patient's chest and inform the candidate that breath sounds are present and equal bilaterally and medical direction has ordered endotracheal intubation. The examiner must now take over ventilation of the patient.		
Directs assistant to pre-oxygenate the patient	1	
Identifies/selects the proper equipment for endotracheal intubation	1	
Checks equipment — Checks for cuff leaks	1	
Checks laryngoscope operation and bulb tightness	1	
Note: The examiner must remove the OPA and move out of the way when the candidate is prepared to intubate the patient.		
Positions the patient's head properly	1	
Inserts the laryngoscope blade into the patient's mouth while displacing the patient's tongue laterally	1	
Elevates the patient's mandible with the laryngoscope	1	
Introduces the endotracheal tube and advances the tube to the proper depth	1	
Inflates the cuff to the proper pressure	1	
Disconnects the syringe from the cuff inlet port	1	
Directs assistant to ventilate the patient	1	
Confirms proper placement of the endotracheal tube by auscultation bilaterally and over the epigastrium	1	
Note: The examiner must ask, "If you had proper placement, what would you expect to hear?"		
Secures the endotracheal tube (may be verbalized)	1	
Total:	21	

Critical Criteria

_____ Did not take or verbalize body substance isolation precautions when necessary

_____ Did not initiate ventilation within 30 seconds after applying gloves or interrupts ventilations for greater than 30 seconds at a time

_____ Did not voice or provide high oxygen concentrations (15 liter/minute or greater)

_____ Did not ventilate the patient at a rate of 10-12 breaths per minute

_____ Did not provide adequate volume per breath (maximum of 2 errors per minute permissible)

_____ Did not pre-oxygenate the patient prior to intubation

_____ Did not successfully intubate the patient within 3 attempts

_____ Used the patient's teeth as a fulcrum

_____ Did not assure proper tube placement by auscultation bilaterally over each lung **and** over the epigastrium

_____ The stylette (if used) extended beyond the end of the endotracheal tube

_____ Inserted any adjunct in a manner that was dangerous to the patient

_____ Did not immediately disconnect the syringe from the inlet port after inflating the cuff

Index

Abandonment, 45, 47
ABCDE acronym, 119
Abnormal skin, 77
Abuse, infant/child, 263
Acceptance, 30
Acetabulum, 62
Adrenal gland, 65
Adrenalin, 66
Adrenals, 65
Advance directives, 46
AED with bystander CPR, 367
Agonal, 63
Airway, 119, 361
Allergies, 187–188
Alveoli, 63
Ambulance operations, 273–276
Anatomical terms, 60
Anger, 30
Answers to review questions
    allergies, 193–194
    ambulance operations, 281–282
    baseline vital signs, 85–87
    behavioral emergencies, 211–213
    bleeding and shock, 235–237
    cardiac emergencies, 176–178
    communications, 139–140
    diabetes, 184–185
    documentation, 146–147
    emergency care, 24–27
    environmental emergencies, 202–204
    head and spine injuries, 258–260
    human body, 72–74
    infants and children, 269–271
    injuries, dealing with, 248–250
    lifting and moving patients, 98–116
    medical, legal/ethical issues, 56–58
    obstetrics and gynecology, 224–227
    patient assessment, 130–132
    pharmacology, 154–155
    poisoning/overdose, 193–194
    respiratory emergencies, 164–166
    SAMPLE history, 85–87
    seizures, 184–185
    well-being of EMT, 41–43

Anterior, 60
Aorta, 64
Apneic patient, 363
Appendix, 359–389
Arteries, 64
Arterioles, 64
Artificial ventilation, 159
Assault, 47
Assessment, 123
Atria, 64
AVPU acronym, 119

Bag-valve mask, 363
Ball-and-socket joint, 63
Bargaining, 30
Baseline vital signs, 76, 78
Basic life support (BLS), 46
Battery, 45, 47
Behavior, 206
Behavioral emergencies, 205–206
Bilateral, 60
Birth complications, 217–218
Bites and stings, 198
Bleeding, 230–231
Bleeding and shock, 229–231
Bleeding control, 365
Blood, 65
Blood pressure, 77–78
Blood vessels, 64–65
BLS. *See* basic life support (BLS)
Body mechanics, 90–91
Brachial arteries, 64
Brachial pulse, 119
Brain, 65
Breach of duty, 48
Breathing, 119, 158–159
Breathing rates, 63, 76–77
Bronchi, 63
Bronchioles, 63
BSI, 17, 32, 37

Capillaries, 63, 65
Capillary beds, 63
Capillary refill, 77

Cardiac arrest management, 367
Cardiac emergencies, 167–171
Cardiac muscle, 66
Cardiac patients, 170–171
Carotid arteries, 64
Carotid pulse, 77
Casualties, 276
Central nervous system, 65
Cervical collar (c-collar), 91
Cervical section, 61
Circulation, 119–120
Circulatory system, 64, 230
CISD. *See* critical incident stress debriefing
        (CISD)
Coccyx section, 61
Cold injuries, 196
Comfort measures only, 46
Communications, 133–135
Complications of birth, 217–218
Confidentiality, 48
Consent, 47
Constricted eyes, 77
Coronary arteries, 64
Correct anatomical position, 60
CPR, 119
Cricoid cartilage, 64
Cricoid cartilage larynx, 63
Crime scene evidence, 49
Criminal assaults, 48
Critical incident stress debriefing (CISD),
        32
Cyanosis, 63

DCAPBTLS acronym, 121, 125
Delivery, 216
Denial, 30
Depression, 30
Dermis, 66
Developmental phases, 262
Diabetes, 179–180
Diaphragm, 63
Diastolic pressure, 65, 77
Dilated eyes, 77
Disability, 120
Disasters, 276
Distal, 60
DNR. *See* do not resuscitate orders (DNR)
Do not resuscitate orders (DNR), 45–46
Documentation, 141–142
Dorsal position, 60
Dorsalis pedis, 64
Drowning, 197
Dual lumen device insertion, 387
Duty to act, 45, 48–49

Emergency care
    for cardiac patients, 170–171
    for practitioners, 13–17, 30
Emergency Medical Responder (EMR), 15
Emergency medical services (EMS), 14
Emergency Medical Technician (EMT)
    ethical responsibilities, 46
    personal attributes, 16
    quality improvement, 16
    roles and responsibilities, 15–16
    scope of practice, 46
    standards and attributes, 14–15
    well-being of, 29–33
Emergency moves, 91
EMR. *See* Emergency Medical Responder (EMR)
EMS. *See* emergency medical services (EMS)
EMT. *See* Emergency Medical Technician (EMT)
EMT exam
    exam content, 2–3
    exam difficulty, 3
    information sources, 4
    key terms, 10
    learning styles, 4
    preparing for, 8–9
    purpose of testing, 1–2
    study habits, 4–5
    studying for, 3–4
    test anxiety, 7–8
    testing, computer-based, 6
    testing, paper-and-pencil, 6–7
    written exam, preparing for, 2–3
Endocrine system, 65–66
Environmental emergencies, 195–198
Epidermis, 66
Epiglottis, 63
Esophagus, 63
Ethical issues, 45–49
Exposure, 120
Expressed consent, 47

Face, 60
Female anatomy, 216
Femoral arteries, 64
Fibula, 62
Final exam 1
    answer key, 307
    answer sheet, 285
    answers, 308–316
    questions, 287–306
Final exam 2
    answer key, 337
    answer sheet, 317
    answers, 338–345
    questions, 319–336

Final exams, about, 283
Flexible stretcher, 90, 92
Fowler's position, 60
Friends and family, 31

Glossary, 347–357
Greater trochanter, 62
Guardian consent, 47
Gunshot, 48
Gynecology and obstetrics, 215–218

Hazardous Materials, The Emergency Response Handbook
    (HAZMAT), 33, 118
Hazards, 276
HAZMAT. *See Hazardous Materials, The Emergency
    Response Handbook* (HAZMAT)
Head and spine injuries, 251–253
Health care system, 14
Heart, 64
Heart anatomy and physiology, 169–170
Heat exposure, 196–197
HEPA. *See* High Efficiency Particulate Air (HEPA)
High Efficiency Particulate Air (HEPA), 32
Hinge joint, 63
History and physical exam, 120–122
Human body, 59–66
Human skeleton, 61
Humerus, 62
Hypoperfusion, 65
Hypothalamus, 65
Hypothermia, 196

Immobilization skills, 369, 371, 373
Implied consent, 47
Infants and children, 261–263
Inferior position, 60
Inferior vena cava, 65
Inhalers, 159–160
Initial assessment, 118–120
Injuries, 239–242
Inspiration, 63
Involuntary muscle, 66

Joint, 63
Joint injury, 369

Labored breathing, 77
Lateral, 60
Learning objectives, 11
Legal issues, 17, 45–49
Legal subpoena, 48
Lifting and moving equipment, 92
Lifting and moving patients, 89–93
Long bone injury, 371

Lower extremities, 62–63
Lumbar section, 61

Mandible, 60
Maxilla, 60
Medial, 60
Medical direction, 17
Medical identification insignia, 49, 78
Medical issues, 45–49
Medical patients, 121–122
Mentally incompetent adults, 47
Metacarpals, 62
Mid-axillary line, 60
Mid-line, 60
Motor nerves, 65
Motor vehicle collision (MVC), 37
Mouth to mask with supplemental oxygen, 375
Moving and lifting equipment, 92
Moving and lifting patients, 89–93
Muscular system, 66–67
Musculoskeletal injuries, 241–242
MVC. *See* motor vehicle collision (MVC)

Nasopharyngeal airway, 119
Nasopharynx, 63
National Highway Traffic Safety Administration, 14
National Registry, 8–10
National Registry of Emergency Medical Technicians,
    1, 10, 359
Negligence, 45, 48
Nervous system, 65, 252
Nonurgent moves, 92
Norepinephrine, 66

Objectives
    allergies, 187–188
    ambulance operations, 273–275
    behavioral emergencies, 205–206
    bleeding and shock, 229–230
    cardiac emergencies, 167–169
    communications, 133–134
    diabetes, 179
    documentation, 141
    emergency care, 13
    environmental emergencies, 195
    hazards, casualties, and disasters, 276
    head and spine injuries, 251–252
    human body, 59–60
    infants and children, 261–262
    initial assessment, 118–119
    injuries, dealing with, 239–240
    lifting and moving patients, 89–90
    medical, legal/ethical issues, 45–46
    mental status, 179

musculoskeletal injuries, 241
obstetrics and gynecology, 215–216
ongoing assessment, 123
pharmacology, 149
physical exam, 122
poisoning and overdose, 188–189
respiratory emergencies, 157–158
sample history, 75–76
scene size-up, 117
trauma patients, 120
vital signs, 75–76
well-being of EMT, 29–30
Obstetrics and gynecology, 215–218
Occupational Safety and Health Administration
    (OSHA), 32
Off-line medical direction, 17
Olecrenon, 62
Ongoing assessment, 123
Online medical direction, 17
OPQRST acronym, 122
Organ donors, 48
Oropharyngeal airway, 119
Oropharynx, 63
OSHA. *See* Occupational Safety and Health
    Administration (OSHA)
Overdose, 188–189
Oxygen administration, 377
Oxygen skills, 361

Palmar, 60
Pancreas, 65
Parasthesia, 65
Parental consent, 47
Patella, 62
Patient assessment, 117–123
Patient assessment/management, 379–380
Patient positioning, 93
Pelvis, 61
Peripheral nervous system, 65
PERL acronym, 79, 120
Personal protection, 33
Phalanges, 62–63
Pharmacology, 149–150
Physical exam, 120–122
Pineal gland, 66
Pituitary gland, 65
Plantar, 60
Platelets, 65
Poisoning, 188–189
Posterior, 60
Posterior tibia, 64
Postural hypotension, 93
Power lift position, 90

Proximal, 60
Public safety personnel, 14
Pulse, 77

Radial arteries, 64
Radial pulse, 77
Rape, 48
Red blood cells, 65
Refusal of care, 47
Rescue, 33–34
Respiration, inadequate, 63
Respiratory emergencies, 157–160
Respiratory system, 63–64
Review questions
    allergies, 190–193
    ambulance operations, 277–280
    baseline vital signs, 79–85
    behavioral emergencies, 208–211
    bleeding and shock, 232–235
    cardiac emergencies, 172–175
    communications, 136–138
    diabetes, 182–184
    documentation, 143–146
    emergency care, 18–23
    environmental emergency, 199–202
    head and spine injuries, 254–257
    human body, 67–71
    infants and children, 265–268
    injuries, dealing with, 244–248
    lifting and moving patients, 94–98
    medical, legal/ethical issues, 50–55
    obstetrics and gynecology, 219–223
    patient assessment, 125–129
    pharmacology, 150–151
    poisoning/overdose, 190–193
    respiratory emergencies, 161–164
    SAMPLE history, 79–85
    seizures, 182–184
    well-being of EMT, 35–40

Sacral section, 61
Sacrococcygeal spine, 61
SAMPLE history, 75–78, 121
Scenarios
    allergies, 189–192
    ambulance operations, 276–277
    baseline vital signs, 79
    behavioral emergencies, 207
    bleeding and shock, 231–232
    cardiac emergencies, 171–172
    communications, 135
    diabetes, 181
    documentation, 142–143

emergency care, 17
environmental emergencies, 198
head and spine injuries, 253–254
human body, 66–67
infants and children, 264
injuries, dealing with, 242–243
lifting and moving patients, 93
medical, legal/ethical issues, 49–50
obstetrics and gynecology, 218
patient assessment, 123–125
pharmacology, 150–151
poisoning and overdose, 189–192
respiratory emergencies, 160
SAMPLE history, 79
seizures, 181
well-being of EMT, 34
Scene safety, 32
Scene size-up, 117–118
Scoop stretcher, 92
Seizures, 180–181
Sensory nerves, 65
Shallow breathing, 77
Shock, 65, 229–231
Shock management, 365
Shock position, 60
Skeletal muscle, 66
Skeletal system, 60–63
Skin, 77, 241
Skull, 60
Smooth muscle, 66
Soft tissue injuries, 239–241
Special needs children, 263
Special reporting situations, 49–50
Special situations, 48–49
Spinal cord, 65
Spinal column, 61
Spinal immobilization, 383, 385
Spine and head injuries, 251–253
Spine board, 91, 93
Squat lift position, 90
Stings and bites, 198
Stress management, 31
Stressful situations, 31
Subcutaneous layer, 66

Superior position, 60
Superior vena cava, 65
Supine patient, 92
Supine position, 60
Symptoms, 78
Systolic pressure, 65, 77

Tarsals, 63
Termination of care, 47
Thoracic section, 61
Thorax, 61
Thymus, 66
Thyroid, 65
Thyroid gland, 65
Tibia, 62
Tissue perfusion, 77
Torso, 60
Tourniquets, 231
Trachea, 63–64
Traction splinting, 373
Transferring a supine patient, 92
Trauma, infant/child, 263
Trauma patients, 120–121
Trendelenburg, 60
Type I & II diabetes, 180

Ulna, 62
Unilateral, 60
Upper airway adjustments/suction, 361
Upper extremities, 61–62

Veins, 65
Ventilation skills, 361
Ventilatory management, 387, 389
Ventral position, 60
Ventricles, 64
Venules, 65
Vital signs, 76–77
Voluntary muscle, 66

Wheeled ambulatory stretcher, 90
White blood cells, 65

Zygoma, 60

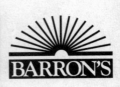
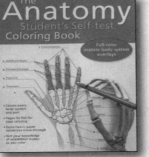 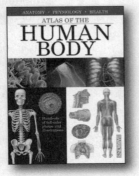 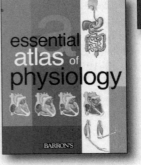 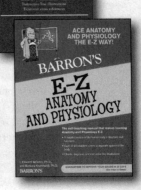

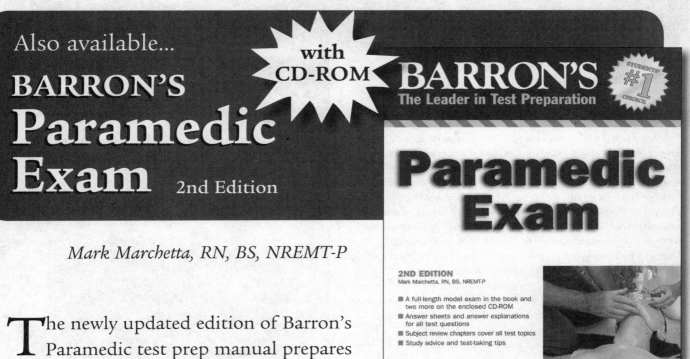
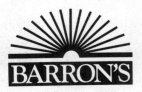

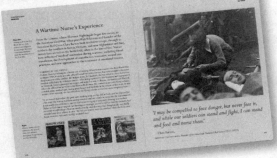